made INCREDIBLY EASY!

Fundamentals of Nursing

dapted for the UK by

**at Berridge MA (Ed), PG Dip Ed,
Sc (Hons), RGN, RNT**

enior Lecturer,
eputy Programme Director (RTP)
irmingham City University

nd

**atherine Liddle MA (Ed),
G Dip Ed, BSc (Hons),
GN, RNT**

enior Lecturer,
rogramme Director (RTP)
irmingham City University

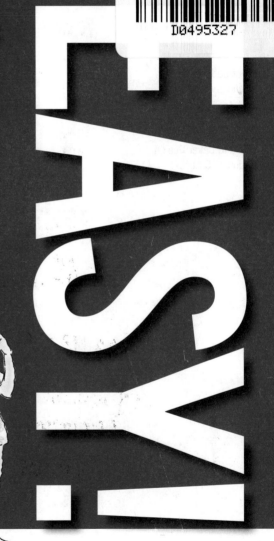

First UK Edition

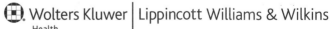

Wolters Kluwer | Lippincott Williams & Wilkins
Health
Philadelphia · Baltimore · New York · London
Buenos Aires · Hong Kong · Sydney · Tokyo

Staff

Acquisitions Editor
Rachel Hendrick

Academic Marketing Executive
Alison Major

Production Editor
Kevin Johnson

Proofreader
Helena Engstrand

Illustrator
Bot Roda

Text and Cover Design
Designers Collective

Printed and bound by Euradius in the Netherlands
Typeset by MPS Limited, A Macmillan Company
For information, write to Lippincott Williams & Wilkins, 250 Waterloo Road, London SE1 8RD.

British Library Cataloging-in-Publication Data. A catalogue record for this book is available from the British Library

ISBN-13: 978-1-901831-13-9
ISBN-10: 1-901831-13-2

Contents

Acknowledgements   *v*

Foreword   *vi*

Contributors and consultants   *viii*

Part I   Foundational concepts

1   Overview of nursing   3

2   Basics of health and illness   21

3   Ethical and legal considerations   29

4   Nursing process   43

Part II   General nursing skills

5   Communication   59

6   Nursing assessment   73

7   Taking vital signs   82

8   Asepsis and infection control   101

9   Medication basics   116

10   Medication administration   145

11   I.V. therapy   196

Part III Physiological needs

12   Oxygenation   219

13   Skin integrity and wound healing   249

14   Mobility, activity, and exercise   315

15   Self-care and hygiene   339

16   Comfort, rest, and sleep   365

17   Pain management   383

18   Nutrition   415

19   Urinary elimination   448

20   Bowel elimination   471

Appendices and index

Glossary 496

Selected references 500

Index 503

Acknowledgements

Reviewers of the UK edition

Michele Board, RGN, DPSN, BA (HONS), MSC
Senior Lecturer Nursing Older people, School of health and Social Care, Bournemouth University

Lorna McInulty, MN, RGN, PGCHERP, ONC
Senior lecturer, Emergency and Unscheduled Care, University of Central Lancashire

Maxine Pryce-Miller, MA Ed PGDip PGCE BSc (Hons) RSCN Rgn
Senior Lecturer-Child Health, School of Health & Well Being, University of Wolverhampton

Stephen David Searby, RGN, BSc (Hons), PGCert Ed
Adult Nurse Tutor, Faculty of Health and Medical Sciences, University of Surrey

Hannele Weir, MSc., BA (Hons.), PGCE, SCPHN, RN
Lecturer in Applied Sociology, Department of Interdisciplinary Studies in Professional Practice, City University

Firstly, we would like to thank the reviewers of this book for giving us valuable feedback; it must have taken hours of their time! Secondly, we would like to express our gratitude to our colleagues in the clinical skills division for keeping us sane throughout this experience.

Foreword

This book is intended to introduce the student nurse to a brief overview of nursing and clinical nursing skills that may be encountered on clinical placement. It may also be useful for those who want to return to nursing, or even those who have been nursing for some time and need a refresher!

Fundamentals of Nursing Made Incredibly Easy, 1st UK edition has been adapted from the American version, taking into account UK legal and professional aspects of nursing. The content is logically organized into three parts. The first, "Foundational concepts," provides an overview of nursing and offers information on health care, ethical and legal considerations, and the nursing process. The second part, "General nursing skills," covers communication, health assessment, vital signs, infection and key medication information. The final part, "Physiological needs," contains information on oxygenation, patient self-care, mobility, skin integrity, pain management, nutrition, and urinary and bowel elimination.

Each chapter starts with a brief outline of its content, allowing readers to quickly determine where they should focus. A quiz at the end of each chapter serves to challenge readers on how much information they absorbed. *Memory joggers* offer simple tricks to help readers remember key information. Fun illustrations and cartoons make learning fun—the surest way to keep readers interested!

In addition, icons draw your attention to important issues:

Teacher's lounge—provides patient-teaching tips on such topics as procedures, equipment, and home care

Ages and stages—identifies areas and procedures in which age could impact the nurse's care

Stay on the ball—focuses on critical areas involving possible dangers, risks, complications, contraindications, or ways to ensure safety

 Take note!—offers tips on documentation.

Fundamentals of Nursing Made Incredibly Easy is a welcome edition to the *Incredibly Easy* series! It will prove invaluable to nursing students as they prepare for their nursing career. Practicing nurses will find this a handy review of content they've already mastered. A handy reference for all, this book proves how interesting and crucial basic foundational material can be!

Pat Berridge MA (Ed), PG Dip Ed, BSc (Hons), RGN, RNT
Faculty of Health, Birmingham City University
Senior Lecturer
Deputy Programme Director (RTP)

Catherine Liddle MA (Ed), PG Dip Ed, BSc (Hons), RGN, RNT
Faculty of Health, Birmingham City University
Senior Lecturer
Programme Director (RTP)

Contributors and consultants to the US edition

Elizabeth A. Archer, RN, EdD
Associate Professor
Baptist College of Health Sciences
Memphis

Rita Bates, RN, MSN
Assistant Professor
University of Arkansas
Fort Smith

MaryAnn Edelman, RN, MS, CNS
Assistant Professor
Kingsborough Community College
Department of Nursing
Brooklyn, NY

Erica Fooshee, RN, MSN
Nursing Instructor
Pensacola (FL) Junior College
Department of Nursing

Sally Gaines, RN, MSN
Nursing Instructor
West Texas A&M University
Canyon

Rebecca Crews Gruener, RN, MS
Associate Professor of Nursing
Louisiana State University at Alexandria

Mari S. Hunter, RN, APN-C, MSN
Nursing Instructor
Great Basin College
Elko, NV

Rosemary Macy, RN, PhD(C)
Assistant Professor
Boise (Idaho) State University

Susan O'Dell, RN, APRN-BC, MSN, FNP
Assistant Professor of Nursing
Mercy College of Northwest Ohio
Toledo

Rhonda M. Sansone, RN, MSN, CRNP
Assistant Professor
Community College of Allegheny County
Pittsburgh

Sandra Waguespack, RN, MSN
Clinical Instructor
Louisiana State University Health Sciences Center
School of Nursing
New Orleans

Part I

Foundational concepts

1	Overview of nursing	3
2	Basics of health and illness	21
3	Ethical and legal considerations	29
4	Nursing process	43

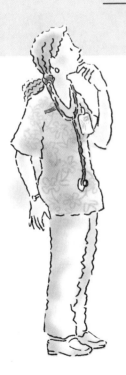

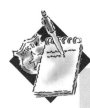

Just the facts

In this chapter, you'll learn:

♦ the historical roots of nursing and its emergence as a profession

♦ the practice guidelines and the educational background required for nursing

♦ the functions and roles of nurses in various care settings

♦ the guiding principles behind nursing theories and patient care.

Historical evolution of nursing

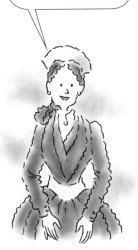

Florence Nightingale challenged traditional views of nursing by emphasising critical thinking, patients' needs and respect.

As we progress through the 21st century, the role of the nurse continues to expand. The increasing reliance on technology in nursing education and practice and the pressures of health-care reforms have combined to make nursing practice more complex than ever.

The delivery of health care has changed which has led to the progression of the nurses' role. Contributing factors include the reduction of junior doctors' hours, the move to deliver care for those with chronic illnesses into the community and the desire of nurses to expand their roles and knowledge to accommodate the increased workload. Patients now have access to more information regarding their illness and this can lead to increased pressure on the nurses because a better informed patient may well challenge the nurse's practice!

The birth of nursing

Nursing's origins lie in religious and military traditions that demanded unquestioning obedience to authority. Florence Nightingale challenged these traditions by emphasising critical thinking, attention to patients' individual needs and respect for patients' rights.

Go with Flo

The first school of nursing based on Nightingale's model opened in 1860 following her return from the Crimean War. Her aim was to train nurses to work in hospitals, to work with the poor and to teach.

A specialist emerges

After World War II major scientific discoveries and technological advancements altered the nature of hospital care. Increasingly, the care of hospitalised patients required experienced, skilled nurses. The development of intensive and coronary care units gave rise to the concept of the advanced clinician: a nurse qualified to give specialised care and the forerunner of today's clinical nurse specialist. The nurse specialist role has now been developed in most areas of nursing, for example in tissue viability, stoma care and pain control. Nursing also responded to greater public interest in health promotion and disease prevention. Today, nurses play an active role in health promotion examples of these include stress management, anger management, dietary advice, smoking cessation and exercise programmes. Health promotion can be used in all areas of nursing, looking after the mental and physical welfare of people.

Question, analyse and argue

Another crucial change in nursing stemmed from a midcentury shift in attitudes about education for women. The practice of extending full educational opportunities to women has significantly altered the role that nurses play in today's health-care system. Armed with a strong educational base, nurses have the confidence necessary to question, analyse and argue for family-centred health care—and to secure a major role for nursing in delivering that care.

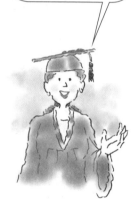

A strong educational base gives me the confidence to question, analyse, argue for and deliver quality patient care.

Nursing as a profession

Florence Nightingale believed that a nurse's goal should be 'to put the patient in the best condition for nature to act upon him.' Definitions of nursing change, but nursing itself has retained a common focus: providing humanistic and holistic care to each patient.

In the 1960s Virginia Henderson discussed the nurses' role in illness and in health as follows: 'The unique function of the nurse is to assist the individual, sick or well, in the performance of those activities contributing to health or its recovery (or to peaceful death) that he would perform unaided if he had the necessary strength, will or knowledge.'

This definition is still widely used in nursing literature today but has its critics, as it does not encompass the wider issues of including the family.

Henderson does however emphasise the independent nature of nursing and the importance of working with other health-care professionals.

Defining

The Royal College of Nursing has now defined nursing in order that lay people can understand the role of the nurse and also contribute to and influence policies and educational issues.

Definition of nursing (RCN 2008)

Nursing is . . . the use of clinical judgement in the provision of care to enable people to improve, maintain, or recover health, to cope with health problems and to achieve the best possible quality of life, whatever their disease or disability, until death.

The six defining characteristics are:

- **A particular purpose:** the purpose of nursing is to promote health, healing, growth and development, and to prevent disease, illness, injury and disability. When people become ill or disabled, the purpose of nursing is, in addition, to minimise distress and suffering, and to enable people to understand and cope with their disease or disability, its treatment and its consequences. When death is inevitable, the purpose of nursing is to maintain the best possible quality of life until its end.

- **A particular mode of intervention:** nursing interventions are concerned with empowering people, and helping them to achieve, maintain or recover independence. Nursing is an intellectual, physical, emotional and moral process which includes the identification of nursing needs: therapeutic interventions and personal care; information, education, advice and advocacy; and physical, emotional and spiritual support. In addition to direct patient care, nursing practice includes management, teaching, and policy and knowledge development.

- **A particular domain:** the specific domain of nursing is people's unique responses to and experience of health, illness, frailty, disability and health-related life events in whatever environment or circumstances they find themselves. Peoples' responses may be physiological, psychological, social, cultural or spiritual, and are often a combination of all of these. The term 'people' includes individuals of all ages, families and communities, throughout the entire life span.

- **A particular focus:** the focus of nursing is the whole person and the human response rather than a particular aspect of the person or a particular pathological condition.

- **A particular value base:** nursing is based on ethical values which respect the dignity, autonomy and uniqueness of human beings, the privileged nurse–patient relationship and the acceptance of personal accountability for decisions and actions. These values are expressed in written codes of ethics, and supported by a system of professional regulation.

- **A commitment to partnership:** nurses work in partnership with patients, their relatives and other carers, and in collaboration with others as members of a multidisciplinary team. Where appropriate they will lead the team, prescribing, delegating and supervising the work of others; at other times they will participate under the leadership of others. At all times, however, they remain personally professionally accountable for their own decisions and actions.

Reproduced by kind permission of RCN, London.

> **The Role of the NMC (Nursing and Midwifery Council)**
> - Sets standards for professional conduct, practice and education.
> - Maintains the register of registered nurses and midwives for all branches.
> - Considers cases of misconduct.
> - Provides advice.

> The face of nursing continues to change with the times, growing more autonomous and more professional.

Not just a job

Most people use the term 'nursing professionals' to describe a group of people who practice nursing. However, not everyone agrees that nursing has the full autonomy that it needs to distinguish itself as a profession rather than an occupation. The debate still continues today!

Practice guidelines

Nursing has already achieved some degree of autonomy. It exercises control over its education and practice. In 2002 The Nursing and Midwifery Council (NMC) replaced the United Kingdom Central Council (UKCC) as the regulatory body for nurses and midwives which sets standards that nurses must adhere to.

Standards of nursing care

These standards of care set minimum criteria for your proficiency on the job, enabling you and others to judge the quality of care you and your nursing colleagues provide. They help to ensure high-quality care and, in the legal arena, they serve as criteria to help determine whether adequate care was provided to a patient.

> No part of standards of nursing care is pie-in-the-sky. Professional standards help us all deliver the best care.

Code of conduct

In 2007 the NMC invited all stakeholders to contribute to an online consultation regarding the revision of the Code to reflect the changes in health care. In 2008 the Code was renamed *The Code: Standards of Conduct, Performance and Ethics for Nurses and Midwives*. The Code is comprehensive and reflects current professional practice. It therefore allows nurses and midwives to know what is expected of them and informs the public and other professionals.

Following on from the Code, the NMC have produced clear guidance for student nurses and midwives. *Guidance on professional conduct for nursing and midwifery students* (2009) identifies the personal and professional conduct expected from all nursing and midwifery students to ensure that they are fit for practise whilst undertaking their programmes. The guidance is based upon the Code which governs the conduct of registered nurses and midwives. Students may be given a copy of this, but copies of this can be obtained from the NMC website: www.nmc-uk.org.

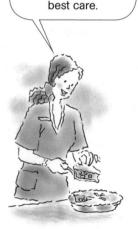

NMC: The Code

Standards of conduct, performance and ethics for nurses and midwives

The people in your care must be able to trust you with their health and wellbeing. To justify the trust, you must:

- make the care of people your first concern, treating them as individuals and respecting their dignity
- work with others to protect and promote the health and wellbeing of those in your care, their families and carers, and the wider community
- provide a high standard of practice and care at all times
- be open and honest, act with integrity and uphold the reputation of your profession
- be personally accountable for actions and omissions in your professional practice and must always be able to justify your decisions
- always act lawfully, whether those laws relate to your professional practice or personal life
- comply with this Code, else it may question your fitness to practise and endanger your registration
- consider this Code together with the Nursing and Midwifery Council's rules, standards, guidance and advice available at www.nmc-uk.org.

Make the care of people your first concern, treating them as individuals and respecting their dignity

Treat people as individuals

- You must treat people as individuals and respect their dignity
- You must not discriminate in any way against those in your care
- You must treat people kindly and considerately
- You must act as an advocate for those in your care, helping them to access relevant health and social care, information and support

Respect people's confidentiality

- You must respect people's right to confidentiality
- You must ensure people are informed about how and why information is shared by those who will be providing their care
- You must disclose information if you believe someone may be at risk of harm, in line with the law of the country in which you are practising

Collaborate with those in your care

- You must listen to the people in your care and respond to their concerns and preferences
- You must support people in caring for themselves to improve and maintain their health
- You must recognise and respect the contribution that people make to their own care and wellbeing
- You must make arrangements to meet people's language and communication needs
- You must share with people, in a way they can understand, the information they want or need to know about their health

(continued)

NMC: The Code (continued)

Ensure you gain consent

- You must ensure that you gain consent before you begin any treatment or care
- You must respect and support people's rights to accept or decline treatment and care
- You must uphold people's rights to be fully involved in decisions about their care
- You must be aware of the legislation regarding mental capacity, ensuring that people who lack capacity remain at the centre of decision-making and are fully safeguarded
- You must be able to demonstrate that you have acted in someone's best interests if you have provided care in an emergency

Maintain clear professional boundaries

- You must refuse any gifts, favours or hospitality that might be interpreted as an attempt to gain preferential treatment
- You must not ask for or accept loans from anyone in your care or anyone close to them
- You must establish and actively maintain clear sexual boundaries at all times with people in your care, their families and carers

Work with others to protect and promote the health and wellbeing of those in your care, their families and carers, and the wider community

Share information with your colleagues

- You must keep your colleagues informed when you are sharing the care of others
- You must work with colleagues to monitor the quality of your work and maintain the safety of those in your care
- You must facilitate students and others to develop their competence

Work effectively as part of a team

- You must work co-operatively within teams and respect the skills, expertise and contributions of your colleagues
- You must be willing to share your skills and experience for the benefit of your colleagues
- You must consult and take advice from colleagues when appropriate
- You must treat your colleagues fairly and without discrimination
- You must make a referral to another practitioner when it is in the best interests of someone in your care

Delegate effectively

- You must establish that anyone you delegate to is able to carry out your instructions
- You must confirm that the outcome of any delegated task meets required standards
- You must make sure that everyone you are responsible for is supervised and supported

Manage risk

- You must act without delay if you believe that you, a colleague or anyone else may be putting someone at risk
- You must inform someone in authority if you experience problems that prevent you working within this Code or other nationally agreed standards
- You must report your concerns in writing if problems in the environment of care are putting people at risk

Provide a high standard of practice and care at all times

Use the best available evidence

- You must deliver care based on the best available evidence or best practice
- You must ensure any advice you give is evidence based if you are suggesting health-care products or services
- You must ensure that the use of complementary or alternative therapies is safe and in the best interests of those in your care

Keep your skills and knowledge up to date

- You must have the knowledge and skills for safe and effective practice when working without direct supervision
- You must recognise and work within the limits of your competence
- You must keep your knowledge and skills up to date throughout your working life
- You must take part in appropriate learning and practice activities that maintain and develop your competence and performance

Keep clear and accurate records

- You must keep clear and accurate records of the discussions you have, the assessments you make, the treatment and medicines you give and how effective these have been
- You must complete records as soon as possible after an event has occurred
- You must not tamper with original records in any way
- You must ensure any entries you make in someone's paper records are clearly and legibly signed, dated and timed
- You must ensure any entries you make in someone's electronic records are clearly attributable to you
- You must ensure all records are kept securely

Be open and honest, act with integrity and uphold the reputation of your profession

Act with integrity

- You must demonstrate a personal and professional commitment to equality and diversity
- You must adhere to the laws of the country in which you are practising
- You must inform the NMC if you have been cautioned, charged or found guilty of a criminal offence
- You must inform any employers you work for if your fitness to practise is called into question

Deal with problems

- You must give a constructive and honest response to anyone who complains about the care they have received
- You must not allow someone's complaint to prejudice the care you provide for them
- You must act immediately to put matters right if someone in your care has suffered harm for any reason
- You must explain fully and promptly to the person affected what has happened and the likely effects
- You must co-operate with internal and external investigations

Be impartial

- You must not abuse your privileged position for your own ends
- You must ensure that your professional judgment is not influenced by any commercial considerations

(continued)

NMC: The Code (continued)

Uphold the reputation of your profession

- You must not use your professional status to promote causes that are not related to health
- You must co-operate with the media only when you can confidently protect the confidential information and dignity of those in your care
- You must uphold the reputation of your profession at all times

Reproduced by kind permission of NMC, London.

Educational preparation

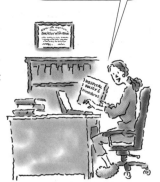

Today's nurses need to keep up to date with policies, procedures and nursing trends.

Pre-registration nurse education has been delivered by higher education institutions since the 1990s; it consists of the need to complete 50% in practice and 50% in academic work and this was identified by the UKCC in the Fitness for Practice and Purpose report. The NMC continued to apply this to pre-registration programmes by identifying this in their Standards of Proficiency for Pre-registration Nursing Education, which is currently being updated.

One other important document is the Essential Skills Clusters (ESCs) for Pre-registration Nursing Programmes; these are competencies students must achieve in practice in order for them to gain registration, some by the end of the common foundation programme and others by the end of the branch programmes. (See *The domains of the essential skills clusters*.) Each domain is broken down into subsections, which detail the expected competence to be achieved, mainly in the placement area or by the use of simulation in some situations. Students currently undertake a three-year programme of study guided by principles relevant to the standards to ensure they are fit for purpose at the end of their programme.

NMC Standards of Proficiency for Pre-registration Nursing Education

Guidelines for nursing programmes

- Length and structure of the programme
- Teaching and learning strategies used
- Academic standard and types of assessment
- Balance of theory and practice
- Course content and range of experiences
- Types of knowledge underpinning practice
- Support available
- Supernumerary status

(NMC, 2004)

> **The domains of the essential skills clusters (ESCs)**
>
> - Care, compassion and communication
> - Organisational aspects of care
> - Infection prevention and control
> - Nutrition and fluid management
> - Medicines management
>
> (NMC, 2007)

Lifelong Learning

Nurses are encouraged to advance their education following their registration. There is also the need to complete the post-registration education and practice (PREP) requirements, which are currently five days (35 hours) of learning, relevant to their practice, over a three-year period. It is the nurses' responsibility to ensure that the knowledge gained should be used to inform practice, through reflection and examining their own practice.

Nursing organisations and unions

The main nursing professional organisation is the Royal College of Nursing (RCN); it provides current information and resource material and allows you a voice in your profession. Members now include registered nurses and midwives, student nurses and midwives, and health-care assistants. Their aim is to promote excellence in nursing and midwifery by being involved in the shaping of government policies.

The main trade union that nurses join, Unison, also has an influence on health-care issues.

Functions of nurses

Recent changes in health care reflect changes in the population that require nursing care and a philosophical shift towards health promotion rather than treatment of illness. The role of the nurse has broadened in response to these changes. Nurses are caregivers, as always, but now they're also educators, advocates, leaders and managers, change agents and researchers.

Caregiver

Nurses have always been caregivers, but the activities this role encompasses changed dramatically in the 20th century. Increased education of nurses, expanded nursing research and the consequent recognition that nurses are autonomous and informed professionals has caused a shift from a dependent role for the nurse, being seen as a doctor's aide, to one of independence by now being accountable and responsible for their actions or omissions. This has led to greater collaboration with other health-care professionals.

A model of independence

Unlike earlier models, some nurses, for example nurse consultants and clinical nurse specialists, now conduct independent assessments and implement patient care based on their knowledge and skills. They also collaborate with other members of the health-care team to implement and evaluate that care.

Teacher

With greater emphasis on health promotion and illness prevention, the nurse's role as teacher has become increasingly important. The nurse assesses learning needs, plans and implements teaching strategies to meet those needs and evaluates the effectiveness of the teaching. To be an effective teacher, the nurse must have excellent interpersonal skills and be familiar with the appropriate developmental stages of children, adolescents and adults, as well as the principles of learning for each age group.

The teaching role encompasses student nurses, patients and family members, as well as other health professionals.

Before you go

Patient teaching is also a major part of discharge planning. Along with teaching come responsibilities for making referrals, identifying community and personal resources, and arranging for necessary equipment and supplies for home care.

Advocate

As an advocate, the nurse helps the patient and their family members interpret information from other health-care providers and make decisions about their health-related needs. The nurse must accept and respect a patient's decision, even if it differs from the decision the nurse would make.

Leader

All nurses practice leadership and manage time, people, resources and the environment in which they provide care. They carry out these tasks by directing, delegating and co-ordinating activities.

Although all health-care team members, including the nurse, provide patient care, the nurse plays an important role in coordinating the efforts of all team members to meet the patient's goals and contributes to a patient's case conference to facilitate communication among team members.

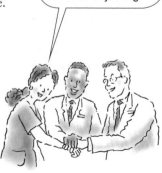

Sometimes it's necessary to huddle up, especially when the game plan—the patient's care plan—needs adjusting.

Change agent

As a change agent, the nurse works with the patients to address their health concerns and with staff members to address organisational and community concerns. This role demands knowledge of change theory, which provides a framework for understanding the dynamics of change, human responses to change and strategies for effecting change.

Discharge planner

As a discharge planner, the nurse assesses the patient's needs at discharge, including the patient's support systems and living situation. The nurse also links the patient with available community resources.

Remember! Discharge planning should start as soon as the patient is admitted to prevent delays in discharge.

Researcher

The primary tasks of nursing research are to promote growth in the science of nursing and to develop evidence-based nursing practice. Every nurse should be involved in nursing research and apply research findings to their nursing practice.

Identify and incorporate

Although not all nurses are trained in research methods, each nurse can participate by remaining alert for nursing problems and asking questions about care practices. Many nurses who give direct care identify such problems, which then serve as a basis for research. Nurses can improve nursing care by incorporating research findings into their practice and communicating the research to others.

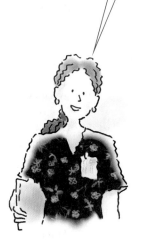

Every nurse should be involved in nursing research and apply research findings to their nursing practice.

Roles of nurses

In today's nursing profession, nurses have a broad area of opportunity. They may be staff nurses, nurse-managers, case managers, clinical nurse specialists, nurse practitioners, nurse educators and nurse researchers.

Staff nurse

The staff nurse is the first level of nursing following registration with the NMC. They are the primary caregivers by independently making assessments, planning and implementing patient care, and providing direct nursing care. For example, a staff nurse may make clinical observations and execute interventions, such as administering medications and treatments and promoting such activities of daily living as bathing and toileting.

Ward manager/sister or charge nurse

This role involves managing staff, budget, patient care and staff development to ensure that effective and quality nursing care is being provided in a timely and fiscally managed environment.

Case manager

To counter the trend towards fragmented, depersonalised nursing care in the community the role of case manager has been developed. This role enables the nurse to manage comprehensive care of an individual patient.

Clinical nurse specialist

The clinical nurse specialist has acquired expertise in a clinical specialty; they provide clinical expertise in the area and are involved in teaching and research.

Nurse practitioner

A nurse practitioner has obtained, at least, a first-level degree and specialises in a clinical area. They provide primary health care to patients and families and can function independently. They may obtain histories and conduct physical examinations, order laboratory and diagnostic tests and interpret results, diagnose disorders, treat patients, counsel and educate patients and family members, and provide continual follow-up care after patients are discharged.

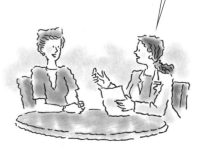

As your nurse practitioner, I thought we should take a few minutes to go over your medical history.

Nurse educator

The nurse educator works in a higher education institute and teaches on pre- and post-registration nursing programmes. They will also have a minimum of a first-level degree and also need to hold a teaching qualification.

Nurse researcher

The nurse researcher promotes the science of nursing by investigating problems related to nursing. The goal is to develop and refine nursing knowledge and practice.

Nursing theories

Many nursing leaders believe that the profession must establish itself as a scientific discipline to enhance its reputation. To do that, nursing needs a theoretical base that simultaneously shapes and reflects its practice. Nursing models combine concepts and theories, and were developed to guide nurses in the way they plan and deliver patient care in an organised fashion.

Concepts common to nursing theories

Four themes guide the development of nursing theory:

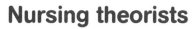 principles and laws that govern life processes, wellbeing and optimal functioning of people—sick or well

principles and laws that govern life processes, wellbeing and optimal functioning of people—sick or well

patterns of human behaviour that describe how people interact with the environment in critical life situations

processes for bringing about positive changes in the health status of individuals

nursing's key role as the central focus of all nursing theories.

> I think I'm on to something here!

> Even the theory of gravity had to start somewhere.

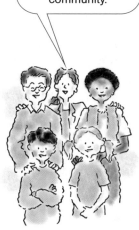

Nursing theorists

Theorists and researchers are now collaborating with practicing nurses in the development, testing and refining of nursing theory. (See *Comparing nursing theories*, page 16.)

Non-nursing theories

Many theories not specifically developed for nursing have been adopted by the nursing profession to provide guidelines for practising excellent patient care.

Systems theories

In systems theory, a system can be an individual, a family or a community. System theories are the basis for holistic nursing when the patient is viewed not as a whole but as many parts that are interrelated.

> A system can be an individual, a family or a community.

The sum of its parts

In general, system theories include a purpose (or goal), content (the information obtained from the system) and a process used to achieve the goal. The whole (be it an individual, family or community) is broken down, and all of the parts are examined. System theories integrate each part of the whole and examine how each part affects the whole.

Comparing nursing theories

Model or approach	Aims	Branch of nursing most commonly used in	Components of the model or approach
Peplau's person-centred approach	• Promotes the nurse–patient relationship • To explore and understand the patient's feelings • Involves the patient in their care	• Mental health	• Orientation • Identification • Exploitation • Resolution
Roper, Logan and Tierney's model	• To promote independence and individuality of the patient	• The most widely used model in nursing in the UK (referred to as ADLs or ALs).	**Activities of living (ADLs):** • Maintaining a safe environment • Communicating • Breathing • Eating and drinking • Eliminating • Personal cleansing and dressing • Controlling body temperature • Mobilising • Working and playing • Expressing sexuality • Sleeping • Dying
Orem's Self-care model	• To enable the patients to make their own decisions about their care thus promoting self-care	• Rehabilitation and older people • Learning disability nursing	• Universal requisites • Developmental • Health deviation
Roy's adaptation model	• To promote adaptation and coping strategies	• Mental Health	• Physiological mode • Self-concept mode • Role function mode • Independence mode
Neuman's model	• A profession concerned with the variables that affect the person's responses to stressors	• Mental health	• The relationship to stress and coping mechanisms
Casey's model	• The model focuses on working with children and their families as a partnership. The best people to care for the child are the family with professional guidance	• Child	• The child • The family • The nurse • Health • Environment
Rogers' humanist approach or person-centred approach	• A learned profession that promotes and maintains health and that includes professionals who care for and rehabilitate the sick and disabled	• Mental Health	• We all have the potential to grow just like all organisms have the potential to grow. The role of the nurse is to create this growth-promoting environment. Non-judgemental positive regard

Maslow's hierarchy of needs

You must know your patient's needs and values. Of course, physiologic needs—represented by the base of the pyramid in the diagram below—must be met first.

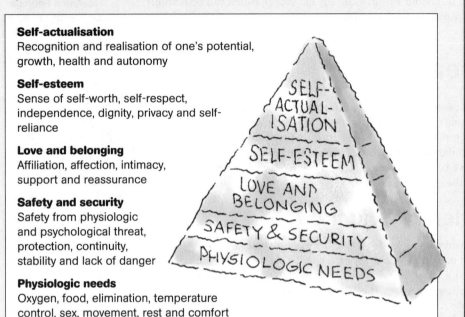

Self-actualisation
Recognition and realisation of one's potential, growth, health and autonomy

Self-esteem
Sense of self-worth, self-respect, independence, dignity, privacy and self-reliance

Love and belonging
Affiliation, affection, intimacy, support and reassurance

Safety and security
Safety from physiologic and psychological threat, protection, continuity, stability and lack of danger

Physiologic needs
Oxygen, food, elimination, temperature control, sex, movement, rest and comfort

Human need theories

Human needs are the physiologic or psychological factors that must be met for an individual to have a healthy existence. These are basic needs that were categorised by Maslow according to importance. Lower-level physiologic needs, such as the need for oxygen, food, elimination, temperature control, sex, rest and comfort, must be met before higher-level needs, such as a sense of self-worth and self-respect, can be met. However, it is not everyone's choice to move beyond the lower levels, where they may feel safe, but for others it might provide the opportunity to broaden their experiences and ultimately realise self-actualisation! There are five levels of human needs in ascending order. (See *Maslow's hierarchy of needs*.)

Developmental theories

Developmental theories classify an individual's behaviour or tasks according to their age or development. These theories use categories to describe characteristics associated with the majority of individuals at periods when

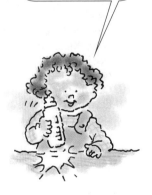

According to one developmental theory, I'm working on developing my sense of autonomy by banging this bottle on the table right now.

distinctive developmental changes occur. However, they don't take into account individual differences. These types of theories focus on only one type of development, such as cognitive, psychosocial, psychosexual and moral or faith development. Even so, developmental theories do allow the nurse to describe typical behaviour within a certain age group, which can be helpful during patient teaching and counselling.

Nursing research

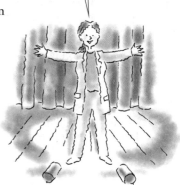

Good evening, ladies and germs. I'd like to share with you my latest research findings on the importance of humour in the clinical setting . . .

Research is the foundation on which all sciences are based. Its reliance on observations made in a controlled setting limits confusion over which factors actually produce the results. Health-care professionals have long recognised the importance of research in the laboratory setting, but recently have begun to develop ways to make research information more useful in the clinical setting.

Supported by evidence

The goal of research is to improve the delivery of care and, thereby, improve patient outcomes. Nursing care is commonly based on evidence that's derived from research. Evidence can be used to support current practices or to change practices. (See *Research and nursing*.)

Research and nursing

All scientific research is based on the same basic process.

Research steps

The research process consists of these steps:

1. **Identify a problem.** Identifying problems in the critical-care environment isn't difficult. An example of such a problem is skin breakdown.
2. **Conduct a literature review.** The goal of this step is to see what has been published about the identified problem.
3. **Formulate a research question or hypothesis.** In the case of skin breakdown, one question is, 'Which type of adhesive is most irritating to the skin of a patient on bed rest?'
4. **Design a study.** The study may be experimental or non-experimental. The nurse must decide what data are to be collected and how to collect that data.
5. **Obtain consent.** The nurse must obtain consent to conduct research from the study participants. Most facilities have an internal review board that must approve such permission for studies.
6. **Collect data.** After the study is approved, the nurse can begin conducting the study and collecting the data.
7. **Analyse the data.** The nurse analyses the data and states the conclusions derived from the analysis.
8. **Share the information.** Lastly, the researcher shares the collected information with other nurses through publications and presentations.

The best way to get involved in research is to be a good consumer of nursing research. You can do so by reading nursing journals and being aware of the quality of research and reported results.

Share and share alike

Don't be afraid to share research findings with colleagues. Sharing promotes sound clinical care, and all involved may learn about easier and more efficient ways to care for patients.

Evidence-based care

One way to make research results more useful in clinical practice is by delivering evidence-based care. Evidence-based care isn't based on traditions, customs or intuition. It's derived from various concrete sources, including:
- formal nursing research
- clinical knowledge
- scientific knowledge.

An evidence-based example

Research results may provide insight into the treatment of a patient who, for example, doesn't respond to a medication or treatment that seems effective for other patients.

In this example, you may believe that a certain drug should be effective for pain relief based on previous experience with that drug. The trouble with such an approach is that other factors can contribute to pain relief, such as the route of administration, the dosage and the concurrent treatments.

First, last and always

Regardless of the value of evidence-based care, you should always use professional clinical judgement when dealing with critically ill patients and their families. Remember that each patient's condition ultimately dictates treatment.

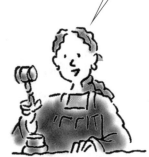

Always remember to use sound clinical judgement when providing patient care.

Quick quiz

1. The standards of nursing care are administered by the:
    A. National Patient Safety Agency (NPSA).
    B. General Medical Council (GMC).
    C. Nursing and Midwifery Council (NMC).
    D. National Institute of Health and Clinical Excellence.

    Answer: C. The standards of nursing care are administered by the NMC.

2. A nurse who can obtain histories, conduct physical examinations, order laboratory and diagnostic tests, interpret results, diagnose disorders and treat patients has what nursing credentials?
    A.   Clinical nurse specialist.
    B.   Case manager.
    C.   Nurse practitioner.
    D.   Ward manager.

Answer: C. The nurse practitioner may obtain histories, conduct physical examinations, order laboratory and diagnostic tests, interpret results, diagnose disorders and treat patients.

3. The easiest way to participate in research is to:
    A.   be a good consumer of research.
    B.   do a meta-analysis of related studies.
    C.   conduct a research study.

Answer: A. Nurses should start by reading research articles and judging whether or not they're applicable to their practice. Research findings aren't useful if they aren't incorporated into actual practice.

4. The purpose of evidence-based practice is to:
    A.   validate traditional nursing practices.
    B.   improve patient outcomes.
    C.   dispute traditional nursing practices.
    D.   establish a body of knowledge unique to nursing.

Answer: B. Although evidence-based practices may validate or dispute traditional practice, the purpose is to improve patient outcomes.

Scoring

☆☆☆   If you answered all four questions correctly, fantastic! You're building a good nursing foundation.

☆☆   If you answered two questions correctly, super! Your foundation is getting strong.

☆   If you answered fewer than two questions correctly, don't worry! With a little review, your foundation will be strong before you know it.

2 Basics of health and illness

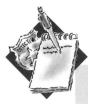

Just the facts

In this chapter, you'll learn:

♦ how different people define health and illness

♦ common factors affecting health and illness

♦ the effects of illness on the family and aging.

The health-illness continuum

How people view themselves, as individuals and as part of the environment, affects the way health is defined. Many people view health as a continuum, with wellness, the highest level of function at one end, and illness and death at the other. All people are somewhere on this continuum, and as their health status changes, their location on the continuum also changes.

Health defined

Throughout history, the definition of health has changed depending on the knowledge and beliefs of the time. Some cultures have regarded health and disease as reward or punishment for their actions. Others have viewed health as soundness or wholeness of the body.

What is it?

Although health is a commonly used term, definitions abound. No single definition is universally accepted. A common one describes health as a disease-free state, but this definition describes an either-or situation—a person as healthy or ill.

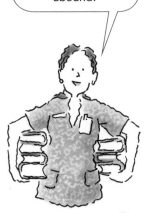

Although health is a commonly used term, definitions abound!

WHO says…?

The World Health Organization (WHO, 1992) calls health 'a state of complete physical, mental, and social well-being and not merely the absence of disease or infirmity'. This definition doesn't allow for degrees of health or illness. It also fails to reflect the concept of health as dynamic and constantly changing.

It's about culture

Sociologists view health as a condition that allows the pursuit and enjoyment of desired cultural values. These values include the ability to carry out activities of daily living, such as working and carrying out self-care with regard to maintaining standards of hygiene.

It's about levels

Many people view health as a level of wellness. According to this definition, people strive to attain their full potential. This definition allows a more holistic, subjective view of health.

Factors affecting health

One of the nurse's primary functions is to assist patients in reaching an optimal level of wellness. When assessing patients, the nurse must be aware of factors that affect their health status and plan to tailor interventions accordingly. Such factors include:

- genetics (biological and genetic makeup that causes illness and chronic conditions)
- cognitive abilities (which affect a person's view of health and their ability to seek out resources which may improve their health)
- demographic factors, such as age and gender (because certain diseases are more prevalent in a certain age group or gender)
- geographic locale (which predisposes a person to certain conditions)
- culture (which determines a person's perception of health, the motivation to seek care and the types of health practices performed)
- lifestyle and environment (such as diet, level of activity and exposure to toxins)
- health beliefs and practices (which can affect health positively or negatively)
- previous health experiences (which influence reactions to illness and the decision to seek care)
- spirituality (which affects a person's view of illness and health care)
- support systems (which affect the degree to which a person adapts and copes with a situation).

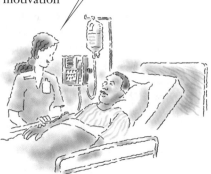

Because so many factors have a bearing on your health, we'll need to consider each one carefully and tailor interventions accordingly.

Illness defined

Nurses must understand the concept of illness, particularly how illness may affect the patient. Illness may be defined as a sickness or deviation from a healthy state. It's considered a broader concept than disease. Disease commonly refers to a specific biological or psychological problem that's supported by clinical manifestations and results in a body system or organ malfunction. (See *Disease development*.) Illness, on the other hand, occurs when a person is no longer in a state of perceived 'normal' health. A person may have a disease but not be ill all the time because their body has adapted to the disease.

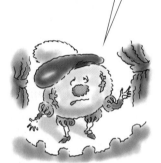

To be ill or not to be ill… That is the question!

What does it mean to you?

The meaning of illness also depends on how the patient interprets the disease's source and importance, how the disease affects their behaviour and relationships with others and how they try to remedy

---

Disease development

A disease is usually detected when it causes a change in metabolism or cell division, which, in turn, causes signs and symptoms. How the cells respond to disease depends on the causative agent and the affected cells, tissues and organs. In the absence of intervention, resolution of the disease depends on many factors functioning over a period of time, such as the extent of disease and the presence of other diseases. Manifestations of disease may include hypofunction, hyperfunction or increased or decreased mechanical function.

Disease stages

Typically, diseases progress through these stages:

exposure or injury—target tissue exposed to a causative agent or injury

latency or incubation period—no evident signs or symptoms

prodromal period—generally mild, non-specific signs and symptoms

acute phase—disease at its full intensity, possibly with complications; called the subclinical acute phase if the patient still functions as though the disease weren't present

remission—second latency phase that occurs in some diseases and is commonly followed by another acute phase

convalescence—progression towards recovery

recovery—return to health or normal functioning; no remaining signs or symptoms of disease.

the problem. Another significant component is the meaning that a person attaches to the experience of being ill. For example, if a person only receives attention from others when they are ill, they may take on the sick role more frequently!

Types of illness
Illness may be acute or chronic. Acute illness usually refers to a disease or condition that has a relatively abrupt onset, high intensity and short duration. If no complications occur, most acute illnesses end in a full recovery, and the person returns to the previous or a similar level of functioning.

Regain and maintain

Chronic illness refers to a condition that typically has a slower onset, less intensity and a longer duration than acute illness. The goal is to help the patient regain and maintain the highest possible level of health, although some patients fail to return to their previous level of functioning.

Effects of illness
When a person experiences an illness, one or more changes occur that signal its presence. These may include:
- changes in body appearance or function
- sensory changes
- changes in emotional status
- changes in relationships.

Perception and reaction

People's reactions to feeling ill vary. Some people seek action immediately, and others take no action. Some may exaggerate their symptoms, and others may deny that their symptoms exist. A patient's perception of and reaction to illness are unique and are usually based on their culture, knowledge, view of health and previous experiences with illness and the health-care system.

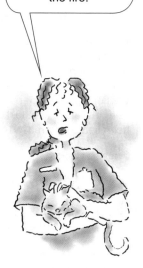

I can't quite put my finger on it, but something's not right. I think I'll need to stay home and cuddle up in front of the fire!

Effects of illness on family
The presence of illness in a family can have a dramatic effect on the functioning of the family as a unit. The type of effect depends on these factors:
- which member is ill (e.g. primary breadwinner, single parent, self employed)
- the seriousness and duration of the illness (e.g. short or long term illness. Is the person able to work part time?)
- the family's social and cultural customs (family members' roles might change to fill the void left by the ill person).

Health promotion

Research shows that poor health practices contribute to a wide range of illnesses, a shortened life span and increased health-care costs. Good health practices have the opposite effect: fewer illnesses, a longer life span and lower health-care costs.

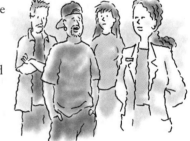

The earlier in life good practices are started, the fewer poor habits have to be overcome.

Better late than never

Good health practices can benefit most people no matter when they're started. Of course, the earlier in life good practices are started, the fewer poor habits have to be overcome. Even so, later is better than never. For example, stopping cigarette smoking has immediate and long-term benefits. Immediately, the patient will experience improved circulation, pulse rate and blood pressure. After 10 years without smoking, they will cut their risk of dying from lung cancer by half.

What is health promotion?

Quite simply, health promotion is teaching good health practices and finding ways to help people correct their poor health practices.

The government plan, Our Healthier Nation 1999, sets forth comprehensive health goals for the nation with the aim of reducing mortality and morbidity in all ages. These objectives make a useful teaching plan. (See *Our Healthier Nation: Selected objectives*.) This plan has yet to be reviewed, and since its publication it has been followed by various other initiatives including *Choosing Health: Making health choices easier* (DH, 2004); this white paper sets out key principles to support the public in making informed choices about their health.

Our Healthier Nation: Selected objectives

- Launched in 1999 by the U.K. government, Our Healthier Nation sets forth a comprehensive government plan focused on four main killers: cancer, coronary heart disease and stroke, accidents and mental illness.

By 2010

- **Cancer:** to reduce the death rate in people under *75 by at least a fifth*
- **Coronary heart disease and stroke:** to reduce the death rate in people under 75 *by at least two fifths*
- **Accidents:** to reduce the death rate by *at least a fifth* and serious injury *by at least a tenth*
- **Mental illness:** to reduce the death rate from suicide and undetermined injury *by at least a fifth*.

In 2007 the banning of smoking in enclosed public places including restaurants and work places was implemented throughout the whole of the United Kingdom. The minimum age for purchasing tobacco was also raised from 16 to 18 years.

The uptake of the 'flu jab' is encouraged and offered to the following people at risk of seasonal flu:

- aged 65 or over
- have a serious medical condition
- live in a residential or nursing home
- are the main carer for an older person or disabled person whose welfare may be at risk if you fall ill
- are a health-care or social-care professional directly involved in patient care.

Some other health promotional activites include access to clean needles for intravenous drug users, immunising children and encouraging the use of weight loss programmes.

National Service Frameworks

National Service Frameworks have been introduced to enable professional health-care workers to follow standard guidelines for particular care groups, which incorporates health promotion as an action, to promote the well-being of the individual. Some areas included in the programme are:

- diabetes
- coronary heart disease
- care of older people
- cancer care
- mental health
- long-term conditions
- children and young people.

Adult health care

Adults may fall victim to a variety of health problems, including heart disease and cancer. Although some of these problems stem from genetic predisposition, many are linked to unhealthy habits, such as overeating, smoking, lack of exercise, and alcohol and drug abuse. Your teaching can help an adult recognise and correct these habits to ensure a longer, healthier life.

Older adults

Today, people live longer than ever before. Life expectancy is now 80 for women and 75 for men. Fortunately, most older people can maintain their independence, with few needing to be cared for providing

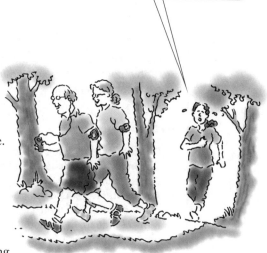

Wait for me, Grandma and Granddad! How much further is it to the ice cream van?

they remain active (WHO, 2002). Following on from this, in July 2009, the Department of Health launched a 'Prevention Package for Older People' to increase their independence by utilising health- and social-care services.

Active Aging! WHO...?

WHO identified the need for the older people to keep active.

The aim of keeping active is to lengthen life expectancy and maintain quality of life for everyone, including those who are weak, disabled and need to be cared for. It's not only being physically able or having the ability to continue to work, but the ability to continue to take an active part in all social and civic activities when they wish to. The Active Aging Framework also highlights the need to care for the older person when they are frail and need assistance (WHO, 2002).

Cope and avoid

Even so, most older people suffer from at least one chronic health problem. With the nurse's help, they can be taught to cope better with existing health problems and learn to avoid new ones. Doing so will improve their quality of life and allow them to continue contributing to society.

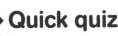

Quick quiz

1. Which of the following is an example of health promotion?
    A.   Administering antibiotics to a patient
    B.   Splinting a patient's fractured bone
    C.   Assisting a patient in stopping smoking
    D.   Inserting an I.V. catheter

Answer: C. Health promotion involves teaching good health practices as well as helping people correct their poor health practices. Helping a patient stop smoking helps him to correct a poor health practice.

2. One of the goals of Our Healthier Nation is to decrease cancer death rates in the under 75s by:
    A.   1/5
    B.   1/15
    C.   1/20
    D.   1/25

Answer: C. One of the goals of Our Healthier Nation is to decrease cancer deaths in the under 75s by 1/5 by 2010.

3. When describing disease development, which disease stage is described as producing generally mild, non-specific signs and symptoms?
  A.   Latent
  B.   Acute
  C.   Second latency
  D.   Prodromal

Answer: D. The prodromal period is described as producing generally mild, non-specific signs and symptoms.

Scoring

☆☆☆ If you answered all three questions correctly, super! Your understanding of the spectrum of health and illness is spectacular.

☆☆ If you answered two questions correctly, great! You sure have been practising your nursing practice.

☆ If you answered fewer than two questions correctly, don't despair! Keep 'continuum' to review, and you'll soon have a healthy understanding of the chapter.

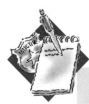

Just the facts

In this chapter, you'll learn:

♦ the significance of values and ethics in providing nursing care

♦ how to approach ethical dilemmas in patient care

♦ the nurse's role and responsibilities in ensuring patients' rights

♦ the difference between intentional and unintentional torts.

Values

Values are strongly held personal and professional beliefs about worth and importance. The word value derives from the Latin valere (worth). Values are key to developing ethical consciousness and guide us in making important life decisions. Because values are highly individualised yet subject to influence from outside sources, it isn't surprising that value conflicts are common among nurses, doctors, patients and families.

Personal values

Clarifying your own values is an important part of developing a professional ethic. A person may become more aware of their values by consciously examining their own statements and behaviour.

Values clarification

Each nurse and patient brings values to the health-care system. These values include beliefs about such concepts as life, death, a higher power and who should and shouldn't receive health care as well as such complex issues as

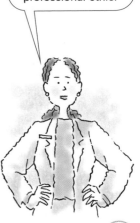

Clarifying your values is an important part of developing a professional ethic.

organ transplantation and the right to die. The patient's values may change when they are faced with illness, injury and possible death.

Values clarification refers to the process of raising consciousness so that value conflicts can be resolved. You're likely to encounter many conflicting sets of values in the course of your professional career. To provide optimal support to the patient, you must undergo your own values clarification process.

First reflect . . .

Exercises, such as analysing conversations between colleagues, offer one way to clarify values. Reflecting on one's own statements and actions is another way.

. . . then choose . . .

You must choose among competing values to establish your own. Then you need to incorporate chosen values into your everyday thoughts and actions. You'll then be better prepared to act on chosen values when you're confronted with difficult choices.

. . . and, finally, clarify

Making values decisions need not be haphazard. By clarifying your own values and checking to see if they're consistent with the established standards of the nursing profession, you can enhance your ability to make responsible judgements.

Ethics

Understanding ethics plays an important part in decision-making.

Ethics is defined as a code of moral principles which nurses and other health-care workers apply to their decision-making. Health-care workers today deal with many ethical issues, for example the withdrawal of treatment or, sometimes, the cost and availability of treatments. To enable us to make these decisions we rely on applying the four principles of ethics as described by Beauchamp and Childress (2001) which are:

*   non-maleficence (to prevent harm to the patient)
*   beneficence (in the patient's best interest)
*   respect for autonomy (the right to make own decisions)
*   justice (treating patients in a fair and equitable way).

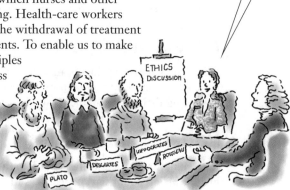

OK, how would you handle a hypothetical situation like this . . .?

International Council of Nurses Code of Ethics (2005)

According to the ICN, the fundamental responsibility of the nurse is fourfold:

1. promote health
2. prevent illness
3. restore health
4. alleviate suffering.

The ICN further states that the need for nursing is universal. Inherent in nursing is respect for life, dignity and the rights of humanity. It's unrestricted by considerations of nationality, race, colour, age, gender, politics or social status. The code has five principal elements that outline the standards of ethical conduct.

Nurses and people

- The nurse's primary responsibility is to people who require nursing care.
- The nurse, in providing care, respects the beliefs, values and customs of the individual.
- The nurse holds in confidence personal information and uses judgement in sharing this information.

Nurses and practice

- The nurse carries personal responsibility for nursing practice and maintaining competence by continual learning.
- The nurse maintains the highest standards of nursing possible within the reality of a specific situation.

- The nurse uses good judgement in relation to individual competence when accepting and delegating responsibilities.
- The nurse, when acting in a professional capacity, should at all times maintain standards of personal conduct that would reflect credit upon the profession.

Nurses and society

- The nurse shares with other citizens the responsibility for initiating and supporting actions to meet the health and social needs of the public.

Nurses and colleagues

- The nurse sustains a co-operative relationship with colleagues in nursing and other fields.
- The nurse takes appropriate actions to safeguard the patient when their care is endangered by a colleague or another person.

Nurses and the profession

- The nurse plays the major role in determining and implementing desirable standards of nursing practice and nursing education.
- The nurse is active in developing a core of professional knowledge.
- The nurse, acting through the professional organisation, participates in establishing and maintaining equitable social and economic working conditions in nursing.

Code of ethics

A code of ethics is a group of fundamental beliefs about what's morally right or wrong, along with reasons for maintaining those beliefs. (See *ICN code of ethics for nurses* (2005) and *NMC the code* (2008), page 7.) Both of these codes contain fundamental statements which represent the beliefs and values of the nursing profession, and they assist in judging the standard of nursing given at any one time.

Confidentiality!

The need for confidentiality also forms part of the NMC Code. Patients and their family expect all health-care professionals to maintain confidentiality and share information with only relevant personnel.

The move to computerise patient records has its own problems. It may increase the risk of more people being able to access them. Therefore, it is essential that staff understand the importance of not sharing computer log in codes, and to remember to log out when leaving a computer screen.

The Caldicott Guardian

The Caldicott Guardian is a senior member of the NHS Trust (usually a clinician) who is responsible for maintaining the confidentiality of all identifiable health-care records in that setting. All groups delivering health care were required to appoint a Caldicott Guardian to ensure the protection of patient records and who may view them.

For your eyes only

Patient records with identifiable health information must be secured so that they aren't accessible to those who don't have a need for them. Identifiable health information may include the patient's name, national health number, hospital number, birth date, admission and discharge dates, and health history.

Accessing health records

Under the Data Protection Act 1998 and the Access to Health Records Act 1990, all patients have a right to access their medical records. The Data Protection Act 1998 governs access to health records of living people while the Access to Health Records Act 1990 governs the access to records of the deceased.

A request for access to a health record is dealt with by the 'data controller', who may be the manager of the medical records or another nominated person. The data controller can refuse the request or limit the amount of information released if they feel that this would cause serious harm, physically or mentally, to the patient or their relatives. Revealing sensitive information to a relative may cause more distress to them, especially when the patient did not disclose the information to them.

Ethical decisions

Every day, nurses make ethical decisions in their nursing practice. These decisions may involve patient care, actions related to colleagues, or nurse-doctor relationships. At times, you may find yourself trapped in the middle of an ethical dilemma, pulled in every direction by your duties and responsibilities to your patient, your employer and yourself. Even after you make a decision, you may ask yourself, 'Did I make the right decision?'

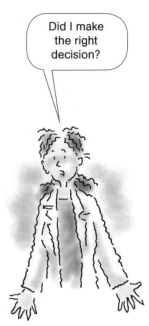

Did I make the right decision?

It isn't automatic

There are no automatic solutions to all ethical conflicts. Although such conflicts may be painful and confusing, particularly in nursing, you don't have to be a philosopher to act ethically or to make decisions that fall within nursing's ethical codes. Nonetheless, you need to understand the principles of ethics that guide your nursing practice. Legally, nurses are responsible for using their knowledge and skills to protect the comfort and safety of their patients. Ethically, nurses, in their role as patient advocates, are responsible for safeguarding their patients' rights.

Being an advocate

Although a nurse isn't legally responsible for obtaining a patient's informed consent, the nurse is ethically responsible as the patient's advocate for reporting to the doctor a patient's misunderstanding about treatment. To be an effective advocate, a nurse must understand the ethical and legal principles of informed consent. In order to consent the patient must understand their condition, the proposed treatment, treatment alternatives, potential risks and benefits, and relative chances of success or failure.

Ethical conflicts

Rapid advances in medical research have outpaced society's ability to solve the ethical problems associated with new health-care technology. For nurses, ethical decision-making in clinical practice is complicated by socio-cultural factors, legal controversies, growing professional autonomy and consumer involvement in health care.

Decisions, decisions

Major areas of ethical conflict may include end-of-life decisions, withholding or withdrawing treatment, advance directives and organ donation. No matter what your nursing specialty, you'll probably encounter at least one of these conflicts during your nursing career.

End-of life decisions

End-of-life decisions are almost always difficult for patients, families and health-care professionals to make. Nurses are in a unique position as patient advocates assisting patients and their families through the process of death.

Unsolvable mysteries

Your primary role as a patient advocate is to promote the patient's wishes. When the patient is unable to make their wishes known (they may be unconscious or too ill) ethical decision making takes priority. Decisions aren't always easy to make, and the answers aren't usually clear-cut. At times, such ethical dilemmas may seem unsolvable.

Question of quality

It's sometimes difficult to determine what can be done to achieve a good quality of life and what can simply be achieved, technologically speaking.

Years ago, death was considered a natural part of life and most people died at home, surrounded by their families. Today, most people die in hospitals, and death is commonly regarded as a medical failure rather than a natural event. Sometimes it's hard to know whether you're assisting in extending the patient's life or merely delaying the patient's death. The decision to keep a patient comfortable at the end of life by the use of I.V. fluids is an example, and relatives may see the withdrawal of this as hastening the patient's death.

Consulting the committee

Some NHS trusts have clinical ethical committees that advise on ethical dilemmas; they also provide advice and guidance for policy making and staff education. (See *The ethics committee*.)

The committee members may include doctors, nurses, therapists, a lawyer, a representative of a religious body, a trust board member and a lay person.

Determining medical futility

Medical futility refers to treatment that isn't likely to benefit the patient even though it may appear to be effective. For example, a patient with a terminal illness who's expected to die experiences cardiac arrest.

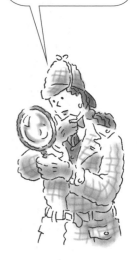

Deducing the patient's wishes isn't always easy. In fact, at times, it may seem unsolvable.

The ethics committee

The ethics committee addresses ethical issues regarding the clinical aspects of patient care. It provides a forum for the patient, their family and health-care providers to resolve conflicts.

The functions of an ethics committee include:

- policy development (such as developing policies to guide deliberations over individual cases)
- education (such as inviting guest speakers to visit your health-care facility and discuss ethical concerns)
- case consultation (such as debating the prognosis of a patient who's in a persistent vegetative state).

Approaching ethical decisions

When faced with an ethical dilemma, consider these questions:

- What health issues are involved?
- What ethical issues are involved?
- What further information is necessary before a judgement can be made?
- Who will be affected by this decision? (Include the decision-maker and other caregivers if they'll be affected emotionally or professionally.)
- What are the values and opinions of the people involved?

- What conflicts exist between the values and ethical standards of the people involved?
- Must a decision be made and, if so, who should make it?
- What alternatives are available?
- For each alternative, what are the ethical justifications?
- For each alternative, what are the possible outcomes?

Cardiopulmonary resuscitation (CPR) may be effective in restoring a heartbeat but may be deemed futile because it doesn't change the patient's outcome. CPR must be initiated unless written otherwise by the patient or doctor's order.

Withholding or withdrawing treatment

The issue of withholding or withdrawing treatment can certainly present some ethical dilemmas. When withdrawing treatment from a patient, even at the patient's request, controversy over the principle of non-maleficence (to prevent harm) exists.

Harm alarm

Such controversy revolves around the definition of harm. Some feel that removing a patient from a ventilator and allowing death is an intentional infliction of harm. Others argue that keeping a person on a ventilator against the patient's will, thus prolonging death, is an intentional infliction of harm. (See *Approaching ethical decisions*.)

Cardiac arrest

A patient can refuse CPR and the health-care team must follow the patient's wishes. These wishes must be recorded in the patient's notes, or they may be included in an advance directive. (See *Advance directives or living wills*.)

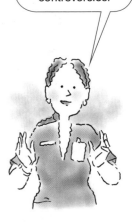

Be advised . . . ethical dilemmas are full of controversies.

Note! Do not resuscitate (DNR) relates only to CPR; other types of life-saving treatments will be given and the patient can change their mind at any time about their decision.

If the patient has not made their wishes known about CPR, doctors will decide if it's in the patient's best interests to be resuscitated. Family and friends don't have the right to decide, but they will be involved in discussions about what to do.

If the patient wants to be resuscitated regardless of the outcome, medical staff will arrange for a second medical opinion if they have concerns that CPR wouldn't be successful.

If the patient still wants to be revived, medical staff will attempt resuscitation if it's best for the patient at the time, but they will not go against their clinical judgement.

In Scotland, people over 16 can appoint a 'proxy'; a partner, relative or friend who has the legal power to give consent to medical treatment when the patient can't make decisions. (Crown copyright.)

Who decides?

The wishes of a competent, informed patient should always be honoured. However, when a patient can't make decisions, the health-care team—consisting of the patient's family, nursing staff and doctors—may have to make end-of-life decisions for the patient.

Advance directives or living wills

These are written statements made and signed by the patient determining their wishes to undergo medical treatment if they become incapable of making a decision later, due to them losing their mental capacity. Although witnessed verbal instructions may be respected, written decisions avoid any doubt about the patient's wishes.

Most people prefer to make their own decisions regarding end-of-life care. It's important that patients discuss their wishes with their loved ones; however, many don't. Instead, total strangers may be asked to make important health-care decisions when a patient can't do so. That's why it's important for people to make choices ahead of time and to make these choices known by developing advance directives. It is important to note that there are no government laws or acts of parliament governing advanced directives or living wills, so currently this is covered under common law and a judge interprets the wishes of the patient. The Law Commission has drafted guidance which includes that the patient should be able to refuse specific medical treatments but they should not state which treatment they want.

> Remember to ask whether your patient has an advance directive or living will.

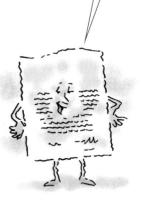

Note! They cannot ask for their life to be ended, force doctors to act against their professional judgement or nominate someone else to decide about their treatment.

The Mental Capacity Act 2005

The Mental Capacity Act 2005 came into force in April 2007 and forms the legal basis for advance decisions.

Valid advance decisions

To be valid an advance decision needs to:

- be made by a person who is 18 or over and has the capacity to make it
- specify the treatment to be refused (it can do this in lay terms)
- specify the circumstances in which this refusal would apply
- not have been made under the influence or harassment of anyone else
- not have been modified verbally or in writing since it was made.

Refusal of life-sustaining treatment

Advance decisions refusing life-sustaining treatment must:

- be in writing (it can be written by a family member, recorded in medical notes by a doctor or on an electronic record)
- be signed and witnessed (it can be signed by someone else at the person's direction—the witness is to confirm the signature, not the content of the advance directive)
- include an express statement that the decision stands 'even if life is at risk'.

When might an advance decision not be followed?

A doctor might not act on an advance decision if:

- the person has done anything clearly inconsistent with the advance decision which affects its validity (e.g. a change in religious faith)
- the current circumstances would not have been anticipated by the person and would have affected their decision (e.g. a recent development in treatment that radically changes the outlook for their particular condition)
- it is not clear about what should happen
- the person has been treated under the Mental Health Act.

A doctor can also treat if there is doubt or a dispute about the validity of an advance decision and the case has been referred to the court.

Crown copyright

Organ donation

When asked, most people say that they support organ donation. However, only a small percentage of qualified organs are ever donated. Thousands of names are on waiting lists for organs in the United Kingdom alone. Organ transplantation is successful for many patients, giving them additional, high-quality years of life.

The next of kin are asked to make the organ donation. This can be a very difficult time for them and should be handled by experienced health-care personnel.

These conditions usually preclude any organ or tissue donation:
- advanced age
- metastatic cancer
- history of hepatitis, human immunodeficiency virus or acquired immune deficiency syndrome
- sepsis.

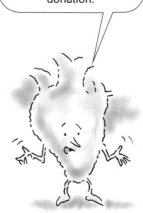

With so many people needing transplants, it's a shame to let a healthy fella like me go to waste. Learn all you can about organ donation.

Organ donation

If the death has to be reported to the coroner, the coroner's consent may be necessary before the organs or body can be donated. A medical certificate must be issued before any organs can be removed.

It is essential for heart, lungs, liver and pancreas, to be removed only from donors:

- who have been certified to be brain stem dead and
- whose breathing, and hence heartbeat, are maintained by a ventilator in a hospital intensive care unit.

Kidneys can, very rarely, be removed up to an hour after heart death. Other organs can be removed up to the following times after heart death:

- skin and the corneas from the eyes—up to 24 hours
- bone—up to 36 hours
- heart valves—up to 72 hours.

Crown copyright

Discuss among yourselves

When ethical problems arise, discuss them candidly with other members of the health-care team, especially the patient's doctor. Also, consider calling on social workers, psychologists, the clergy and ethics committee members to help you resolve difficult ethical problems. By learning as much as possible, you can facilitate the decision-making process for the patient, their family, the doctor and yourself. When patients or relatives sometimes ask 'what would you do?' in these situations, you must take care to give the positive and negative aspects of the treatment and not to give your own opinion, which may be difficult.

Laws

Laws are binding rules of conduct enforced by authority. Ideally, laws are based on what's right and good. Realistically, though, the relation between laws and ethics is complex. When a law is challenged as unjust or unfair, the challenge usually reflects some underlying clinical principle. Even so, there's a strong connection between ethics and laws regarding the nurse's role as a patient advocate.

Torts

Torts are personal civil injuries that reside outside a contractual relationship. Torts result in a civil trial to assess compensation for the plaintiff. Torts can be intentional or unintentional.

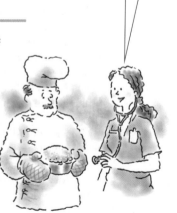

No, that's a lovely tart, but I said 'tort'! You know, an injury that resides outside a contractual relationship.

Intentional torts

Intentional torts include fraud, assault and battery, invasion of privacy, false imprisonment and defamation of character.

Unintentional torts

Unintentional torts include negligence and malpractice. Negligence is a mistake or the failure to be careful. Malpractice is defined as a professional person's wrongful conduct, improper discharge of professional duties or failure to meet standards of care that results in harm to another person.

Regulation of nursing practice

The practice of nursing requires rules and regulations to ensure patient safety and a competent level of behaviour in the professional role as a nurse. Your nursing registration allows you to practice as a professional nurse. Standards of nursing practice help ensure high-quality care and serve as criteria in legal questions of whether adequate care was rendered. These standards are clearly defined by the *NMC the Code* (2008). (See Chapter 1.)

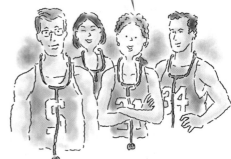

Becoming a registered nurse makes you part of an elite health-care team—and that's an awesome responsibility!

Registration

Your registration entitles you to practise as a professionally qualified nurse. However, like most privileges, your registration imposes certain responsibilities. As a registered nurse, you're responsible for providing quality care to your patients. To meet this responsibility and protect your right

---

The NMC recommends that a registered nurse, midwife or specialist community public health nurse, in advising, treating and caring for patients/clients, has professional indemnity insurance. This is in the interests of clients, patients and registrants in the event of claims of professional negligence.

- Employers have vicarious liability for the negligent acts and/or omissions of their employees.
- It is the individual registrant's responsibility to establish their insurance status and take appropriate action.
- In situations where an employer does not have vicarious liability, the NMC recommends that registrants obtain adequate professional indemnity insurance.
- If unable to secure professional indemnity insurance, a registrant will need to demonstrate that all their clients/patients are fully informed of this fact and of the implications this might have in the event of a claim for professional negligence.

Reproduced with kind permission of NMC, London.

to practice, you must understand the professional and legal significance of your registration.

PREP

In order to maintain registration, nurses must achieve the post-registration education and practice standards (PREP). These are separated into two standards:

* The PREP (practice) standard.

   Registered nurses or midwives must have worked in their relative profession during the previous three years for a minimum of 450 hours. This work can include paid or unpaid work.

   If these hours have not been achieved in the timeframe you must undertake a return to practice programme at an approval institution.

* The PREP (continuing professional development) standard.

   The registered nurses must demonstrate that they have undertaken at least 35 hours of learning activity relevant to their practice within the 3-year period. This must be recorded in their personal and professional profile which all nurses must maintain throughout their career (NMC, 2008). The PREP handbook contains more detailed information and gives examples; this can be obtained from www.nmc-uk.org.

Legal issues affecting nursing

Nurses are faced with legal issues that may affect their nursing care. Patient rights and documentation are two of the most common issues nurses face.

Patient rights

At one time, nurses were forbidden to give patients even the most basic information about their care or health, but patients began demanding more information about their care and turned to nurses to assist them in getting the information. In 1991 *The Patients' Charter* was published, outlining standards which all patients could expect; it no longer exists but has been replaced with a variety of care improvement initiatives at government and local levels. These, for example, include waiting time initiatives, privacy and dignity issues, and provision of information.

Informed consent

Being adequately informed about proposed treatment, procedures, surgery or research in order to properly consent is a patient's legal right. So, it isn't surprising that the topic of informed consent appears in all current medical and nursing texts and that a signed informed consent form must be in the patient's records when invasive or experimental procedures, treatment or surgery is contemplated.

Note! The Mental Health Act cannot be used to enforce people to receive treatment for any physical interventions.

In the know

Informed consent basically means that the patient, or someone acting on their behalf, has enough information to know what's at risk in undergoing the proposed treatment, and the possible consequences should consent to the treatment be refused or withdrawn. Nurses may provide patients and their families with information that's within a nurse's scope of practice and knowledge base. However, it is the responsibility of the medical staff to explain the risks and benefit of treatments. The nurse may then support what has been said by providing literature or a referring to a relevant specialist nurse who will be able to support the patient more fully.

Capacity to consent

Under certain circumstances, people with mental disorders may be held incompetent to consent.

When there's a question about an individual's ability to give consent, the Mental Health Act 1983 (revised 2007) can be used to ensure the person receives the treatment they need for their own mental health or to protect others from harm. Section 29 of the Mental Health Act (2007) clarifies the position when a patient is deemed unable to understand the effects, nature and purpose of their treatment. A second doctor (who must be approved for this purpose) is needed to confirm treatment and needs to provide a certificate to this effect. They certify that treatment is needed and can be given even though the patient can't consent.

Documentation

Accurate documentation is a record of the care given to a patient throughout their stay; it also includes reasons for not delivering care. For example if a patient refuses a wash in the morning this is documented in order that this aspect of care can be offered again later in the day. This is also important in case a complaint is made by the patient or their relatives at a later time. It also proves that you're following the accepted standards of nursing care mandated by the law, your profession and your employer. Always document your nursing care and your patient's response to that care. *The NMC record keeping: Guidance for nurses and midwives* (2009) gives clear guidance for standards of all documentation including:

- principles of good record-keeping
- confidentiality
- access
- disclosure of information
- information systems
- personal and professional knowledge and skills.

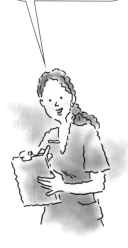

By all means, provide your patients with the information they need to give an informed consent— only, make sure it's within your scope of practice and nursing knowledge base.

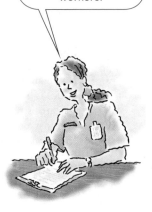

Proper documentation communicates crucial information to other health-care workers.

The evidence speaks for itself

Proper documentation communicates crucial information to caregivers so they make fewer errors. How and what you document can determine whether you or your employer wins or loses a legal dispute. Medical records are used as evidence; poor documentation is the pivotal issue in many malpractice cases.

Quick quiz

1. The Code of Ethics for Nurses provides information that's necessary for the practicing nurse to:
 A. document their nursing care appropriately.
 B. make ethical decisions about patient care.
 C. use their professional skills in providing the most effective holistic care possible.
 D. strengthen and protect patient privacy.

Answer: C. The Code of Ethics for Nurses provides information that's necessary for the practicing nurse to use their professional skills in providing the most effective holistic care possible.

2. Which of the following is a type of unintentional tort?
 A. Invasion of privacy
 B. Malpractice
 C. Assault and battery
 D. Defamation of character

Answer: B. Unintentional torts include negligence and malpractice. Intentional torts include invasion of privacy, fraud, assault and battery, invasion of privacy, false imprisonment and defamation of character.

3. Which part of the medical record can be used as evidence in court?
 A. Entire record
 B. Medical orders
 C. Care plan
 D. Nursing notes

Answer: A. The entire medical record is a legal document that's admissible in court.

Scoring

☆☆☆ If you answered all three questions correctly, bravo! Your understanding of ethics is beyond reproach.

☆☆ If you answered two questions correctly, way to go! You've judged correctly on most legal issues in this chapter.

☆ If you answered fewer than two questions correctly, don't fret! It isn't grounds for malpractice. Review the chapter, and try again.

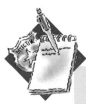

Just the facts

In this chapter, you'll learn:

♦ guidelines for performing an assessment based on the nursing process

♦ ways to write nursing care plans with expected outcomes and appropriate interventions

♦ how to evaluate and document nursing interventions and outcomes.

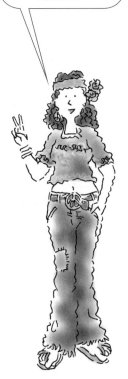

Peace and love weren't the only good things to come out of the 1960s. The nursing process was another!

A look at the nursing process

The nursing process is a problem-solving approach to nursing care. It's a systematic method for assessing the patient's health problems, devising a plan to address them, implementing the plan and evaluating the effectiveness of the care provided.

The nursing process emerged in the 1960s as team health care came into wider practice and nurses were increasingly called upon to define their specific roles. The roots of the nursing process can be traced to World War II, however, when technology, medical advances and a growing need for nurses began to change the nursing profession.

Going through the phases

The nursing process consists of four distinct phases:

Assessment. Identifying problems and their causes with the patient.

Plan. Making an action plan to eliminate the problems.

Implementation. Carry out the plan.

Evaluation. Determine if the plans have had an effect.

These four phases are dynamic, and they commonly overlap. Together, they resemble similar steps that many other professionals take to identify and correct problems.

Assessment

The first step in the nursing process is assessment, and this begins when you first see the patient. Information gathered should accurately reflect the patient's life experiences and their patterns of living. Assessment continues through the patient's care as you obtain more information about their changing condition.

Getting the whole picture

During assessment, you collect relevant information from various sources and analyse it to form a complete picture of your patient. As you collect this information, you need to document it accurately for two reasons:

It guides you through the rest of the nursing process, helping you formulate nursing care plans, expected outcomes and nursing interventions.

It serves as a vital communication tool for other team members— as a baseline for evaluating a patient's progress and for use as legal documentation.

First impressions

In your initial assessment, consider the patient's immediate and emerging needs, including not only their physical needs but also their psychological, spiritual and social concerns. The initial assessment helps you determine what care the patient needs and sets the stage for further assessments. Remember that a patient's family, culture and religion are important factors in the patient's response to illness and treatment.

Assessment types

Assessment is usually undertaken by using an appropriate model of nursing; for example using the Roper, Logan and Tierney's activities of living will enable you to make a systematic assessment in order to plan the care of the patient. It is important to involve the patient and to remember that assessment is an ongoing process which changes the plan of care throughout the patient's illness.

Initial assessment

An initial, or admission, assessment occurs when the patient first comes to the health-care facility. The initial assessment helps you determine what care the patient needs and sets the stage for further assessments.

Emergency assessment

An emergency assessment occurs during a life-threatening situation. Rapid identification of and interventions for the patient's immediate health problem is foremost. These difficulties usually centre on the patient's ABCs (airway, breathing and circulation). An emergency assessment isn't a comprehensive assessment.

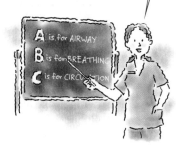

An emergency assessment usually focuses only on the basics. Remember your ABCs!

Health history

A health history includes physical, psychological, cultural, spiritual and psychosocial data. It's the main source of information about the patient's health status and guides the physical examination that follows.

A nursing history is different from a medical history. A medical history guides diagnosis and treatment of illnesses; a nursing history focuses holistically on the human response to illness.

The nursing history you collect helps you:
- plan health care
- assess the impact of illness on the patient and members of their family. Remember! this will include physical, mental, social and spiritual aspects.
- evaluate the patient's health education needs
- initiate discharge planning.

Effective techniques

To obtain the most benefit from an assessment, try to ensure that the patient feels comfortable and respected and believe they can trust you. Use effective interview techniques to help the patient identify resources and improve problem-solving abilities. Remember, however, that successful techniques in one situation may not be effective in another. Your attitude and the patient's interpretation of your questions can vary. In general, you should:
- allow the patient time to think and reflect
- encourage the patient to talk
- encourage the patient to describe a particular experience
- indicate that you've listened to the patient such as by paraphrasing the patient's response.

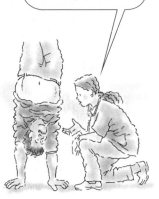

I think you might be a little more comfortable completing your assessment in one of the chairs behind me.

Know right from wrong

Although there are many right ways to communicate with a patient, there are also some wrong ways that can hamper your interview. (See *Interview techniques to avoid*.)

Conducting the interview

The physical surroundings, psychological atmosphere, interview structure and questioning style can all affect the interview flow and outcome. So can your ability to adopt a communication style that fits your patient's needs and the situation at hand. To enhance the interviewing process, close the door to help prevent interruptions and try to arrange yourself so that you're facing the patient, slightly offset from them, to create a friendly feeling.

Start at the very beginning

Begin by introducing yourself. Establish an interview time frame, and ask whether the patient has questions about the interview procedure. Spend a few minutes chatting informally before beginning the interview.

A note on notes

Lengthy note taking may distract the patient, who may wonder whether you're listening. If you must take notes, tell the patient before the interview starts.

Short and sweet

A patient who's ill, experiencing pain or sedated may have difficulty completing the assessment. In such instances, obtain only the information pertaining to the immediate problem. To avoid tiring a seriously ill patient, obtain the information in several sessions or ask a close family relative or friend to supply essential information.

Two types

Typically, the assessment includes two types of questions: open-ended, which permit more subtle and flexible responses, and closed-ended, which require only a yes-or-no response. Open-ended questions usually result in the most useful information and give patients the feeling that they're actively participating in and have some control over the interview. Closed-ended questions help eliminate rambling conversations. They're also useful when the assessment requires brevity—for example when a patient reports extreme pain or digresses frequently.

Interview techniques to avoid

Some interview techniques cause problems between the nurse and the patient. Avoid:
- asking 'why' or 'how' questions
- asking probing or persistent questions
- using inappropriate language
- giving advice
- giving false reassurance
- changing the subject or interrupting
- using clichés or stereotypical responses
- giving excessive approval or agreement
- jumping to conclusions
- using defensive responses.

Logical and patient

Whatever question type you use, move logically from one assessment section to the next. Allow the patient to concentrate and give complete information on a subject before moving on.

Obtaining assessment data

There are two sources of data: primary and secondary. The patient is the source of primary data. These data are considered the most reliable unless circumstances prevent you from obtaining information directly from the patient, as when the patient has an altered level of consciousness, impending surgery or severe pain. The patient would also be an unreliable source if they are confused or suffers from a mental condition that alters thinking, judgement and memory.

Secondary sources provide information that supports, validates, clarifies and supplements the information gathered from the patient. These sources include family members or significant others, laboratory results, health-care record, diagnostic procedures and health team members.

Personal information

Begin obtaining the patient's health history by collecting personal information. This data section identifies the patient and provides important demographic information. By filling out a form, you usually gather such facts as the patient's address, telephone number, age, sex, date of birth, race, nationality, marital status, occupation, education, religion, cultural background and emergency contact person.

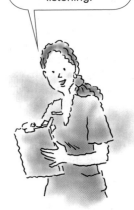

> Lengthy note-taking may distract the patient or make them wonder whether you're listening.

Planning the care

After you have identified the problems with the patient, you will develop a written care plan. A written care plan serves as a communication tool among health-care team members that helps ensure continuity of care. The plan consists of two parts:

- patient outcomes, or expected outcomes, which describe behaviours or results to be achieved within a specified time frame

- nursing interventions needed to achieve those outcomes.

Measure and observe

Be sure to state both parts of the care plan in measurable, observable terms and dates. The statement 'The patient will perceive himself with greater

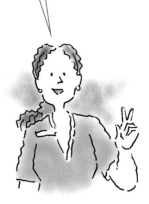

> Remember, a nursing care plan contains two important parts: measurable, achievable goals and specific interventions for effecting change and achieving the goals.

Ensuring a successful care plan

Your care plan must rest on a solid foundation of carefully identified problems. It also must fit your patient's needs, age, developmental level, culture, strengths and weaknesses and willingness and ability to take part in their care. Your plan should help the patient attain the highest functional level possible while posing minimal risk and not creating new problems. If complete recovery isn't possible, your plan should help the patient cope physically and emotionally with their impaired or declining health.

Using the following guidelines will help ensure that your care plan is effective.

Be realistic

Avoid setting a goal that's too difficult for the patient to achieve. The patient may become discouraged, depressed and apathetic if they can't achieve expected outcomes. Start with short-term goals.

Tailor your approach

Individualise your care plan and the nursing interventions. Keep in mind that each patient is unique; no two patients' problems are exactly alike.

Avoid vague terms

Use precise, quantitative terms rather than vague ones. For example to indicate that the patient's vital signs are stable, document specific measurements, such as 'heart rate 80 beats per minute' rather than 'heart rate stable'.

self-worth' is too vague, lacks a time frame and offers no means to observe the patient's self-perception. A patient outcome such as 'The patient will describe himself in a positive way within 1 week' provides an observable means to evaluate the patient's behaviour and a time frame for the behavioural change. (See *Ensuring a successful care plan*.)

Implementation

The implementation phase is when you put your care plan into action. Implementation encompasses all nursing interventions directed at solving the patient's problems and meeting health-care needs. While you co-ordinate implementation, you also seek help from the patient, the patient's family and other caregivers.

Now, I've got a job for you...and you...and you...and you...

Monitor and gauge

After implementing the care plan, continue to monitor the patient to gauge the effectiveness of interventions and adjust them as the patient's condition changes. Documentation of outcomes achieved should be reflected in the care plan. Expect to review, revise and update the entire care plan regularly, according to local policy. Keep in mind that the care plan is a permanent part of the patient's medical record. (See *Writing excellent outcome statements*.)

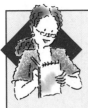

Note!

Writing excellent outcome statements

These tips will help you write clear, precise outcome statements:

- When writing expected outcomes in your care plan, always start with a specific action verb that focuses on your patient's behaviour. By telling your reader how your patient should look, walk, eat, drink, turn, cough, speak or stand, for example you give a clear picture of how to evaluate progress.
- Avoid starting expected outcome statements with allow, let, enable or similar verbs. Such words focus attention on your own and other health-care team members' behaviour—not the patient's.
- With many documentation formats, you won't need to include the phrase 'The patient will' with each expected outcome statement. However, you'll have to specify to which person the outcome refers when family, friends or others are directly involved.

Evaluation

After the stated time has elapsed for the care plan to effect the desired changes, you're ready for evaluation, the next step in the nursing process. During evaluation, you must decide whether the interventions carried out have enabled the patient to achieve the desired outcomes. (See *Effective evaluation statements*, page 50.)

Start with the finish

Begin by reviewing the patient outcomes stated for each problem. Then observe your patient's condition and judge how well they meet the outcomes related to them. Does the patient's condition match the outcomes or fall short of them?

Consider the evaluation to be positive if the patient's condition has changed as expected, if the outcomes have been accomplished or if progress has occurred. Failure to meet these criteria constitutes a negative evaluation and requires new interventions.

A successful resolution

The evaluation phase also allows you to judge the effectiveness of the nursing process as a whole. If the process has been applied successfully, the patient's

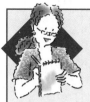

Note!

Effective evaluation statements

These evaluation statements clearly describe common outcomes. Note that they include specific details of the care provided and objective evidence of the patient's response to care:

- Able to describe the signs and symptoms of hyperglycaemia (response to patient education)
- Able to walk to the chair with a steady gait, unassisted for approximately 5 metres (tolerance of change or increase in activity)
- Unable to tolerate removal of O_2, became dyspnoeic on room air, even at rest (tolerance of treatments)

health status will improve. Their health problems will have been solved, or progress will have been made toward achieving their resolution. They will also be able to perform self-care measures with a sense of independence and confidence, and you'll feel reassured that you've fulfilled your professional responsibility.

Nursing care plans

The nursing care plan is a vital source of information about the patient's problems, needs and goals. It contains detailed instructions for achieving the goals established for the patient and is used to direct care. (See *Tips for top-notch care plans*.)

Your patient's nursing care plan may be in one of two styles: traditional or standardised.

Traditional care plan

The traditional care plan is written from scratch for each patient. Most have three main columns:

 patient's problem

 goals

 interventions.

Tips for top-notch care plans

Use a traditional or standardised method for recording your care plan. A traditional care plan is written from scratch for each patient. A standardised care plan saves time because it's pre-determined based on the patient's problems.

No matter which method you use, follow these tips to write an accurate and useful plan:

- Write in black ink, and sign your name.
- Use clear, concise language, not vague terms or generalities.
- Use agreed abbreviations to avoid confusion.
- Review all your assessment data before selecting an approach for each problem; if you can't complete the initial assessment, immediately write insufficient information on your records.
- Write an agreed goal and a target date for each problem you identify.

- Set realistic goals.
- When writing nursing interventions, consider what to watch for and how often, what nursing measures to take and how to perform them, and what to teach the patient and their family before discharge.
- Make each nursing intervention specific.
- Be creative; include a drawing or an innovative procedure if doing so makes your directions more specific.
- Record all of the patient's problems and concerns so they won't be forgotten.
- Make sure your care plan is implemented correctly.
- Evaluate the results of your plan, and discontinue problems that have been resolved; select new approaches, if necessary, for problems that haven't been resolved.

Documenting marathon

When using the traditional care plan, there may be other columns for the date when the care plan was initiated, target dates for agreed goals, and dates for review, revisions and resolutions. Most forms also have a place for you to sign or initial whenever you make an entry or revision. Although this type of care plan allows you to individualise the care of each patient, it requires lengthy documentation.

Standardised care plan

More commonly, your patient will have a standardised care plan that's pre-printed to save documentation time. Most standardised plans are specifically designed for one particular problem; therefore, some patients will require several plans, one for each problem identified.

Using standardised care plans frees you up to spend more time caring for your patients—after all, isn't that why you chose to become a nurse in the first place?

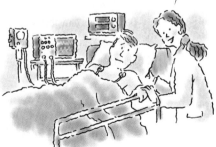

Individualising care plans

Even though these care plans are standardised, they allow you to individualise the plan for each of your patients by adding:

- *frequency of interventions*. To an intervention, such as 'Perform passive range-of-motion exercises', you might add 'twice daily: 1 × each morning and evening'.
- *specific instructions for interventions*. For the standard intervention 'Elevate patient's head', you might specify 'before sleep, on three pillows'.

Care pathways

Care pathways are care plans developed by multidisciplinary teams, not just nurses. They include assessment criteria, interventions, treatments and agreed goals for specific conditions according to a time line. These allow the patient to have a summary of their care and the goals and time frame.

Most care pathways have been developed in line with National Institute for Health and Clinical Excellence (NICE) guidelines to enable a more structured and uniform approach to care, which then allows for more in-depth analysis of the outcomes.

Examples of local and national care pathways which have been developed include:

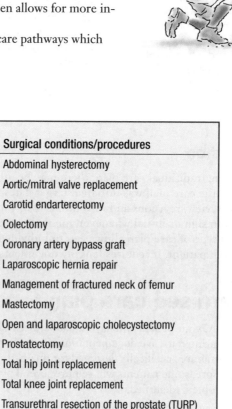

I was so sure the care pathway would be just past that last banana tree! Dr. Livingstone, where are you?

Medical conditions	Surgical conditions/procedures
Acute exacerbation of chronic obstructive lung disease	Abdominal hysterectomy
Acute myocardial infarction	Aortic/mitral valve replacement
Acute pneumonia	Carotid endarterectomy
Asthma	Colectomy
Chest pain	Coronary artery bypass graft
Deep venous thrombosis	Laparoscopic hernia repair
Depression in the elderly	Management of fractured neck of femur
Inflammatory bowel disease	Mastectomy
Stroke	Open and laparoscopic cholecystectomy
Varicose veins	Prostatectomy
	Total hip joint replacement
	Total knee joint replacement
	Transurethral resection of the prostate (TURP)

Complete coverage

Think of the pathway as a pre-determined checklist describing the tasks you and the patient must accomplish. Unlike a nursing care plan, its focus is multidisciplinary, covering all of the patient's problems, not just those identified during a nursing assessment. (See *Care pathways*.)

Care pathways cover the key events that must occur before the patient's target discharge date. These events include:
- consultations
- diagnostic tests
- treatments
- medications
- procedures
- activities
- diet
- patient teaching
- discharge planning
- achievement of agreed goals.

Multidisciplinary team

Nurses aren't the only health-care professionals involved in patient care. You'll need to collaborate with the multidisciplinary team to meet the diverse needs of your patients.

Share and share alike

The focus of a multidisciplinary team is on the patient and patient outcomes. Each team member shares the responsibility for achieving them. To provide more effective and comprehensive care, you need to understand each team member's role.

Members of the health-care team include the:
- registered dietician, who assesses and monitors nutritional needs, makes nutritional recommendations and provides patient education
- social worker, who provides support and counselling to patients and their families, and helps with financial difficulties
- occupational therapist, who assists the patient in performing activities of daily living, participating in recreation and working to their highest functional level
- physiotherapist, who provides therapy to improve or restore physical functioning and prevent deterioration
- pharmacist, who reviews, prepares and dispenses the patient's medications; provides information and guidance in the preparation and administration of medications; and provides patient education.

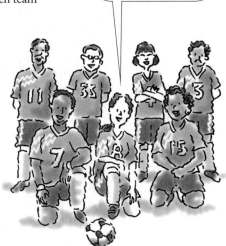

Multidisciplinary teamwork gets the job done!

Passing notes is permitted!

When you're reviewing the patient's chart, be sure to read the progress notes written by other members of the health-care team. These notes will provide you with important information about your patient.

If you have questions about the patient's condition or treatment, contact the appropriate team members for more information. For example, the pharmacist can provide information about how to space medications to eliminate drug or food interactions, whereas the physiotherapist can provide guidelines on how to transfer a patient with fractures safely from the bed to a chair.

Work well with others

You'll also need to co-ordinate care with other team members. For example medicating your post-operative patient before respiratory exercises helps the patient cough and deep-breathe more effectively with the physiotherapist. When working with the other team members, remember to use good communication skills. Above all, treat all team members with respect, and they'll respect you in turn!

> Thanks for reviewing the patient with me. It's so busy today. I appreciate your taking the time!

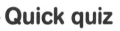

Quick quiz

1. When assessing a patient, ask first about:
    A.   their main problem.
    B.   personal information.
    C.   family history.

Answer: B. Take care of the personal information first; otherwise, you might get involved in the patient history and forget to ask basic questions.

2. Expected outcomes are defined as:
    A.   goals the patient should reach as a result of planned nursing interventions.
    B.   goals set by the medical team for each patient.
    C.   goals a little higher than what the patient can realistically reach to help motivate him.
    D.   what a patient and family ask you to accomplish.

Answer: A. Expected outcomes are realistic, measurable goals and their target dates.

3. The primary source of assessment information is:
    A.   the patient's friends.
    B.   the patient's family members.
    C.   the patient.
    D.   the medical records.

Answer: C. The patient should be your primary source of assessment information. However, if the patient is sedated, confused, hostile, angry, dyspnoeic or in pain, you may have to rely initially on family members or close friends to supply information.

Scoring

☆☆☆   If you answered all three questions correctly, super! You're a nursing process pro.

☆☆   If you answered two questions correctly, great! You've got the nursing process pretty down pat.

☆   If you answered fewer than two questions correctly, chin up! Process this chapter one more time and try again.

Part II

General nursing skills

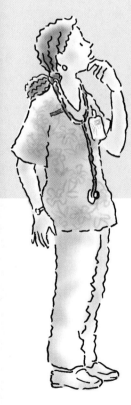

5	Communication	59
6	Nursing assessment	73
7	Taking vital signs	82
8	Asepsis and infection control	101
9	Medication basics	116
10	Medication administration	145
11	I.V. therapy	196

(5) Communication

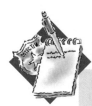

Just the facts

In this chapter, you'll learn:

♦ verbal and non-verbal methods of communication

♦ the phases of a therapeutic relationship

♦ how to incorporate therapeutic use of self

♦ how to identify and handle communication barriers

♦ the importance of communication in documenting patient care.

A look at communication

What is communication? Communication is a way to fulfil a person's basic need to relate to others. Communication is dynamic and ongoing and is a way to interact and develop relationships. It's also a way to effect change.

Nurses encounter many people during the course of their education and nursing career. They communicate with educators, patients, family members and other members of the health-care team. Learning to communicate effectively is a skill that sometimes takes time and effort.

Verbal communication

Verbal communication is the transmission of messages through spoken or written language. For effective verbal communication, five criteria must be met:

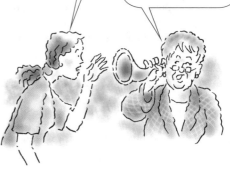

I said, 'Learning to communicate effectively is a skill.'

Ouch! You don't have to shout. Where'd you learn your skills? A barnyard?

simplicity

 clarity

 timing and relevance

 adaptability

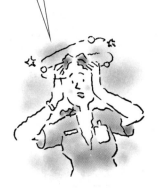 credibility.

Simplicity

In verbal communication, you must state complex information in commonly understood terms. This is especially important when communicating with patients. For instance, when explaining a procedure to the patient, you must be careful to use the most appropriate terminology that the patient will understand. Use short sentences that express the idea completely. Long explanations are sometimes difficult for people to understand because the context of the explanation gets lost.

Avoiding the void

Avoid using medical terminology. For instance, when asking a patient whether they need to use the bathroom facilities, the patient won't understand, 'Do you have to void?' They will better understand what you mean if you ask them if they have to 'pass water' or go to the bathroom.

> I'm sorry. Your explanation was so long and convoluted, you lost me at the beginning!

Clarity

Verbal communication must be clear. You should state exactly what you mean. Don't make the listener guess what you mean or make assumptions.

Say what you mean

For instance, if you're explaining a medication regimen to a patient who has never taken medicine before, don't tell them they must take the medication four times per day. You must be clear and tell them exactly how many hours should elapse before taking the medication.

Timing and relevance

Make sure that the message is communicated at a time when the receiver is ready to receive it. If your patient is in pain, don't try to explain a procedure or do patient teaching. They will be more receptive when their pain subsides.

Score one for format!

Ensure that the message is communicated in an appropriate format. If your patient has trouble visualising what you're saying, try using written materials or diagrams to complement your verbal explanation to help them to understand better.

Adaptability

Communication that's effective is adaptable and states the message that reflects the situation. For instance, as you prepare your teaching plan, you may need to adapt the way you communicate if the patient is hearing or visually impaired or speaks another language.

That suits me just fine

Verbal communication also shows appropriateness to the receiver. If the patient is a young child or an infant, it may be necessary to communicate with the parents or guardian instead of the child.

Credibility

In order for communication to be credible, it must be stated in a trustworthy and believable manner.

Honestly now!

It must also be accurate, consistent and honest. Before you communicate with someone, make sure that you know the content area. Communication commonly spurs continued conversation, so be prepared and well versed in your subject in order to be able to answer any question that arises. If you're asked to explain information that's beyond your scope of practice or your ability, you must be honest with the patient and tell them that you can't answer their question. Explain, however, that you'll convey their concerns to someone who'll be able to answer them.

Verbal communication strategies

Verbal communication strategies range from alternating between open-ended and closed questions to employing such techniques as silence, prompting, confirmation, reflection, clarification, summary and conclusion.

An open . . .

Asking open-ended questions such as 'How did you fall?' lets the patient respond more freely. Their response may provide answers to many other questions. For instance, from the patient's answer, you might learn that they have fallen previously; that they were unsteady on their feet before they fell

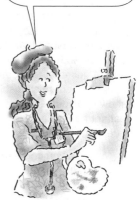

Maybe I can paint a better picture of the procedure this way. Do you prefer watercolours or pastels?

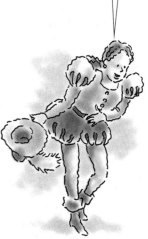

". . . and it must follow, as the night the day, thou canst not then be false to any man" . . . Actually, I honestly don't know the answer!

Two ways to ask

Questions can be characterised as open-ended or closed.

Open-ended questions

Open-ended questions require the patient to express feelings, opinions and ideas. They also help you gather more information than can otherwise be gathered with closed questions. Open-ended questions encourage a good nurse–patient relationship because they show that you're interested in what the patient has to say. Examples of such questions include:

- 'Why did you come to the hospital tonight?'
- 'How would you describe the problems you're having with your breathing?'

- 'What lung problems, if any, do other members of your family have?'

Closed questions

Closed questions elicit 'yes' or 'no' answers or one- to two-word responses. They limit the development of the nurse–patient relationship. Although closed questions can help you 'zoom in' on specific points, they don't provide the patient with an opportunity to elaborate. Examples of closed questions include:

- 'Do you ever get short of breath?'
- 'Are you the only one in your family with lung problems?'

and that they fell just before eating dinner. Armed with this information, you might deduce that the patient had a syncopal episode caused by hypoglycaemia.

. . . and shut case

You may also choose to ask closed questions. Although these questions are unlikely to provide extra information, they may encourage the patient to give clear, concise feedback. (See *Two ways to ask*.)

Silence is golden

Another technique is to allow moments of silence during the interview. In addition to encouraging the patient to continue talking, this technique also gives you a chance to assess his ability to organise thoughts. You may find this technique difficult as most people are uncomfortable with silence, but the more often you use it, the more comfortable you'll become.

Give them a boost

Using such phrases as 'please continue', 'go on' and even 'uh-huh' encourages the patient to continue with his story. Known as prompting, this feedback shows them that you're interested in what they are saying.

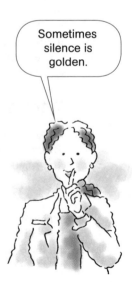

Sometimes silence is golden.

Confirmation conversation

Employing the technique of confirmation (or paraphrasing) helps ensure that you and the patient are on the same track. You might say, 'If I understand you correctly, you said', and then repeat the information the patient gave. Doing so helps to clear up misconceptions that you or the patient might have.

Check and reflect

Try using reflection—repeating something the patient has just said—to help you obtain more specific information. For example, a patient with a stomach ache might say, 'I know I have an ulcer.' If so, you can repeat, 'You know you have an ulcer?' Then the patient might say, 'Yes. I had one before, and the pain is the same.'

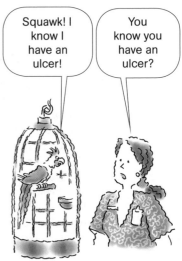

Clear skies

When information is vague or confusing, use the technique of clarification. For example, if your patient says, 'I can't stand this', your response might be, 'What can't you stand?' or 'What do you mean by "I can't stand this"?' Doing so gives the patient an opportunity to explain their statement.

Put the landing gear down . . .

Get in the habit of restating the information the patient gave you. Known as summarisation, this technique ensures that the data you've collected are accurate and complete. Summarisation also signals that the interview is about to end.

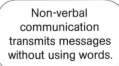

. . . and come in for a safe landing

Signal the patient when you're ready to conclude the interview. This signal gives them the opportunity to gather his thoughts and make any pertinent final statements. You can do this by saying, 'I think I have all the information I need now. Is there anything you would like to add?'

Non-verbal communication

Non-verbal communication transmits messages without using words. It's commonly referred to as body language. Non-verbal communication includes facial expressions, posture, gait, hand gestures, tone of voice, positioning and space, touch, appearance and level of alertness. Non-verbal communication can convey feelings of sadness, joy and anxiety. It reflects self-concept, current mood and health.

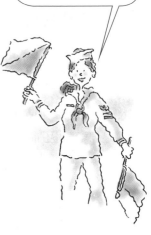

Mixed messages

Non-verbal communication aids interpretation of verbal communication, but also requires acute observation by the receiver for accurate interpretation of the message. For instance, your patient may state that their pain has subsided, but you notice that they are guarded and is clenching the side rails on the bed. Their verbal communication tells you one thing, but their non-verbal actions reveal something else.

Non-verbal communication strategies

To make the most of non-verbal communication, do the following:
• Listen attentively and make eye contact frequently. (See *Overcoming cultural barriers*.)
• Use reassuring gestures, such as nodding your head, to encourage the patient to keep talking.
• Watch for non-verbal clues that indicate the patient is uncomfortable or unsure about how to answer a question. For example, they might lower their voice or glance around uneasily.
• Be aware of your own non-verbal behaviours that might cause the patient to stop talking or become defensive. For example, if you cross your arms, you might appear closed off from them. If you stand while they are sitting, you might appear superior. If you glance at your watch, you might appear to be bored or rushed, which could keep the patient from answering questions completely.
• Observe the patient closely to see whether they understand each question. If they don't appear to understand, repeat the question using different words or familiar examples. For instance, instead of asking, 'Did you have respiratory difficulty after exercising?' ask, 'Did you have to sit down after walking around the block?'

> ### Overcoming cultural barriers
>
> To maintain a good relationship with your patient, remember that their cultural behaviours and beliefs may differ from your own. For example, most people in the United Kingdom make eye contact when talking with others. However, people in several other cultures, including Asians, Afro Caribbean and people from Arabic-speaking countries, may find eye contact disrespectful or aggressive.

Therapeutic relationships

A therapeutic relationship occurs when you interact with a patient in a clinical setting. This interaction is the beginning of the nurse–patient relationship.

The building process

The nurse–patient relationship doesn't just happen; it's created with care and skill and built on the patient's trust of the nurse. The building process follows a natural progression of four distinct phases:

    pre-interaction

    orientation

working

 termination.

Pre-interaction phase

During the pre-interaction phase, you can review the patient data that you might already have, such as the medical or surgical history and information gained from family members. If at all possible, after reviewing this information, try to anticipate any concerns or issues that might arise.

Orientation phase

Orientation is the stage when you first meet the patient. More than likely, it will occur at the bedside when the patient is admitted. This time is the best time for you to talk to the patient and get to know them. However, the meeting commonly isn't leisurely or controlled—especially if the patient is in the emergency department, in pain or apprehensive. Even in difficult situations, though, you must use your verbal and non-verbal communication skills to ease the patient's fears and begin the relationship.

> Do your best to make a good first impression by remaining warm, open and attentive to the patient's needs.

First impressions

During the orientation phase, the patient will be forming a first impression of your meeting. They will be watching you closely and forming an opinion about your interest in their health care. By presenting a warm, caring manner, you'll make this first impression one that helps build a good nurse–patient relationship.

Trust-building

Trust-building is a very important part of the therapeutic relationship you develop with the patient. If the patient doesn't trust you, they won't be open and answer your questions. Take time to sit down with them. Close the curtain so that they feel they have your undivided attention. Sit down in a chair so they don't feel that you're in a hurry to leave. Also, act with integrity so that the patient can develop confidence in you and your abilities.

Role clarification

Patients are becoming increasingly knowledgeable about their bodies. They have access to a wealth of information today via the Internet, newspapers and magazines. As patients learn more about how to stay healthy, they're taking a more active role in their health care. You must recognise this role and respect it. Patients' growing involvement in their own health care is helping to change the approach of many health-care professionals from the authoritarian 'Do as I say' attitude to the more co-operative 'Here's why I recommend this' approach.

Sign here

As you begin to develop the therapeutic relationship with your patient, you develop a contract with them that's built on trust and your mutual desire to see that they receive the treatment they need.

Working phase

The working phase is a team-building phase that includes you, the patient and the entire health-care team. During this phase, you encourage the patient and help them to understand their condition and how to set goals. Using therapeutic communication, you encourage the patient to accomplish their goals.

Let's remember . . . we're a team. By working together, we'll accomplish our goals.

Give and take

This phase is a give-and-take phase because you and the patient have specific roles to play and certain expectations of what will happen during the relationship. You, as the nurse, expect the patient to be willing to participate in their health care by providing accurate information, asking questions about treatments, and participating in treatment procedures as appropriate. The patient, on the other hand, expects that their health-care needs will be met by you and the other members of the health-care team. They expect you, as their health-care advocate, to keep them informed and provide them with the correct treatments and procedures.

Termination phase

As you near the termination phase, you must remind the patient that the termination of the relationship is near. You can do so simply by saying good-bye at the end of your shift. However, termination can be more complex and include discharge planning. At the same time, you may also be paving the way for more relationships to develop with the patient's health-care team as you make necessary referrals for community nurse visits and rehabilitation.

Smooth sailing

By making the termination phase an easy one, you achieve a smooth transition for the patient to other health-care team members.

Therapeutic use of self

Using interpersonal skills in a healing way to help the patient is called therapeutic use of self. Three important techniques enhance therapeutic use of self:

 exhibiting empathy

 demonstrating acceptance

 giving recognition.

Path to empathy

To show empathy, use phrases that address the patient's feelings, such as 'That must have upset you.'

Acceptance acts

To show acceptance, use neutral statements, such as 'I hear what you're saying' and 'I see.' Non-verbal behaviours, such as nodding or making momentary eye contact, also provide encouragement without indicating agreement or disagreement.

I recognise that

To give recognition, listen actively to what the patient says, occasionally providing verbal or non-verbal acknowledgement to encourage them to continue speaking.

Blocks to communication

Various factors contribute to the communication process and directly affect a person's ability to send and receive messages. In some cases, a patient's special needs can be a deterrent to effective communication. However, these needs shouldn't be an excuse for failing to find alternative ways to promote communication. As a nurse, you need to understand which factors influence communication so that you can clear away any barriers. (See *Considering communication barriers*, page 68.)

Obvious communication barriers, such as speaking another language and being hearing or speaking impaired, are obvious communication barriers but aren't insurmountable. What about the

Memory jogger

When it comes to therapeutic interpersonal patient communication skills, lend an EAR! Make sure you show:

Empathy

Acceptance

Recognition.

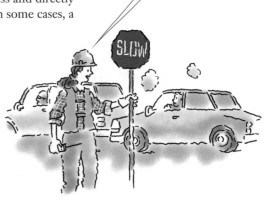

Don't let communication barriers get in your way. There's always another route around a difficult situation.

Considering communication barriers

This diagram shows the components of nurse–patient communication. Note the factors that affect communication, such as orientation, preconceptions and language. Your sensitivity to these factors makes the difference between effective and ineffective communication.

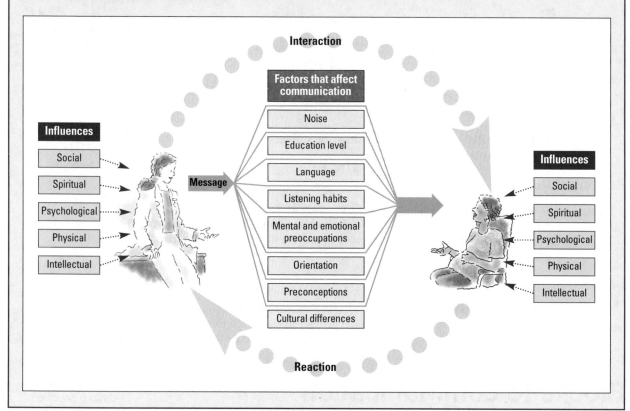

more difficult barriers, such as dealing with a young child, an elderly patient or an unconscious patient?

Children

When dealing with a young patient, it's essential to keep in mind the child's developmental level. And in the case of a very young child, such as an infant, you need to communicate with the infant's parents. Always use a caring and compassionate tone with the parents because, more than likely, they're anxious about having their infant hospitalised.

Let's pretend

Remember that children commonly regress to an earlier stage of development when they're ill. Play is one way to communicate with children to find out how they're feeling.

Always be prepared

When possible, it's ideal to prepare the child for admission to the hospital. The timing of the preparation and the amount of teaching given depend on the child's age, developmental level and personality, as well as the length of the procedure or treatment.

Young children may only need a few hours of preparation, whereas older children may benefit from several days of preparation. The use of developmentally appropriate activities will also help the child cope with the stress of hospitalisation.

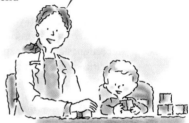

Having developmentally appropriate activities on hand can help a child cope with the stress of hospitalisation.

Keep it in the family

To reduce the fear that accompanies hospitalisation, you can help the child and family cope by:
- explaining procedures
- answering questions openly and honestly
- minimising separation from the parents
- structuring the environment to allow the child to maintain as much control as possible.

Elderly patients

Always address an older patient as Miss, Mrs or Mr, followed by the surname. Experts also recommend the use of touch. For example, shake the patient's hand when you first meet them and say hello; then hold it briefly to convey concern. Use body language, touch and eye contact to encourage participation. Be patient, relaxed and unhurried.

A little talk goes a long way

Talk to the patient, not at them. Tell them how long the process will take. If language poses a problem, enlist the aid of an interpreter, family members or a friend, as appropriate. Early in the interview, try to evaluate the patient's ability to communicate and their reliability as a historian. If you have doubts, before the interview proceeds further, ask them whether a family member or friend can be present.

The more the merrier

Don't be surprised if an older patient requests that someone assist them; they, too, may have concerns about getting through the interview on their own. Having another person present gives you a chance to observe the patient's interaction with this person and provides more data for the history. However, the presence of another person may prevent the patient from speaking freely, so plan a talk with them privately at some time during your assessment.

Be concise and rephrase

Provide carefully structured questions to elicit significant information. Keep your questions concise, rephrase those the patient doesn't understand and use such non-verbal techniques as facial expressions, pointing and touching to enhance your meaning.

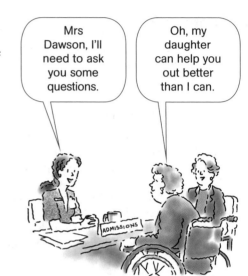

Lose the jargon

Use terms appropriate to the patient's level of understanding; avoid using jargon and complex medical terms. Offer explanations in lay terms, and then use the related medical terms, if appropriate, so the patient can become familiar with them.

To foster your older patient's co-operation, take a little extra time to help them see the relevance of your questions. You may need to repeat an explanation several times during the interview, but don't repeat unnecessarily. Give the patient plenty of time to respond to your questions and directions.

Sound of silence

Remain silent and allow the patient time to collect their thoughts and ideas before responding. Patience is the key to communicating with an older adult who responds slowly to your questions. Even so, don't confuse patience with patronising behaviour. The patient will easily perceive patronisation and may interpret it as your lack of genuine concern.

Unconscious patient

When caring for an unconscious patient, don't assume that you don't need to try to communicate with them. Never assume that they can't hear you. Introduce yourself as you would to a conscious patient. Always explain every procedure you're doing. Don't talk about the patient with other people in the room as if the patient weren't present. Always treat the unconscious patient with kindness, consideration and respect as you would a patient who's conscious.

Communicating by documentation

Patients are cared for by many people who work different shifts, and these various caregivers may speak with one another infrequently. The medical record is the main source of information and communication among nurses, doctors, physiotherapists, social workers and other caregivers. Everyone's notes are important because together they represent a complete picture of the patient's care.

> Everyone's notes are important because together they represent a complete picture of patient care.

Growing team

As health-care facilities continue to streamline and redesign care delivery systems, tasks that were historically performed by nurses are now being assigned to multiskilled workers such as health-care assistants. To deliver highly specialised care, each caregiver must provide accurate, thorough information and be able to interpret what others have written about a patient. Then each can use this information to plan future patient care. Commonly, decisions, actions and revisions related to the patient's care are based on documentation from various team members. A well-prepared medical record shows the high degree of collaboration within the entire health-care team.

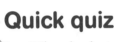

Quick quiz

1. When developing a therapeutic nurse–patient relationship, during what phase do you review the patient's surgical history?
    A. Orientation
    B. Working
    C. Pre-interaction
    D. Termination

Answer: C. During the pre-interaction phase, you can review the patient data that you might already have, such as the medical or surgical history.

2. What's a good way to communicate with a very young child?
    A. Play
    B. Explaining procedures
    C. Showing them pictures
    D. Showing them a movie

Answer: A. Play is an excellent way to communicate with a very young child.

3. What type of behaviour provides encouragement during communication without indicating agreement or disagreement?
    A. Clapping
    B. Sighing

C. Looking away

D. Nodding

Answer: D. Non-verbal behaviours, such as nodding and making momentary eye contact, provide encouragement without indicating agreement or disagreement.

4. What's the main source of information and communication among nurses, doctors, physiotherapists, social workers and other caregivers?

A. Computer

B. Medical record

C. Telephone

D. Word of mouth

Answer: B. The medical record is the main source of information and communication among nurses, doctors, physiotherapists, social workers and other caregivers.

Scoring

☆☆☆ If you answered all four questions correctly, fantastic! You're a communication connoisseur.

☆☆ If you answered three questions correctly, super! You've got a handle on handling communication strategies.

☆ If you answered fewer than three questions correctly, no worries! Reflect on the chapter and try again.

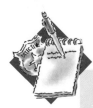

6 Nursing assessment

Just the facts

In this chapter, you'll learn:

♦ reasons for performing a nursing assessment

♦ techniques for effective communication during a nursing assessment

♦ essential steps in a holistic assessment

♦ questions specific to each step of a nursing assessment.

> The nursing assessment is an exploration of your patient's health—past and present. Land ho!

A look at nursing assessment

The first stage of the assessment involves gaining information from the patient or relative/carer if necessary. This information can then be used to identify care and nursing interventions that the patient requires. You may also need to make referrals to other members of the multiprofessional team. The information you will require from the patient will vary depending upon the setting, e.g. a hospital ward, outpatient department or community. The assessment will enable you to plan and deliver individualised care for the patient.

Any assessment involves collecting two kinds of data: objective and subjective. *Objective data* are obtained through observation and assessment and are verifiable. For example a red, swollen arm in a patient who's complaining of arm pain is an example of data that can be seen and verified by someone other than the patient. *Subjective data* can't be verified by anyone other than the patient and are gathered solely from the patient's own account, for example 'My head hurts' or 'I have trouble sleeping at night.'

Exploring past and present

You'll use a nursing assessment to gather subjective data about the patient and explore past and present problems. The assessment should be holistic and therefore you should assess the following needs:
- Physical
- Psychological
- Spiritual
- Emotional
- Sociocultural

Beginning the interview

To help you conduct your assessment the *nursing process* (see Chapter 4) is used, guided by a *nursing model* such as Roper, Logan and Tierney (1998), which is widely used in the UK. This model is based upon the activities of daily living that evolved from Virginia Henderson's work in 1966 and is frequently used as a checklist on admission. This systematic approach to assessment can then be used on a daily basis to review care plans and determine whether there is any improvement or deterioration prior to discharge from hospital.

Keep in mind that the accuracy and completeness of your patient's answers largely depend on your skill as an interviewer. Therefore, before you start asking questions, review the following communication guidelines.

Create the proper environment

To make the most of your patient interview, you'll first need to create an environment in which the patient feels comfortable. Before asking your first question, try to establish a rapport with the patient and explain what you'll cover during the interview. Consider the following when selecting a location for the interview:
- Make the setting as private as possible, choosing a quiet room when able to. This might be difficult on a busy ward and might involve you closing the curtains and not speaking too loudly. Remember that the more at ease the patient is the more interaction you will get.
- Make sure that the patient is comfortable. Sit facing them, 1 to 1.5 m away where possible.
- Introduce yourself, and explain that the purpose of the nursing assessment is to identify key problems and gather information to aid in planning their care.
- You must ensure that the patient is aware that the information that they provide might be shared with other professionals involved in the care, as stated in *The Code* (NMC, 2008).

If your patient has difficulty understanding or speaking English, arrange for an interpreter to sit in on assessment.

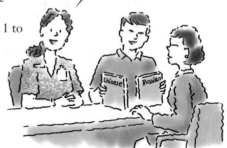

Ages and stages

Overcoming interviewing obstacles

With a little creativity, you can overcome barriers to interviewing. For example if a patient doesn't speak English, there is usually a bank of interpreters you can call on for help. Make sure that you document that an interpreter was used.

A trained medical interpreter, one who's familiar with medical terminology, knows interpreting techniques and understands the patient's rights, would be ideal. Be sure to tell the interpreter to translate the patient's speech verbatim.

Avoid using one of the patient's family members or friends as an interpreter, unless you are unable to get an interpreter. There may be things that the patient might want to say in private.

Breaking the sound barrier

Is your patient hearing impaired? You can overcome this barrier, too. First, make sure the light is bright enough for them to see your lips move. Then face the patient, and speak slowly and clearly. If the patient normally uses a hearing aid, encourage them to use it. If the patient uses sign language, see if there is a sign-language interpreter.

• Assess the patient to see if language barriers exist. For example do they speak and understand English? Can they hear you? (See *Overcoming interviewing obstacles*.)
• Speak slowly and clearly, using easy to understand language. Avoid using medical terms and jargon.
• Address the patient by a formal name, such as Mr Jones, and then find out how they would like to be addressed. Don't call the patient by their first name unless they ask you to. Avoid using terms of endearment, such as 'honey' or 'sweetie'. Treating the patient with respect encourages them to trust you and to provide more accurate and complete information.

Communicate effectively

After you've created a proper environment, you'll want to use various communication strategies to make sure you communicate effectively. Remember that you and the patient communicate non-verbally as well as verbally. Being aware of these forms of communication will aid you in the interview process.

Non-verbal communication strategies

To make the most of non-verbal communication, follow these guidelines:
• Listen attentively, and make eye contact frequently.
• Use reassuring gestures, such as nodding your head, to encourage the patient to keep talking.

• Watch for non-verbal clues that indicate the patient is uncomfortable or unsure about how to answer a question. For example they might lower their voice or glance around uneasily.

• Be aware of your own non-verbal behaviours that might cause the patient to stop talking or become defensive. For example if you cross your arms, you might appear closed off from them. If you stand while they're sitting, you might appear superior. If you glance at your watch, you might appear to be bored or rushed, which could keep the patient from answering questions completely.

• Observe the patient closely to see if they understand each question. If they don't appear to understand, repeat the question using different words or familiar examples. For example instead of asking, 'Did you have respiratory difficulty after exercising?' ask, "Did you have to sit down after walking around the block?"

Asking the right questions

Depending upon which branch of nursing you are involved in you will focus on different areas in more depth.

A complete nursing assessment requires information from each of these categories:

 personal information

 patient's main problem

 medical history

family history

psychosocial history.

activities of daily living.

Personal information

Start the health history by obtaining biographic information from the patient. Do this first so you don't forget about this information after you become involved in details of the patient's health. Ask the patient for their name, address, telephone number, birth date, age, marital status, religion and nationality. Find out whom they live with, and get the name and telephone number of a person to contact in case of an emergency.

Also, ask the patient who their general practitioner is and if they have ever been treated for their present problem. Depending upon the individual and their circumstances the patient may mention or want to discuss a 'living will', known as an *advance decision* or *advance directive*. In this situation a senior member of the medical team should be informed. (See *Advance decisions*.)

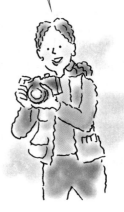

When interviewing a patient, remain focused on the task at hand.

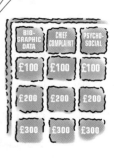

I'll take 'Psychosocial' for £500.00, please.

BIO-GRAPHIC DATA	CHIEF COMPLAINT	PSYCHO-SOCIAL
£100	£100	£100
£200	£200	£200
£300	£300	£300

Ages and stages

Advance decisions

The term 'advance decision' is also referred to as an advance directive or a living will. It indicates instructions provided by the individual, regarding actions to be taken for their health if they are unable to make decisions anymore, due to illness or incapacity. The Mental Capacity Act 2005 forms the legal basis for advance decisions for people in England and Wales. An advance decision gives a person a statutory right to refuse treatment or to state what form of treatment they would like if they were unable to decide for themselves in the future. For example, a person who has dementia may not want life-sustaining treatment if they developed a poor quality of life in the future.

An advance decision to refuse treatment does not have to be in writing; but it is much clearer to have a written decision to avoid any doubt regarding what the patient wants to refuse or uncertainty about the validity of it. When the advance decision is to refuse life-sustaining treatment, for example a patient not being tube fed or hydrated intravenously if they are too ill to feed themselves, it must be written and fulfil certain criteria set out in the Mental Capacity Act.

Some NHS Trusts provide a template for patients who would like to complete an advance decision form, but it is vital that the patient is not being put under pressure by anyone to make an advance decision. Information and factsheets covering the limitations and validity of advance decisions are available from organisations such as Age Concern and the Alzheimer's Society.

Pinpoint your patient's main problem. Remember, accuracy is key to good nursing care.

Main problem

Try to pinpoint the main reason why the patient has been admitted to hospital or referred for nursing care in the community. Document this information in the patient's exact words to avoid misinterpretation. Ask how and when any symptoms developed, what led the patient to seek medical attention and how the problem has affected their life and ability to function.

Medical history

Ask the patient about past and current medical problems, such as hypertension and diabetes. Typical questions include:
- Have you ever been in hospital before? If so, when and why?
- Are you being treated for any problem at the moment?
- Have you ever had surgery? If so, when and why?
- Are you allergic to anything in the environment or any drugs or foods? If so, what kind of allergic reaction do you have?

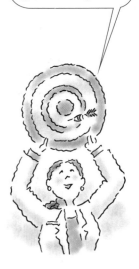

• Are you taking medications, including over-the-counter preparations, such as aspirin, vitamins and cough syrup? If so, how much do you take and how often do you take it? Do you use home remedies such as home-made ointments? Do you use herbal preparations or take dietary supplements? Do you use other alternative or complementary therapies, such as acupuncture, therapeutic massage or chiropractic?

Psychosocial history

Find out how the patient feels about him/her self. Ask about their occupation and responsibilities and whether their illness affect these. Typical questions include:
• How have you coped with medical or emotional crises in the past?
• How adequate is the emotional support you receive from family and friends?

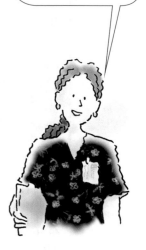

Information about a patient's activities of living will help you plan their care.

Activities of daily living

There are 14 activities of daily living that are considered to be fundamental to maintaining a quality of life. This model will help to plan, assess and evaluate the care of your patient. Find out what's normal for the patient by asking them about the activities of daily living relevant to the patient. Below are some examples of what you might need to discuss:

1. Maintaining a safe environment
Is the patient at risk of injuring themselves from an external factor?

2. Communication
Ask the patient if they have any problems with their sight or hearing? Do they wear glasses? Do they have glaucoma, cataracts, or colour blindness? Do they wear a hearing aid?

3. Breathing
Does the patient have any breathing problems? Have they ever been treated for pneumonia, asthma, emphysema or frequent respiratory tract infections? Do they have shortness of breath on exertion or while lying in bed? Do they need to sleep upright?

4. Eating and drinking
Ask the patient about their appetite, special diets and food allergies. Who cooks and shops at home? Is the patient able to eat independently? Are special utensils required?

5. Elimination
Ask about the frequency of bowel movements and laxative use if relevant. Do they have any problems passing urine?

6. Personal cleansing and dressing
Is assistance needed with washing and dressing? How independent is the patient? Ask the patient's preference regarding showering/bathing/washing.

7. Controlling body temperature
Is the patient sensitive to changes in temperature, especially the young and elderly?

8. *Mobilising*

Do they have difficulty walking, sitting or standing? Are they steady on their feet or do they lose their balance easily? Do they have arthritis, gout, back injury, muscle weakness or paralysis?

9. *Working and playing*

Ask the patient what they do for a living and what they do during their free time. Do they have hobbies?

Ask the patient if they smoke cigarettes. If so, how many do they smoke each day? Do they drink alcohol? If so, how much each day?

Patients may understate the amount they drink because of embarrassment. If you're having trouble getting what you believe are honest answers to such questions, you might try overestimating the amount. For example you might say, 'You told me you drink beer. Do you drink about a six-pack per day?' The patient's response might be, 'No, I drink about half that.'

Ask the patient if he has religious beliefs that affect diet, dress or nursing interventions. Patients will feel reassured when you make it clear that you understand these points.

10. *Expressing sexuality*

Are there any problems related to body image, self-esteem or gender-related issues?

11. *Sleeping*

Ask the patient how well they sleep, if they have any difficulties with sleep. Does the patient take any medication to help them sleep? How many pillows does the patient like to sleep with?

12. *Death and dying*

Be aware of fears about dying and try to deal with these as sensitively as possible, if appropriate. You might need to refer the patient to someone with more relevant experience and knowledge. Is the patient worried about their loss of independence? Do they have a fear that they might not recover from their illness? See *Advance decisions*.

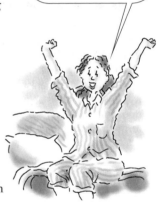

I know I always feel rested after a good night's sleep.

Maintaining a professional attitude

Don't let your personal opinions interfere with this part of the assessment. Maintain a professional, neutral approach, and don't offer advice. Don't use leading questions such as 'You don't do drugs, do you?' to get the answer you're hoping for. This type of question, based on your own value system, will make the patient feel guilty and might prevent him from responding honestly.

When questioning an elderly patient, remember that they may have difficulty hearing or communicating. (See *Overcoming communication problems in elderly patients*, page 80.)

Risk assessment

As part of the assessment process it is frequently necessary to carry out a more in-depth assessment of a patient's need. An assessment tool is used to collect more detailed information and to determine whether a patient

Ages and stages

Overcoming communication problems in elderly patients

An elderly patient may have sensory or memory impairment or a decreased attention span. If your patient is confused or has trouble communicating, you may need to rely on a family member for some or all of the health history.

Single assessment process

Across the UK, health departments are aiming for a single assessment process that can be used, when assessing older people, by any health- or social-care professional or organisation. The idea is to prevent patients being asked the same questions on several occasions and to form a resource for all concerned.

In England the single assessment process (Department of Health, 2002) was introduced by the Department of Health and in Northern Ireland by the Department of Health, Social Services and Public Safety (DHSSPS) and is recognised as the Single Assessment Process (SAP). This was introduced in response to the *National Service Framework for Older People* (Standard 2—Person-centred care) (DH, 2001). In Wales it is known as the Unified Assessment (Welsh Assembly Government, 2006) and Scotland as the Single Shared Assessment (Scottish Executive, 2001).

is at risk. Moving and handling, pressure ulcer risk, oral assessment and nutritional screening are some of the areas of need that might require a risk assessment. Professionals locally may have developed certain risk assessment tools that are used, for example within the trust that you work. Some tools that you will use are more commonly used throughout the UK, such as the Waterlow scale, which is a pressure ulcer risk assessment. (See Chapter 13.) Whichever assessment tool is used in your area it must be appropriate to the patients you care for and it is important that staff are familiar with how to use the tool. The frequency that the assessment tool should be used will be dictated by national or local guidelines, but an assessment should be made as soon as possible and when there is any change in a patient's condition.

Documentation

When documenting any part of the patient assessment, whether it is an electronic version or paper based you should ensure that you are following the NMC's *Record keeping: Guidance for nurses and midwives* (NMC, 2009).

Quick quiz

1. Leading questions may initiate untrue or inaccurate responses because such questions:

    A. encourage short or vague answers.
    B. require an educational level the patient may not possess.
    C. prompt the patient to try to give the answer you're looking for.
    D. confuse the patient.

Answer: C. Because of how they're phrased, leading questions may prompt the patient to give the answer you're looking for.

2. Silence is a communication technique used during an interview to:

    A. show respect.
    B. change the topic.
    C. encourage the patient to continue talking.
    D. clarify information.

Answer: C. Silence allows the patient to collect his thoughts and continue to answer your questions.

3. Data are considered subjective if you obtain them from:

    A. the patient's verbal account.
    B. your observations of the patient's actions.
    C. the patient's records.
    D. X-ray reports.

Answer: A. Data from the patient's own words are subjective.

Scoring

✰✰✰   If you answered all three questions correctly, bravo! You're our intrepid interviewer.

✰✰   If you answered two questions correctly, that's cool! You're our hip historian.

✰   If you answered fewer than two questions correctly, that's OK! Review the chapter and you'll know all the questions—and answers.

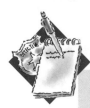

7 Taking vital signs

Just the facts

In this chapter, you'll learn:

♦ types of equipment used in vital signs assessment

♦ skills for performing vital signs assessment

♦ tips to interpret vital signs

♦ abnormalities in vital signs.

What are the vital signs?

Vital signs include pulse/heart rate, temperature, respiration, both rate and effort, and blood pressure.

They can indicate the health or ill health of a person; it is important to remember that they should not be performed in isolation. A holistic assessment will include touch, visual observation, listening and communicating with the person (RCN, 2007).

A look at vital signs assessment

Accurate measurements of your patient's height, weight and vital signs provide critical information about body functions.

The first time you assess a patient, record their baseline vital signs and statistics. Afterwards, take measurements at regular intervals, depending on the patient's condition and your local policies. A series of readings usually provides more valuable information than a single set.

Vital tips

Always analyse vital signs at the same time because two or more abnormal values provide important clues about your patient's problem. For example a rapid, thready pulse along with low blood pressure may signal shock.

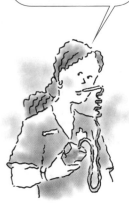

Taking vital signs is a vital part of nursing.

If you obtain an abnormal value, take the vital sign again to make sure it's accurate. Remember that normal readings vary with the patient's age. For example, temperature decreases with age, and respiratory rate may increase with age or with an underlying disease.

Also remember that an abnormal value for one patient may be a normal value for another. Each patient has their own baseline values, which is what makes recording vital signs during the initial assessment so important.

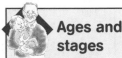

Yes, sir! Stable body temperature helps me and my mates function properly.

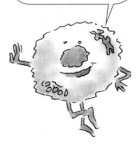

Body temperature

Body temperature represents the balance between heat that's produced by metabolism, muscular activity and other factors and heat that's lost through the skin, lungs and body wastes. A stable temperature pattern promotes proper function of cells, tissues and organs; a change in this pattern usually signals the onset of illness.

Choose one

Oral temperature in adults normally ranges from 36.1 to 37.5°C. Axillary (armpit) temperature, the least accurate reading, is usually 0.6 to 1.1°C lower. Tympanic (in-the-ear) temperature reads 0.3 to 0.6°C higher. Rectal temperature, the most accurate reading, is usually 0.6°C higher; this is only used in certain situations, as it causes embarrassment and is invasive. (See *Types of thermometers*, page 84.)

Normal ups and downs

Temperature normally fluctuates with rest and activity. Lowest readings typically occur between 4 and 5 a.m.; the highest readings, between 4 and 8 p.m. Other factors also influence temperature. (See *Differences in temperature*.)

Consent

Before taking any vital sign you must explain the procedure to the patient and gain consent. Wash your hands. If you're taking an oral temperature and they have had hot or cold liquids or smoked, wait 20 to 30 minutes before getting started.

Taking an oral temperature

What you need
Electronic thermometer ✳ disposable probe cover

Ages and stages

Differences in temperature

Besides activity level, other factors that influence temperature include gender, age, emotional conditions and environment. Keep these principles in mind:

- Women normally have higher temperatures than men, especially during ovulation.
- Normal temperature is highest in neonates and lowest in elderly people.
- A hot external environment can raise temperature; a cold environment lowers it.

Types of thermometers

You can take a patient's oral, rectal or axillary temperature with an electronic digital thermometer. You can take tympanic temperature with a tympanic thermometer.

For adults who are awake, alert, oriented and co-operative, use the oral or tympanic route. For infants, young children and confused or unconscious patients, you may need to use the axillary route.

Oral or rectal route is not recommended for children under the age of 5 (NICE, 2007).

Tympanic thermometer

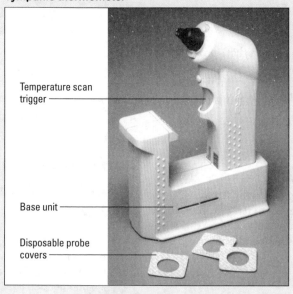

Temperature scan trigger

Base unit

Disposable probe covers

Individual electronic digital thermometer

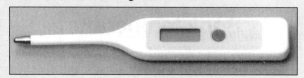

Individual electronic digital thermometer

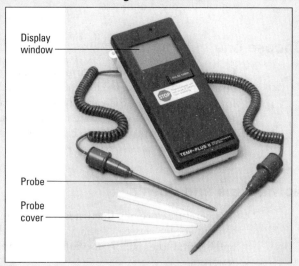

Display window

Probe

Probe cover

How you do it

- Insert the probe into a disposable probe cover.
- Position the tip of the probe under the patient's tongue on either side of the frenulum as far back as possible. Placing the tip in this area promotes contact with superficial blood vessels and ensures a more accurate reading.
- Instruct the patient to close their lips.
- Leave the probe in place until the maximum temperature appears on the digital display. Then remove the probe.
- Read and record the reading on the patient's observations chart or as per local policy.

How temperature readings compare

You can take your patient's temperature in four ways. This chart describes each method.

Method	Normal temperature	Used with
Tympanic (ear)	36.8 to 37.8°C	Adults and children, conscious and co-operative patients and confused or unconscious patients.
Oral	36.5 to 37.5°C	Adults and older children who are awake, alert, oriented and co-operative.
Axillary (armpit)	35.9 to 36.9°C	Infants, young children and patients who are breathless or with impaired immune systems when infection is a concern.
Rectal	37.1 to 38.1°C	Only used in exceptional circumstances, mainly in critical care and emergency care. NOT recommended for use in infants.

Taking an axillary temperature

What you need
Electronic thermometer ✳ facial tissue ✳ disposable probe cover

How you do it
• Position the patient with the axilla exposed, take care to maintain privacy and dignity.
• Gently pat the axilla dry with a facial tissue because moisture conducts heat. Avoid harsh rubbing, which generates heat.
• Position the thermometer in the centre of the axilla.
• Rest the arm against the chest to promote skin contact with the thermometer.
• Leave the thermometer in place for the time recommended by the manufacturer. Axillary temperatures take longer to register than oral or rectal temperature because the thermometer isn't enclosed in a body cavity.
• Remove the thermometer from the axilla.
• Read and record the reading on the patient's observations chart or as per local policy.
• Wash your hands.

With a tympanic thermometer

What you need
Tympanic thermometer ✳ disposable probe cover

How you do it
• Make sure the lens under the probe is clean and shiny. Attach a disposable probe cover.

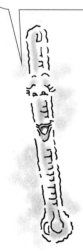

Remember, an armpit isn't an enclosed body cavity, so you'll need to keep me in place a little longer for an accurate reading.

- Stabilise the patient's head; then gently pull their ear straight back (for children up to age 1) or up and back (for adults and children older than age 1).
- Insert the thermometer until the entire ear canal is sealed. The thermometer should be inserted towards the tympanic membrane in the same way an otoscope is inserted.
- Press the activation button, and hold for time recommended by the manufacturer. The temperature will appear on the display.
- Read and record the temperature on the patient's observations chart or as per local policy.

Taking a rectal temperature

What you need
Electronic thermometer ✳ facial tissue ✳ disposable probe cover ✳ gloves ✳ apron ✳ lubricant

How you do it
- Put on gloves and apron.
- Insert the probe into a disposable probe cover. Lubricate tip with lubricating jelly.
- Position the patient on their side with the top leg flexed.
- Cover them to provide privacy and maintain dignity. Fold back the bed clothes to expose the anus.
- Lift the patient's upper buttock, and insert the thermometer about 4 cm for an adult.
- Gently direct the thermometer along the rectal wall towards the umbilicus to avoid perforating the anus or rectum and to help ensure an accurate reading. (The thermometer will register haemorrhoidal artery temperature instead of faecal temperature.)
- Hold the thermometer in place for the time recommended by the manufacturer to prevent damage to rectal tissues caused by displacement.
- Carefully remove the thermometer, wiping it if necessary. Then wipe the patient's anal area to remove any faeces.
- Remove your gloves and apron and wash your hands.
- Read and record the temperature on the patient's observations chart or as per local policy. (See *Tips about temperature*.)

Pulse

The patient's pulse reflects the amount of blood ejected with each heartbeat. The recurring wave, called a pulse, can be palpated (felt) at locations on the body where an artery crosses over bone or firm tissue. To assess the pulse, palpate one of the patient's arterial pulse points and note the rate, rhythm and amplitude of the pulse. A normal pulse for an adult is between 60 and 90 beats per minute.

Stay on the ball

Tips about temperature

Keep these tips in mind when taking a patient's temperature:

- Oral measurement is contraindicated in young children under 5 years old and in patients who are unconscious, disoriented or prone to seizures or those who must breathe through their mouth.
- Rectal measurement is contraindicated in patients with diarrhoea, recent rectal or prostatic surgery or injury (because it may injure inflamed tissue), or recent myocardial infarction (because anal manipulation may stimulate the vagus nerve, causing bradycardia or another rhythm disturbance).
- Rectal measurement is not recommended for use in children under 5 years old.
- Use the same thermometer for repeat temperature taking to ensure consistent results.
- If your patient is receiving nasal oxygen, know that you can still measure their temperature orally because oxygen administration raises oral temperature by only about 0.21°C.

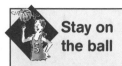

Stay on the ball

Pinpointing pulse sites

You can assess your patient's pulse rate at several sites, including those shown in this illustration.

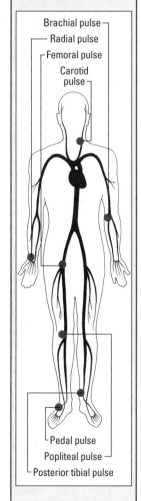

The radial's radical!

The radial pulse is the most accessible. However, in cardiovascular emergencies, you may palpate for the carotid pulse. This vessel is larger and reflects the heart's activity more accurately. (See *Pinpointing pulse sites*.)

Rate, rhythm and volume

Measuring and recording a patient's pulse involves determining the number of beats per minute (the pulse rate), the pattern or irregularity of the beats (the rhythm) and the volume of blood pumped with each beat. (See *Alternate site for taking a pulse*, page 88.)

What you need

Watch with a second hand ✳ stethoscope (for auscultating apical pulse)

How you do it

- Wash your hands and tell the patient that you're going to check their pulse.
- Make sure the patient is comfortable and relaxed because an awkward, uncomfortable position may affect their heart rate.

Ages and stages

Alternate site for taking a pulse

The most common site for taking a pulse is the radial artery in the wrist. This holds true for adults and children older than age 3.

For infants and children younger than age 3, however, the brachial pulse may be easier to locate or listen to the heart with a stethoscope, rather than palpate a pulse. Because auscultation is done at the apex of the heart, the pulse measured is the apical pulse.

Measuring a radial pulse
• Place the patient in a sitting or supine position, with their arms at the side or across their chest.

Keep the thumb out of it

• Gently press your index, middle and ring fingers on the radial artery inside the patient's wrist. You should feel a pulse with only moderate pressure; excessive pressure may obstruct blood flow distal to the pulse site. Don't use your thumb to take the patient's pulse; the thumb has a strong pulse of its own and may be easily confused with the patient's pulse.

One, two, three...sixty

• After locating the pulse, count the beats for 60 seconds to get the number of beats per minute. Counting for a full minute provides a more accurate picture of irregularities.
• While counting the rate, assess pulse rhythm and volume by noting the pattern and strength of the beats. If you detect an irregularity, repeat the count and note whether the irregularity occurs in a pattern or randomly. (See *Identifying pulse patterns*.)
• Document on the patient's observations chart or as per local policy.

Taking an apical pulse
• Help the patient to a supine position.

Warm the scope first, please

• Warm the bell or diaphragm in your hand. Placing a cold stethoscope against the patient's skin may startle them and momentarily increase the heart rate.
• Place the warmed bell or diaphragm over the apex of the heart (normally located at the fifth intercostal space, left of the midclavicular line), and insert the earpieces in your ear.

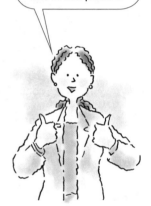

When taking a radial pulse, count for a full minute and keep these thumbs out of the picture.

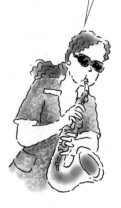

Rhythm and beat go hand-in-hand, daddy-o!

Identifying pulse patterns

This chart lists different types of pulse patterns along with their rates, rhythms and causes and incidence.

Type	Rate	Rhythm	Causes and incidence
Normal	60 to 80 beats/minute; in neonates, 120 to 140 beats/minute	● ● ● ●	• Varies with such factors as age, physical activity and gender (infants and children have higher pulse rates than adults; older adults have lower pulse rates)
Tachycardia	More than 100 beats/minute	●●●●●●●	• Accompanies stimulation of the sympathetic nervous system resulting from emotional stress (such as anger, fear or anxiety) or the use of certain drugs (such as caffeine) • May result from exercise or such health conditions as heart failure, anaemia and fever, which increase oxygen requirements and, thus, pulse rate
Bradycardia	Less than 60 beats/minute	● ● ●	• Accompanies stimulation of the parasympathetic nervous system resulting from drug use, especially cardiac glycosides, and conditions such as cerebral haemorrhage and heart block • May also be present in fit athletes and persons with hypothyroidism
Irregular	Uneven time intervals between beats (e.g. periods of regular rhythm interrupted by pauses or pre-mature beats)	●●●● ●●	• May indicate cardiac irritability, hypoxia, digoxin toxicity, potassium imbalance or a more serious arrhythmia if pre-mature beats occur frequently (occasional pre-mature beats are normal)

• Count the beats for 60 seconds, and note their rhythm, volume and intensity.
• Remove the stethoscope and make the patient comfortable.
• Document on the patient's observations chart or as per local policy.

Taking an apical–radial (A/R) pulse

• Find a colleague to work with you while taking an apical–radial pulse so that they can palpate the radial pulse while you auscultate the apical pulse with a stethoscope, or vice versa.

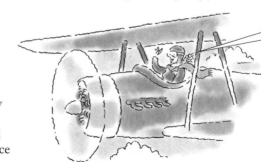

Sometimes, you'll need to fly solo when taking an apical–radial pulse. If that's the case, be sure to keep both hands on the wheel…errr… patient, and watch your timing.

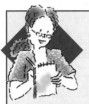

Take note!

Documenting pulse

When documenting a pulse, be sure to record pulse rate, rhythm and volume as well as the time of measurement. 'Full' or 'bounding' describes a pulse of increased volume; 'weak' or 'thready', a pulse of decreased volume. When recording apical pulse, include the intensity of heart sounds. When recording apical–radial pulse, chart the rate according to the pulse site—for example A/R pulse = 80/76.

- Help the patient to the supine position.
- Locate the apical and radial pulses, and then determine a time to begin counting. You should both count beats for 60 seconds.
- Document on the patient's observations chart or as per local policy.

Respiration

Respiration is the exchange of oxygen and carbon dioxide between the atmosphere and the body. External respiration, or breathing, occurs through the work of the diaphragm and chest muscles and delivers oxygen to the lower respiratory tract and alveoli.

Rate, rhythm, depth and sound

Respiration can be measured according to rate, rhythm, depth and sound. These measurements reflect the body's metabolic state, diaphragm and chest muscle condition and airway patency.

Respiratory rate is recorded as the number of cycles per minute, with inspiration and expiration making up one cycle, rhythm, as the regularity of these cycles. Depth is recorded as the volume of air inhaled and exhaled with each respiration; sound is recorded as the audible digression from normal, effortless breathing.

What you need
A watch with a second hand

How you do it
- The best time to assess your patient's respirations is immediately after taking their pulse rate. Keep your fingertips over their radial artery, and don't tell them that you're counting respirations; otherwise, they will become conscious of them, and the rate may change.

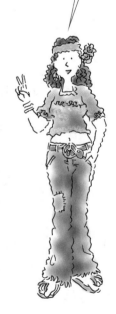

Hey, man, respiration is measured by rate, rhythm, sound and depth. That's deep, sister!

Watch the movement

- Count respirations by observing the rise and fall of the patient's chest as they breathe. Alternatively, position the patient's opposite arm across their chest, and count respirations by feeling its rise and fall. Consider one rise and one fall as one respiration.
- Count for 60 seconds to account for variations in respiratory rate and pattern.
- Observe chest movements for depth of respirations. If the patient inhales a small volume of air, record the depth as shallow; if they inhale a large volume, deep.
- Observe the patient for use of such accessory muscles as the scalene, sternocleidomastoid, trapezius and latissimus dorsi. Such use indicates weakness of the diaphragm and the external intercostal muscles—the major muscles of respiration.

Listen to the sounds

- As you count respirations, watch for and record breath sounds such as stertor, stridor, wheezing and expiratory grunting.
- Stertor is a snoring sound resulting from secretions in the trachea and large bronchi. Listen for it in comatose patients and in patients with a neurologic disorder.
- Stridor is an inspiratory crowing sound that occurs in patients with laryngitis, croup, or upper respiratory tract obstruction with a foreign body. (See *How age affects respiration*.)

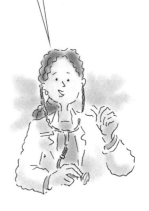

Observing, counting, and listening…assessing respirations is an exercise in multitasking!

Ages and stages

How age affects respiration

When assessing respirations in children and older patients, keep these points in mind:

- When listening for stridor in infants and children with croup, check for sternal, sub-sternal and intercostal retractions.
- In infants, an expiratory grunt indicates imminent respiratory distress.
- In older patients, an expiratory grunt indicates partial airway obstruction.
- A child's respiratory rate may double in response to exercise, illness or emotion.
- Normally, the rate for neonates is 30 to 80 breaths/minute; for toddlers, 20 to 40 breaths/minute; and for children of school age and older, 15 to 25 breaths/minute.
- Children usually reach the adult rate (12 to 20 breaths/minute) at about age 15.

- Wheezing is caused by partial obstruction in the smaller bronchi and bronchioles. This high-pitched, musical sound is common in patients with emphysema or asthma.
- Watch the patient's chest movements and listen to breathing to determine the rhythm and sound of respirations. (See *Identifying respiratory patterns.*)
- Respiratory rates of less than 8 breaths/minute or more than 40 breaths/minute are usually considered abnormal and should be reported promptly.
- Observe the patient for signs of dyspnoea, such as an anxious facial expression, flaring nostrils, a heaving chest wall and cyanosis. To detect

Identifying respiratory patterns

This chart lists types of respirations along with their characteristics, patterns and possible causes.

Type	Characteristics	Pattern	Possible causes
Apnoea	Periodic absence of breathing		• Mechanical airway obstruction • Conditions affecting the brain's respiratory centre in the lateral medulla oblongata
Apneustic	Prolonged, gasping inspiration followed by extremely short, inefficient expiration		• Lesions of the respiratory centre
Bradypnoea	Slow, regular respirations of equal depth		• Normal pattern during sleep • Conditions affecting the respiratory centre, such as tumours, metabolic disorders, respiratory decompensation and the use of opiates or alcohol
Cheyne–Stokes respirations	Fast, deep respirations for 30 to 170 seconds punctuated by periods of apnoea lasting 20 to 60 seconds		• Increased intracranial pressure, severe heart failure, renal failure, meningitis, drug overdose and cerebral anoxia
Eupnoea	Normal rate and rhythm		• Normal respiration
Kussmaul respirations	Fast (more than 20 breaths/minute), deep (resembling sighs), laboured respirations without pause		• Renal failure and metabolic acidosis, particularly diabetic ketoacidosis
Tachypnoea	Rapid respirations, rate rises with body temperature at about 4 breaths/minute for each degree Celsius above normal		• Pneumonia, compensatory respiratory alkalosis, respiratory insufficiency, lesions of the respiratory centre and salicylate poisoning

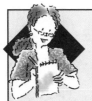

Take note!

Documenting respirations

Record the rate, depth, rhythm and sound of the patient's respirations.

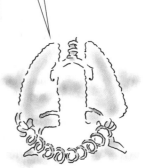

In respiratory disorders, such as COPD, I have to rely on accessory muscles to help me expand.

cyanosis, look for the characteristic bluish discoloration of the nail beds and lips, under the tongue, in the buccal mucosa and in the conjunctiva.
• When assessing a patient's respiratory status, consider personal and family history. Ask if they smoke and, if they do, the number of years and the number of packs per day. (See *Documenting respirations*.)

Accessory to the act...of breathing

Use of accessory muscles can enhance lung expansion when oxygenation drops. Patients with chronic obstructive pulmonary disease (COPD) or respiratory distress may use neck muscles, including the sternocleidomastoid muscles, and abdominal muscles for breathing. Patient position during normal breathing may also suggest such problems as COPD. Normal respirations are quiet and easy, so note any abnormal sounds, such as wheezing and stridor.

Blood pressure

Blood pressure, which is the lateral force that blood exerts on arterial walls, is affected by the force of ventricular contractions, arterial wall elasticity, peripheral vascular resistance and blood volume and viscosity. Blood pressure measurements consist of systolic pressure and diastolic pressure readings.

Systolic (contract) vs. diastolic (relax)

Systolic pressure occurs when the left ventricle contracts. It reflects the integrity of the heart, arteries and arterioles. A normal systolic pressure ranges from 100 to 140 mmHg. *Diastolic pressure* occurs when the left ventricle relaxes. It indicates blood vessel resistance. A normal diastolic pressure ranges from 60 to 85 mmHg. It's generally more significant as it measures the heart at rest. Both pressures are measured in millimetres of mercury (mmHg) with a sphygmomanometer and a stethoscope, usually at the brachial artery.

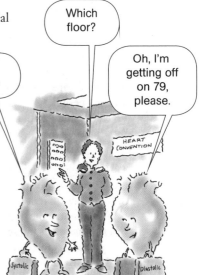

Which floor?

119th, please.

Oh, I'm getting off on 79, please.

Rising

Blood pressure rises with age, weight gain, prolonged stress and anxiety. (See *Effects of age on blood pressure*.)

What you need

Sphygmomanometer ✳ stethoscope ✳ alcohol wipe

Cuffs come in different sizes, ranging from neonate to extra-large adult. Disposable cuffs are available.

The automated vital signs monitor is a non-invasive device that measures, systolic and diastolic pressures, and mean arterial pressure at pre-set intervals. (See *Using an electronic vital signs monitor*.)

The monitor also counts the pulse rate but does not give the important aspects of the strength and rhythm so should not be used for this purpose.

Getting ready

• Carefully choose a cuff of appropriate size for the patient. An excessively narrow cuff may cause a false-high reading; an excessively wide one, a false-low reading.

How you do it

• Wash your hands, and tell the patient that you're going to take their blood pressure.
• The patient can lie in a supine position or sit erect while you measure their blood pressure. Their arm should be extended at heart level and be well supported. If the artery is below heart level, you may get a false-high reading. Make sure the patient is relaxed and comfortable when you measure their blood pressure so it stays at its normal level.

Don't compromise

• Don't take a blood pressure measurement on the same arm of an arteriovenous fistula or haemodialysis shunt because blood flow through the device may be compromised. Don't take a blood pressure measurement on the affected side of a mastectomy because it may compromise lymphatic circulation, worsen oedema and damage the arm. Also, don't take blood pressure on the same arm as a peripherally inserted central catheter because it may damage the device.
• Wrap the deflated cuff snugly around the patient's upper arm.

Estimate!

• Palpate the brachial artery. Estimate the systolic pressure by feeling for the brachial artery, then inflate the cuff rapidly until the pulse disappears, note this level. This gives you the estimated systolic pressure.
• Now centre the diaphragm of the stethoscope over the part of the artery where you detect the strongest beats, and hold it in place with one hand. (See *Using a sphygmomanometer*, page 96.)
• Using the thumb and index finger of your other hand, turn the thumbscrew on the rubber bulb of the air pump clockwise to close the valve.

Ages and stages

Effects of age on blood pressure

Blood pressure changes with age. Below are normal blood pressure values, measured in mmHg at different ages.

Under 1 years

• Systostolic 70–90

1-2 years

• Systolic: 80–95

2-5 years

• Systolic: 80–100

5-12 years

• Systolic: 90–110

16 + years

• Systolic: 100–120

Adult

• Systolic: 100–140
• Diastolic: 60 to 90

Using an electronic vital signs monitor

An electronic vital signs monitor allows you to continually track a patient's vital signs without having to reapply a blood pressure cuff each time. What's more, the patient won't need an invasive arterial line to gather similar data. The steps below can be followed with most monitors.

Some automated vital signs monitors are lightweight and battery-operated and are attached to a stand for continual monitoring, even during patient transfers. Make sure you know the capacity of the monitor's battery, and plug the machine in whenever possible to keep it charged.

Before using any monitor, check its accuracy. Determine the patient's pulse rate and blood pressure manually, using the same arm you'll use for the monitor cuff. Compare your results when you get initial readings from the monitor. If the results differ, call your supply department or the manufacturer's representative.

Preparing the device

- Explain the procedure to the patient. Describe the alarm system so they won't be frightened if it's triggered.
- Squeeze all air from the cuff, and wrap the cuff loosely around the patient's arm, allowing two fingerbreadths between the cuff and the arm or leg. Never apply the cuff to a limb that has an I.V. line in place or to an individual who has had breast or lymph node excision on that side or has an arteriovenous graft, shunt or fistula. Position the cuff's 'artery' arrow over the palpated brachial artery. Then secure the cuff for a snug fit.

Selecting parameters

- When you turn on the monitor, it will default to a manual mode. (In this mode, you can obtain vital signs yourself before switching to the automatic mode.) Press the AUTO button to select the automatic mode. The monitor will give you baseline data for the pulse rate, systolic and diastolic pressures and mean arterial pressure.

- Compare your previous manual results with these baseline data. If they match, you're ready to set the alarm parameters. Press the SELECT button to blank out all displays except systolic pressure.
- Use the HIGH and LOW limit buttons to set the specific parameters for systolic pressure. (These limits range from a high of 240 to a low of 0.) You'll do this three more times for mean arterial pressure, pulse rate and diastolic pressure. After you've set the parameters for diastolic pressure, press the SELECT button again to display all current data. If you forget to do this last step, the monitor will automatically display current data 10 seconds after you set the last parameters.

Collecting data

- You also need to tell the monitor how often to obtain data. Press the SET button until you reach the desired time interval in minutes. If you've chosen the automatic mode, the monitor will display a default cycle time of 3 minutes. You can override the default cycle time to set the interval you prefer.
- You can obtain a set of vital signs any time by pressing the START button. Also, pressing the CANCEL button will stop the interval and deflate the cuff. You can retrieve stored data by pressing the PRIOR DATA button. The monitor will display the last data obtained along with the time elapsed since then. Scrolling backwards, you can retrieve data from the previous 99 minutes.

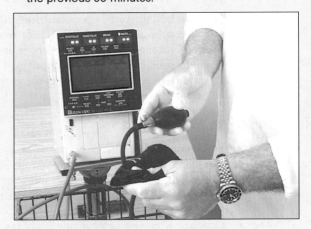

> *Please note.* The radial pulse can be used to estimate the systolic pressure, however, you still need to find the brachial artery in order to perform the manual blood pressure.

Using a sphygmomanometer

Here's how to use a sphygmomanometer properly:

- For accuracy and consistency, position your patient with their upper arm at heart level and their palm turned up.
- Apply the cuff snugly, 2 to 3 cm above the brachial pulse, as shown in the top photo.
- Position the manometer at your eye level.
- Palpate the brachial or radial pulse with your fingertips while inflating the cuff.
- Inflate the cuff to 30 mmHg above the point where the pulse disappears.
- Place the diaphragm of your stethoscope over the point where you felt the pulse, as shown in the bottom photo.
- Release the valve slowly and note the point at which Korotkoff sounds reappear. The start of the pulse sound indicates the systolic pressure.
- The sounds will become muffled and then disappear. The last Korotkoff sound you hear is the diastolic pressure.

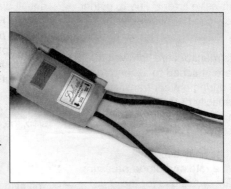

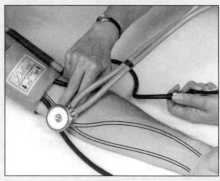

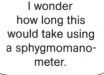

I wonder how long this would take using a sphygmomanometer.

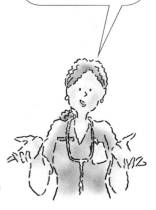

Be aware of pre-existing conditions or problems that can compromise the blood pressure reading or your patient's health.

- Pump air into the cuff while auscultating for the sound over the brachial artery to compress and, eventually, occlude arterial blood flow. Continue pumping air until to 30 mmHg above the estimated systolic pressure.
- Carefully open the valve of the air pump. Then deflate the cuff no faster than 5 mmHg/second, while watching the gauge and auscultating for the sound over the artery.

Tune in to the five sounds

- When you hear the first beat or clear tapping sound, note the pressure on the column or gauge—that is, the systolic pressure. (The beat or tapping sound is the first of five Korotkoff sounds. The second sound resembles a murmur or swish; the third, crisp tapping; the fourth, a soft, muffled tone; and the fifth, the last sound heard.)
- Continue to release air gradually while auscultating for the sound over the artery.

• Note the diastolic pressure—the fourth Korotkoff sound. If you continue to hear sounds as the column or gauge falls to zero (common in children), record the pressure at the beginning of the fourth sound. This step is important because, in some patients, a distinct fifth sound is absent.
• Rapidly deflate the cuff. Record the pressure. After doing so, remove and clean as per local policy, and return it to storage.
• Document the pressure on the pateint's observations chart or as per local policy.
• (For information on situations that can cause false-high or false-low readings, see *Correcting problems of blood pressure measurement, page 98*.)

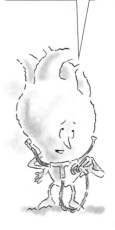

That's one (tap)…two (swish)…three (tap)…four (muffle)…five…

Height and weight

Height and weight are routinely measured when a patient is admitted to a health-care facility. An accurate record of the patient's height and weight is essential for calculating dosages of drugs, assessing the patient's nutritional status and determining the height-to-weight ratio.

Weigh the patient at the same time each day, in similar clothing, and using the same scale. If the patient uses crutches, weigh them with the crutches. Then weigh the crutches and any heavy clothing and subtract their weight from the total to determine the patient's weight.

What weight tells you

Because body weight is the best overall indicator of fluid status, daily monitoring is important for patients receiving a diuretic or a medication that causes sodium retention. Rapid weight gain may signal fluid retention; rapid weight loss, diuresis.

Scales for every position

Weight can be measured with a standing scale or chair scale.

What you need
Scale (sitting or standing) ✳ wheelchair if needed (to transport patient)

Getting ready
Select the appropriate scale—usually, a standing scale for an ambulatory patient or a chair scale for an acutely ill or debilitated patient. Then make sure the scale has been calibrated. If using electronic or battery scales make sure the scales are plugged in or have a working battery.

How you do it
• Tell the patient that you're going to measure weight. Explain the procedure to them, depending on which type of scale you'll use.

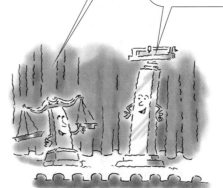

I hear there are fancy new scales at the hospital. I wonder what kinds they have…

Oh, well, you'll have to *weight* and see!

Correcting problems of blood pressure measurement

This chart lists blood pressure measurement problems along with their causes and appropriate nursing actions.

Causes	Nursing actions
False-high reading	
Cuff too small	Make sure the cuff bladder covers 80% of the circumference of the arm or leg being used for measurement.
Cuff wrapped too loosely, reducing its effective width	Tighten the cuff.
Cuff deflated too slowly, causing venous congestion in the arm or leg	Never deflate the cuff more slowly than 2 mmHg per heartbeat.
Sphygmomanometer tilted	Read pressures with the sphygmomanometer vertical.
Measurement poorly timed (e.g. exercised, anxious)	Postpone the blood pressure measurement or help the patient relax before measuring their blood pressure.
False-low reading	
Arm or leg positioned incorrectly	Make sure the patient's arm or leg is in level with their heart.
Sphygmomanometer below eye level	Read the sphygmomanometer at eye level.
Auscultatory gap (sound fades out for 10 to 15 mmHg, and then returns) unnoticed	Estimate systolic pressure by palpation before measuring it. Then check this pressure against measured pressure.
Low-volume sounds inaudible	Before re-inflating the cuff, instruct the patient to raise their arm or leg to decrease venous pressure and amplify low-volume sounds. After inflating the cuff, tell them to lower their arm or leg. Then deflate the cuff and listen. If you still fail to detect low-volume sounds, chart palpated systolic pressure.

Using standing or sitting scales
- Ask the patient to remove heavy clothing and slippers or shoes. If the scale has wheels, lock them. Assist the patient onto the scale and remain close to them to prevent falls.

That's digital

- If you're using a digital scale, make sure the display reads 0 before use.
- Read the display with the patient standing as still as possible.

Height

Height can be measured with the measuring bar on a standing scale or with a tape measure for a patient confined to a supine position.

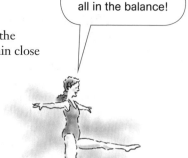

Remember, it's all in the balance!

Raising the bar

• When measuring height, raise the measuring bar above the patient's head tell the patient to stand erect and then lower the bar until it touches the top of the patient's head. Read the patient's height.
• Help the patient off the height scale. Then return the measuring bar to its initial position.
• If the patient is confined to bed then a measuring tape can be used to measure their height.
• Record the measurement on the patient's observations chart or as per local policy.

Quick quiz

1. Which heart rate in a neonate would be considered normal?
   A. 60 to 80 beats/minute
   B. 100 to 120 beats/minute
   C. 120 to 140 beats/minute
   D. 160 to 200 beats/minute

Answer: C. A heart rate of 120 to 140 beats/minute in a neonate is considered normal.

2. The highest temperature reading would be expected to occur during what time of day?
   A. 4 and 5 a.m.
   B. 8 and 9 a.m.
   C. 4 and 8 p.m.
   D. 9 and 11 p.m.

Answer: C. Temperature normally fluctuates with rest and activity. Lowest readings typically occur between 4 and 5 a.m.; the highest readings, between 4 and 8 p.m.

3. Which breath sound is referred to as a snoring sound that results from secretions in the trachea?
   A. Stertor
   B. Stridor
   C. Wheezing
   D. Expiratory grunting

Answer: A. Stertor is a snoring sound that results from secretions in the trachea and large bronchi.

4. Which method for assessing temperature is the least accurate?
   A. Oral
   B. Rectal
   C. Tympanic
   D. Axillary

Answer: D. Axillary temperature, the least accurate reading, is usually 0.6 to 1.1°C lower.

Scoring

☆☆☆ If you answered all four questions correctly, congratulations! You're a vital signs expert.

☆☆ If you answered three questions correctly, great! You've got the pulse on vital signs assessment skills.

☆ If you answered fewer than three questions correctly, don't despair. Take a deep breath, listen to your heart, and know that you still measure up to a good nurse!

8 Asepsis and infection control

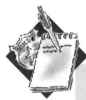

Just the facts

In this chapter, you'll learn:

♦ types of infection

♦ the ways infection is spread

♦ proper hand hygiene

♦ infection control precautions.

A look at infection

Infection is the invasion and multiplication of microorganisms in or on body tissues that produce signs and symptoms as well as an immune response. Such reproduction injures the host by causing cellular damage from microorganism-produced toxins or intracellular multiplication or competing with host metabolism.

Your own worst enemy

The host's own immune response may compound the tissue damage. The damage may be localised (as in infected pressure ulcers) or systemic. The infection's severity varies with the pathogenicity and number of the invading microorganisms and the strength of host defences. The very young and the very old are especially susceptible to infections.

Factor in...

Certain factors contribute to increase the risk of infection. For example, travel can expose people to diseases for which they have little natural immunity.

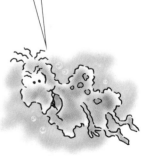

Severity of infection depends on invading organisms and the strength of host defences.

In addition, the expanded use of immunosuppressants, surgery and other invasive procedures increases the risk of infection.

Types of infection

There are three major types of infection:

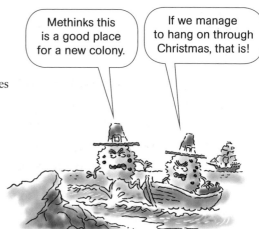

Methinks this is a good place for a new colony.

If we manage to hang on through Christmas, that is!

Subclinical, also called *silent* or *asymptomatic*, is a laboratory-verified infection that causes no signs and symptoms.

Colonised is a multiplication of microbes that produces no signs, symptoms or immune responses.

Dormant, also called *latent*, occurs after a microorganism has been dormant in the host, sometimes for years. An exogenous infection results from environmental pathogens; an endogenous infection, from the host's normal flora (e.g. *Escherichia coli* displaced from the colon, which may cause urinary tract infection).

Pilgrims in a new land

Because a person with a subclinical infection or a colonisation may not have symptoms, this person can be a carrier and transmit infection to others.

Types of infecting organisms

The varied forms of microorganisms responsible for infectious diseases include bacteria, spirochaetes (a type of bacteria), viruses, rickettsiae, chlamydiae, fungi and protozoa. Larger organisms such as helminths (worms) may also cause disease.

Bacteria

Bacteria are single-cell microorganisms with well-defined cell walls that can multiply independently on artificial media without the need for other cells. In developing countries, where poor sanitation heightens the risk of infection, bacterial diseases commonly cause death and disability. Even in industrialised countries, they're still the most common fatal infectious diseases. (See *Bacteria: Oh, the damage they can do!*)

Shaping up

Bacteria can be classified by shape:
- *spherical*—cocci
- *rod-shaped*—bacilli
- *spiral-shaped*—spirilla.

Bacteria: Oh, the damage they can do!

Bacteria and other infectious organisms constantly infect the human body. Some are beneficial, such as the intestinal bacteria that produce vitamins. Others are harmful, causing illnesses ranging from acute otitis media to life-threatening septic shock.

To infect a host, bacteria must first enter it. They do this by adhering to the mucosal surface and directly invading the host cell or attaching to epithelial cells and producing toxins that invade host cells. To survive and multiply within a host, bacteria or their toxins adversely affect biochemical reactions in cells. The result is a disruption of normal cell function or cell death (as shown below). For example, the diphtheria toxin damages heart muscle by inhibiting protein synthesis. In addition, as some organisms multiply, they extend into deeper tissue and eventually enter the bloodstream.

Some toxins cause blood to clot in small blood vessels. The tissues supplied by these vessels may be deprived of blood and damaged (as shown below).

Other toxins can damage the cell walls of small blood vessels, causing leakage. This fluid loss results in decreased blood pressure, which in turn impairs the heart's ability to pump enough blood to vital organs (as shown below).

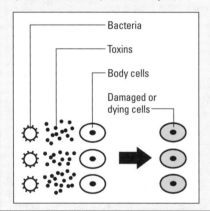

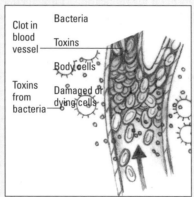

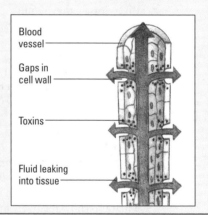

Response, motility, capsulation, spores and oxygen

They also can be classified by:
- response to staining—gram-positive, gram-negative or acid-fast
- motility—motile or non-motile
- tendency towards capsulation—encapsulated or non-encapsulated
- capacity to form spores—sporulating or non-sporulating
- oxygen requirements—aerobic (need oxygen to grow) or anaerobic (don't need oxygen).

Spirochaetes
A type of bacteria, spirochaetes are flexible, slender, undulating spiral rods that have cell walls. Most are anaerobic. The three pathogenic forms in humans include *Treponema*, *Leptospira* and *Borrelia*.

Viruses

Viruses are subcellular organisms made up of only a ribonucleic acid or a deoxyribonucleic acid nucleus covered with proteins. They're the smallest known organisms, so tiny that they're visible only through an electron microscope.

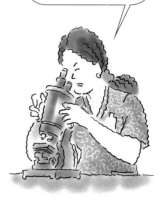

How can such a tiny little thing cause so much trouble?

An invasion occasion

Viruses can't replicate independent of host cells. Rather, they invade a host cell and stimulate it to participate in the formation of additional virus particles. The estimated 400 viruses that infect humans are classified according to their size, shape (spherical, rod-shaped or cubic) or means of transmission.

Rickettsiae

Relatively uncommon in the UK, rickettsiae are small, gram-negative bacteria-like organisms that commonly induce life-threatening infections. Like viruses, they require a host cell for replication. Three genera of rickettsiae include *Rickettsia*, *Coxiella* and *Rochalimaea*.

Chlamydiae

Larger than viruses, chlamydiae have recently been found to be intracellular obligate bacteria. Unlike other bacteria, they depend on host cells for replication. However, unlike viruses, they're susceptible to antibiotics.

Fungi

Fungi are single-cell organisms that have nuclei enveloped by nuclear membranes. They have rigid cell walls like plant cells but lack chlorophyll, the green matter necessary for photosynthesis. They also show relatively little cellular specialisation. Fungi occur as yeasts (single-cell, oval-shaped organisms) or moulds (organisms with hyphae or branching filaments). Depending on the environment, some fungi may occur in both forms. Fungal diseases in humans are called *mycoses*.

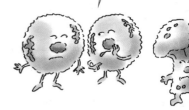

Don't look now, but I think there's a fungus among us.

Protozoa

Protozoa are the simplest single-cell organisms of the animal kingdom, but they show a high level of cellular specialisation. Like other animal cells, they have cell membranes rather than cell walls, and their nuclei are surrounded by nuclear membranes.

Helminths

The three groups of helminths that invade humans include nematodes, cestodes and trematodes. Nematodes are cylindrical, un-segmented, elongated helminths that taper at each end; this shape has earned them the designation *roundworm*. Cestodes, better known as *tapeworms*, have bodies that are flattened front to back with distinct, regular segments. Tapeworms also have heads with suckers or sucking grooves. Trematodes have flattened, un-segmented bodies. They're called *blood*, *intestinal*, *lung* or *liver flukes*, depending on their infection site.

Modes of transmission

Infectious diseases are transmitted directly (by contact) or indirectly. Indirect transmission may occur via airborne transmission, vector-borne transmission or vehicle-borne transmission.

Close contact

In contact transmission, the susceptible host comes into direct contact (as in sexually transmitted diseases) or indirect contact (contaminated inanimate objects) with the source. Direct transmission may also occur via droplet spread—the close-range spray of contaminated droplets into the conjunctiva or mucous membranes.

How's the air?
Airborne transmission results from inhalation of contaminated evaporated saliva droplets (as in pulmonary tuberculosis), which sometimes are suspended in airborne dust particles or vapours.

Hector vector
Vector-borne transmission occurs when an intermediate carrier (vector), such as a flea or a mosquito, transfers an organism. Vehicle-borne transmission occurs when water, food or blood products introduce organisms into a susceptible host via ingestion or inoculation.

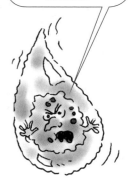

I'll find a way in one way or another!

Health-care-associated infections

Formerly known as *nosocomial infections*, health-care-associated infections (HCAIs) may develop while a patient is in an acute health-care setting (hospital) or in a non-acute setting (community). Most infections of this type result from group A *Streptococcus pyogenes*, *Staphylococcus*, *E. coli*, *Klebsiella*, *Proteus*, *Pseudomonas*, *Haemophilus influenzae*, *Candida albicans* and hepatitis viruses.

HCAIs are usually transmitted by direct contact. Less commonly, they're transmitted by inhalation of or wound invasion by airborne organisms or contaminated equipment and solutions.

Despite best efforts

Despite infection-control projects that include surveillance, prevention and education, HCAIs still remain a problem. Since the 1960s, staphylococcal infections have been declining; however, fungal infections and infections caused by gram-negative bacilli have been steadily increasing. During the

> ## Preventing health-care-associated infections
>
> Here's how to help prevent HCAIs
>
> - Follow good hand-washing techniques and encourage other staff members to do the same.
> - Follow strict infection-control procedures.
> - Document hospital infections as they occur.
> - Identify outbreaks early and take steps to prevent their spread.
> - Eliminate unnecessary procedures that contribute to infection.
> - Strictly follow necessary isolation techniques.
> - Observe all patients for signs of infection, especially patients who are at high risk for infection.
> - Keep staff members and visitors with obvious infection as well as known carriers away from susceptible patients.
> - Staff should change out of their uniform before leaving work and laundering guidance should be followed.
> - Ask patients' visitors to use hand gel on entering and leaving the clinical area. Visitors' chairs should also be used instead of sitting on the patient's bed or chair.

1960s and 1970s, the problem of antibiotic resistance emerged giving rise to meticillin-resistant *Staphylococcus aureus* (MRSA), which remains a problem today. MRSA has received vast amounts of media coverage causing the public to become anxious and with the exposure of dirty hospitals and poor compliance with infection control, it has become high on the political agenda. It is thought that 20% to 30% of the population carries *S. aureus* and this poses a threat to vulnerable patients and plays a large part in HCAIs. To reduce the MRSA bacteraemia rates, Trusts have had to put procedures in place for screening high-risk patients, isolation of colonised patients, decontamination of equipment, hand-hygiene programmes and cleaning of the clinical areas. The basic principles of infection control should be applied to reduce the transmission of MRSA to other patients and advice sought from infection control teams when staff are unsure about dealing with MRSA. (See *Preventing health-care-associated infections*.)

Many risks for many reasons

HCAIs continue to pose a problem because most patients are older and more debilitated than in the past. The advances in treatment that increase longevity in patients with diseases that alter immune defences also create a population at high risk for infection. Moreover, the growing use of invasive and surgical procedures, immunosuppressants and antibiotics predisposes patients to infection and superinfection and helps create new strains of antibiotic-resistant bacteria. The growing number of hospital personnel who come in contact with each patient increases the risk of exposure. (See *Infection control precautions*.)

Infection control precautions

Various government led initiatives have been published due to the high concern about HCAI, with recommendations for infection control. Below are some of the key publications.

Saving Lives: Reducing Infection, Delivering Clean and Safe Care (DH, 2007). This programme consists of 'high impact interventions' (HII) for key invasive procedures, that clinical staff should undertake in order to reduce HCAI. The tools provided are intended to increase the reliability of key clinical procedures, thus preventing HCAI, such as urinary tract and surgical site infections and pneumonia.

The Health Act 2006: Code of Practice for the Prevention and Control of Healthcare-associated Infections (DH, 2006a). The aim of the code is to help National Health Service (NHS) providers plan and implement actions in order to prevent and control HCAI. The criteria must be met by the NHS organisations and the Healthcare Commission monitors compliance with the Code. A failure to comply with the Code can result in an 'improvement notice' or 'special measures' being issued.

Epic2: National Evidence-based Guidelines for Preventing Healthcare-associated Infections in NHS England (Pratt et al., 2007). These DH updated guidelines are referred to as EPIC 2. These evidence-based guidelines should be adhered to when providing care to all patients, to prevent the spread of HCAI.

Standard precautions

Standard precautions, previously more commonly termed as 'universal precautions' describe the infection-preventive actions, which all health-care workers in any environment where health care is provided take to reduce the risk of HCAI. These precautions are: hand hygiene, the safe handling and disposal of sharps, the disposal of waste, the use of personal protective equipment and clothing, isolation of patients and decontamination of equipment and the environment. The precautions are based on the principle that the following may contain infectious agents that can be transmitted between patients and health-care workers:

- blood
- all body fluids, secretions and excretions, except sweat, regardless of whether they contain visible blood
- skin that isn't intact
- mucous membranes.

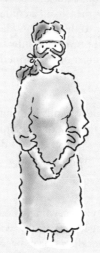

Always take precautions, and wear personal protective clothing when warranted!

Preventing infection

Nurses have a duty legally and ethically to protect their patients from infection. The national infection control policies mentioned earlier are implemented at a local level by infection control teams. The teams consist of infection control nurses and doctors who are responsible for planning, implementing and monitoring infection controls programmes and policies. If you are unsure about anything relating to infection control you should seek advice from the team.

What YOU can do

Individual health-care professionals can also prevent infection by:
- employing drug prophylaxis when necessary
- using strict hand-hygiene technique
- following standard precautions
- using correct personal protective equipment.

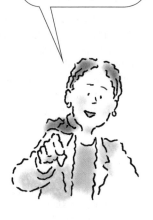

Immunisations and improved living conditions are great, but there's a lot YOU can do to prevent infection, too!

Drug prophylaxis

Although prophylactic antibiotic therapy may prevent certain diseases, the risk of superinfection and the emergence of drug resistant strains may outweigh the benefits. So prophylactic antibiotics are usually reserved for patients at high risk for exposure to dangerous infection.

Hand hygiene

The hands are the conduits for almost every transfer of potential pathogens from one patient to another, from a contaminated object to the patient, or from a staff member to the patient. Hand hygiene is the single most important procedure in preventing infection. To protect patients from HCAIs, hand hygiene must be performed routinely and thoroughly.

Keep it real

In effect, clean and healthy hands with intact skin; short, natural fingernails and no rings minimise the risk of contamination. Artificial nails may serve as a reservoir for microorganisms, and microorganisms are more difficult to remove from rough or chapped hands.

Soap for most

Follow your local policy concerning when to wash with soap and when to use an antiseptic cleaning agent. Typically, you'll wash with soap before coming on duty; before and after direct or indirect patient contact; before and after performing any bodily functions, such as blowing your nose or using the toilet; before preparing or serving food; before preparing or administering medications; after direct or indirect contact with a patient's excretions, secretions or blood; and after completing your shift.

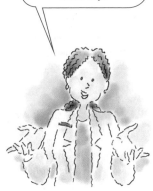

Think of your hands as healing tools. Always keep them clean, healthy and ready to assist... naturally!

Antiseptic when susceptible

An antiseptic solution and water is used to decontaminate hands before performing surgery or highly invasive procedures.

Hold the alcohol

If your hands aren't visibly soiled, an alcohol-based hand rub is preferred for routine decontamination. Don't use alcohol-based hand sanitiser if you might come in contact with items contaminated with *Clostridium difficile* or *Bacillus anthracis* (Anthrax). These organisms can form spores and alcohol will not kill spores. Wash hands with soap and water if either of these organisms is known or suspected to be present.

Care and contact

Wash your hands before and after performing patient care or procedures or having contact with contaminated objects, even though you may have worn gloves. Always wash your hands after removing gloves. The World Health Organization launched *My 5 Moments for Hand Hygiene* in 2009. The approach, which is now used in many Trusts, identifies when health-care workers should clean their hands and can be found at www.who.int/gpsc/5may/background/5moments/en/.

Home sweet home

If you're providing care in the patient's home, bring your own supply of soap and disposable paper towels or alcohol hand rub.

What you need

Hand washing
Liquid soap ✳ warm running water ✳ paper towels

Hand rub
Alcohol-based hand rub

How you do it
You should follow your local policy guidelines for specific hand-washing technique. There are national hand-hygiene campaigns running to improve hand-hygiene compliance. The National Patient Safety Agency (NPSA) campaign can be found at www.npsa.nhs.uk/cleanyourhands and in Scotland the campaign by Health Protection Scotland is available at www.washyourhandsofthem.com.

Hand washing
• *Long natural nails may harbour more microorganisms*; keep nails naturally short.
• Wet your hands and wrists with warm water and apply soap from a dispenser. Don't use bar soap *because it allows cross-contamination.*
• Hold your hands below elbow level *to prevent water from running up your arms and back down, thus contaminating clean areas.*
• Work up a generous lather by rubbing your hands together vigorously following the hand-washing technique adopted as local policy, for a minimum of 10 to 15 seconds. *Soap and warm water reduce surface tension and this reduced tension, aided by friction, loosens surface microorganisms, which wash away in the lather.*

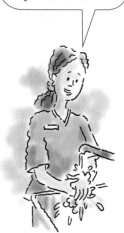

Hand washing should be such an automatic part of your daily routine that, after a while, you'll feel like your hands are leading you to the sink!

Effective hand-washing technique

An effective hand-washing technique involves three processes: preparation, washing and drying (Pratt et al., 2007).

Preparation

To minimise the spread of infection, follow these basic hand-washing instructions. With your hands angled downwards, adjust the water temperature until it's comfortably warm and wet hands before applying hand-washing solution.

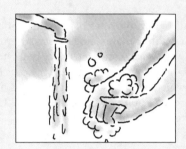

Lather up

You should wash your hands for a minimum of 10 to 15 seconds, making sure that the hand-washing solution covers all surfaces of your hands, including the wrists. Attention should be paid to in between the fingers, the thumbs and the tips of the fingers.

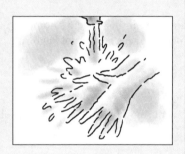

Pat dry

Rinse your hands completely to wash away suds and microorganisms. Pat dry with paper towels and use a foot operated pedal bin to dispose of towels to prevent re-contamination.

- Pay special attention to the tips of fingers, the thumbs, knuckles and the areas between the fingers *because microorganisms thrive in these protected or overlooked areas.* If you don't remove your wedding band, move it up and down your finger to clean beneath it.
- Avoid splashing water on yourself or the floor *because microorganisms spread more easily on wet surfaces and because slippery floors are dangerous.* Avoid touching the sink or taps *because they're considered contaminated.*
- Rinse hands and wrists well *because running water flushes suds, soil, and microorganisms away.*
- Pat hands and wrists dry with paper towels. Avoid rubbing, *which can cause abrasion and chapping.*
- If the sink isn't equipped with elbow-operated taps, turn them off by gripping them with a dry paper towel *to avoid recontamination of your hands.*
- Because frequent hand washing strips the skin of natural oils, this simple procedure can result in dryness, cracking and irritation. However, these effects are probably more common after repeated use of antiseptic cleaning agents, especially in people with sensitive skin. *To help minimise*

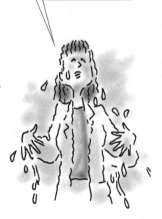

Just being clean isn't enough... it's all in the technique!

irritation, rinse your hands thoroughly, making sure they're free from residue.
• *To prevent your hands from becoming dry or chapped*, apply an emollient hand cream after each washing or switch to a different cleaning agent. Make sure that the hand cream or lotion you use won't cause the material in your gloves to deteriorate. If you develop dermatitis, you may need to be evaluated by occupational health *to determine whether you should continue to work until the condition resolves*.

Hand sanitising with alcohol hand rub
You should follow your local policy for applying alcohol hand rub. The National Patient Safety Agency and Health Protection Scotland also have step-by-step techniques for using hand rub, available at the websites.

Personal protective equipment
The EPIC 2 guidelines (Pratt et al., 2007) state that a risk assessment should be made of the risk of transmission of microorganisms to the patient or carer and the risk of contamination with blood, body fluids, secretions and excretions. The health-care worker can then select protective equipment (gloves, aprons, gowns, face masks and eye protection) based upon this assessment.
• Gloves are worn to protect the health-care workers' hands from contamination with organic matter or microorganisms and to prevent transmission of microorganisms to patients and staff. The EPIC 2 guidelines (Pratt et al., 2007) recommend gloves are worn where there is a risk of exposure to blood, body fluids, secretions and excretions; when touching mucous membranes or broken skin of all patients; contact with sterile sites; handling sharp or contaminated instruments; and when performing invasive procedures.
• Change gloves in between patients and after each episode of care on the same patient. Wash hands before and after contact with each patient, and when gloves are removed.
• Wear a mask and protective eyewear or a face shield to protect mucous membranes of the mouth, nose and eyes during procedures that may generate drops of blood or other body fluids. Respiratory protection equipment must be worn when caring for a patient with some airborne respiratory infections.
• Wear a disposable apron if you are in direct contact with a patient, when there is a risk that clothing may become contaminated with microorganisms or blood, body fluids, secretions and excretions. Wear a full body gown during procedures that are likely to generate extensive splashing of blood, body fluids, secretions or excretions.
• After removing gloves, thoroughly wash hands and other skin surfaces that may be contaminated with blood or other body fluids.
• If you perform or assist in vaginal or caesarean deliveries, wear gloves and a gown when handling the placenta or the infant and during umbilical cord care.

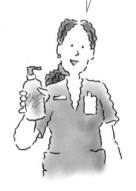

Use hand cream to avoid dry, chapped hands caused by frequent hand washing. But make sure that the lotion you use won't deteriorate your gloves.

Safe handling and disposal of sharps

• Prevent injuries caused by needles, scalpels and other sharp instruments or devices when cleaning used instruments, disposing of used needles and handling sharp instruments after procedures.

• To prevent needle-stick injuries, don't recap used needles, bend or break needles, remove them from disposable syringes or manipulate them. They should not be passed directly from hand to hand. Use safety-protected needles and needleless I.V. systems whenever possible.

• Place disposable syringes and needles, scalpel blades and other sharp items in sharps containers at the point of use for disposal, making sure these containers are located near the area of use. They must not be filled above the marked filled line and should be placed out of reach of children and confused patients.

• If a needle-stick injury or splashes to eyes, mouth or broken skin occurs, follow your local policy. Following a needle-stick injury, encourage the site to bleed and wash with soap and water. For splashes to eyes, mouth or broken skin, rinse thoroughly with running water. Seek help and cover puncture site with a waterproof dressing. Promptly report injuries and mucous-membrane exposure to your manager. Complete an accident or incident form and identify the patient source if possible. Report to the occupational health department or if closed, report to accident and emergency.

Additional precautions

• Make sure mouthpieces, one-way valve masks, resuscitation bags or other ventilation devices are available in areas where the need for resuscitation is likely. *Note*: saliva hasn't been implicated in HIV transmission.

• If you have exudative lesions or weeping dermatitis, refrain from direct patient care and handling patient-care equipment until the condition resolves.

Using isolation equipment

Isolation procedures may be implemented to prevent the spread of infection from patient to patient, from the patient to health-care workers or from health-care workers to the patient. This type of isolation is referred to as *source isolation*. They may also be used to reduce the risk of infection in immunocompromised patients and this is known as *protective isolation*. Central to the success of these procedures is the selection of proper equipment and adequate training of those who use it.

What you need

Materials required for isolation typically include protective clothing, all items and equipment to care for the patient, alcohol hand rub and a door card stating that isolation precautions are in effect.

Barrier clothing: Disposable aprons ✳ impermeable gowns (for heavy contamination) ✳ disposable gloves ✳ goggles/safety glasses/visors (where risk of splashing) ✳ masks (where risk of airborne contamination) (each staff member must be trained in their proper use.)

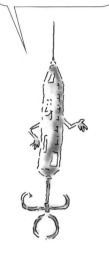

Handling syringes is sticky business. Take all necessary precautions to avoid injury and infection.

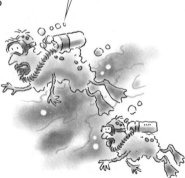

I wouldn't have guessed in a million years it would be so easy breaking in through all that armour…

Isolation supplies for inside the room: Red alginate polythene bag for laundry ✳ yellow clinical waste bag ✳ sharps container ✳ equipment for performing vital signs ✳ disposable gloves

A trolley outside the room needs to be set up with disposable aprons and alcohol hand rub.

How you do it

- Wash your hands with an antimicrobial cleaning agent to prevent the growth of microorganisms under gloves.

Putting on protective clothing

- Put on disposable plastic apron or impermeable gown if heavy contamination is expected.
- Place the mask snugly over your nose and mouth if there's a risk of airborne contamination.
- Wear protective eye glasses/visors/goggles if blood or body fluids are present.
- Apply alcohol hand rub and put on disposable gloves as per local policy.

Removing protective clothing

- Remember that the outside surfaces of your barrier clothes are contaminated.
- If wearing gloves, remove and put in yellow clinical waste bag.
- Remove apron, discard in clinical waste bag and clean hands with alcohol hand rub.
- Gowns (if worn) should not be reused.

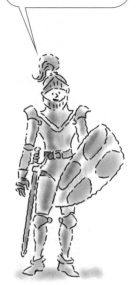

Barrier clothing isn't what it used to be, thank goodness! Now you need gowns, gloves, goggles, and masks—a bit more comfortable if you ask me!

Removing contaminated gloves

Proper removal techniques are essential for preventing the spread of pathogens from gloves to your skin surface. Follow these steps carefully:

Using your left hand, pinch the right glove near the top. Avoid allowing the glove's outer surface to buckle inwards, against your wrist.

Pull downwards, allowing the glove to turn inside out as it comes off. Keep the right glove in your left hand after removing it.

Now insert the first two fingers of your ungloved right hand under the edge of the left glove. Avoid touching the glove's outer surface or folding it against your left wrist.

Pull downwards so that the glove turns inside out as it comes off. Continue pulling until the left glove completely encloses the right one and its uncontaminated inner surface is facing out.

Hospital environmental hygiene

Hospital hygiene is very important as poor standards of cleanliness lead to the harbouring of organisms such as MRSA and *C. difficile*, which lead to cross-infection. Correct decontamination of medical devices and instruments is also vital and is highlighted alongside hospital hygiene, in various published documents. Single-use equipment should be used where possible, and where multi-use equipment is used it needs to be decontaminated appropriately after use. It is necessary to be aware of the difference between single-use equipment and single patient use. Single-use means that the equipment must be discarded after it has been used once; single patient use equipment can be decontaminated and used again for the same patient.

Disposal of waste

The Department of Health (2006b) published a detailed guide highlighting how legislation has changed procedures regarding the management of health-care waste. Recommendations are made for identifying and classifying infectious and clinical waste, a new colour-coded system for identification and segregation of waste, the use of European Waste Catalogue Codes (EWC) and an offensive/hygiene waste stream to include non-infectious human hygiene waste.

Quick quiz

1. What's the most effective method of infection control?
    A. Isolation precautions
    B. Hand-washing
    C. Neutropenic precautions
    D. Wearing sterile gloves

Answer: B. Hand-washing with soap and water or an alcohol-based hand sanitiser is the most effective infection control method.

2. Which type of bacteria depends on host cells for replication?
    A. Rickettsiae
    B. Spirochaetes
    C. Fungi
    D. Chlamydiae

Answer: D. Unlike other bacteria, chlamydiae depend on host cells for replication.

3. What type of transmission occurs when an intermediate carrier, such as a flea or mosquito, transfers an organism?
    A. Vector-borne transmission
    B. Vehicle-born transmission
    C. Contact transmission
    D. Airborne transmission

Answer: A. Vector-borne transmission occurs when an intermediate carrier (vector), such as a flea or mosquito, transfers an organism.

4.   What's the name for a laboratory-verified infection that causes no signs or symptoms?
>   A.   Colonised
>   B.   Sub-clinical
>   C.   Latent
>   D.   Dormant

Answer: B. A laboratory-verified infection that causes no signs and symptoms is called a *subclinical*, *silent* or *asymptomatic infection*.

Scoring

☆☆☆   If you answered all four questions correctly, bravo! You're super at preventing superinfection.

☆☆   If you answered three questions correctly, great! There are no spirochaetes on you.

☆   If you answered fewer than three questions correctly, chin up! Review the chapter and you'll be discarding this quiz properly in no time.

9 Medication basics

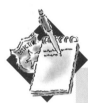

Just the facts

In this chapter, you'll learn:

♦ legal and professional aspects

♦ basics of medication administration

♦ drug administration routes

♦ key concepts of pharmacokinetics and pharmacodynamics

♦ dosage and administration considerations

♦ common medication errors.

A look at medication

When you care for a patient in your day-to-day nursing practice, one of the most crucial skills you bring to the bedside is your ability to administer medications. From legal, ethical and practical standpoints, medication administration is much more than simply a delivery service. It's a highly technical skill that requires you to exercise wide-ranging knowledge, analytical skill, professional judgement and clinical expertise. Indeed, some would consider the safe, effective administration of medications the foundation of your success as a professional nurse.

Legal aspects

You need to be aware that there are a number of government legislations related to the whole process of medication management, including the prescribing, labelling, storage and sale of medication. (See *Some relevant legislation*.)

Changing times! Changes are made to legislation, so it is important to follow the most recent regulation.

Some relevant legislation

The Medicines Act 1968	Controls the sales and labelling of all medicines.
	Prescription-only medicines (POM). A medicine that can be sold by a pharmacist if it has been prescribed by a doctor.
	Pharmacy-only medicines (P). Medicines that don't need a prescription but can only be sold when a pharmacist is present.
	General sales list (GSL). Medicines that are readily available from shops, e.g. paracetamol (although the amount of this medicine is restricted).
The Misuse of Drugs (Safe Custody) Regulations 1973	Controls the manufacture, supply and possession of controlled drugs. (The Class of a drug A, B and C)
The Misuse of Drugs Regulations 2001	Defines the professional duties of those who are authorised to supply and possess controlled drugs, while carrying out their work. (The Schedules 1 to 5)

Professional aspects

You also have professional guidelines which will help guide you. The NMC's Standards for Medicines Administration (2008) is a comprehensive guide which you should obtain. Following this will ensure you stay safe.

> Remember! Student nurses must always be directly supervised by a registered nurse when supplying and administering medication.

The basics

To deliver medications accurately, you need a sound working knowledge of:
- drug terminology
- routes by which drugs are delivered
- effects that drugs produce after they're inside the body.

Pharmacology is the scientific study of the origin, nature, chemistry, effects and uses of drugs. This chapter reviews some concepts basic to pharmacology, which is essential to your ability to administer drugs safely, starting with the most basic of all: drug names.

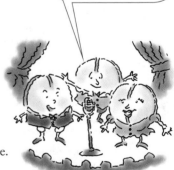

And now, ladies and gentlemen, let's get back to basics.

The name game

The typical drug has three or more names:
- The chemical name describes the drug's atomic and molecular structure.
- The generic name is a shorter, simpler version of the drug's chemical name. These are also called non-proprietary or approved names.
- The trade name (also known as the brand name or propriety name) is the name selected by the drug company that sells it. Trade names are protected by copyright laws. (See *What's in a name?*, page 118)

What's in a name?

Most drugs have three names—chemical, generic and trade—as this example demonstrates. Some drugs may have more than one trade name. The best way to avoid confusion is to use the generic name when speaking or writing about a drug.

Chemical name

7-chloro-1,3-dihydro-1-methyl-5-phenyl-2H-1,4-benzodiazepin-2-one

Generic name

diazepam

Trade name

Valium

A class act

Drugs that share similar characteristics are grouped together into pharmacological classes, or families. For example, the class known as beta-adrenergic blockers contains several drugs with similar properties such as atenolol and celiprolol.

Drugs can also be grouped according to their therapeutic class, which classifies drugs according to their use. For example, thiazide diuretics and beta-adrenergic blockers are both antihypertensives, but they belong to different pharmacological classes because they share few characteristics.

Routes of administration

A drug's administration route influences the quantity given and the rate at which the drug is absorbed and distributed. These variables in turn affect the drug's action and the patient's response. Routes of administration that involve the gastro-intestinal (GI) tract are known as enteral routes. Those that don't involve the GI tract are known as parenteral routes. Parenteral routes can be useful for treating a patient who can't take a drug orally. Compare the advantages and disadvantages of the following routes.

Topical route

The topical route is used to deliver a drug via the skin or a mucous membrane. The drug is applied directly onto the unbroken skin or mucous membrane. The advantages of delivering drugs by this route include:

- easy administration
- few allergic reactions
- fewer adverse reactions than drugs administered by systemic routes.

You can make a real mess of it

Delivering precise doses can be difficult with the topical route. These medications can be messy to apply; they also may stain the patients' clothing and linen and may have a distinctive smell.

Ophthalmic administration

Ophthalmic administration involves drugs, such as creams, ointments and liquid drops that are placed in the conjunctival sac or directly onto the surface of the eye. For all types of ophthalmic administration, take care to avoid contaminating the medication container or transferring organisms to the patient's eye.

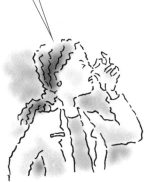

Besides being messy, some topical medications have a very distinctive smell...phew!

Ear drops

Solutions placed into the ear can be used to treat infection or inflammation of the external ear canal, produce local anaesthesia or soften built-up cerumen (earwax) for removal.

Bring ear drops to room temperature before administering them because cold solutions can cause pain or vertigo.

Nasal administration

Nasal administration involves drugs that are placed directly into the patient's nostrils. Medicated solutions can be placed into the patient's nostrils from a dropper or as an atomized spray from a squeeze bottle or pump device. Creams and ointments can also be applied.

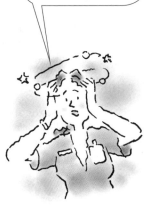

Make sure that ear drops are at room temperature before administration. Otherwise, they can cause pain or vertigo.

Bypassing the first-pass effect

The highly vascular nasal mucosa allows systemic absorption while avoiding first-pass metabolism by the liver. The liver changes the drug to a more water-soluble form for excretion before it enters circulation.

Respiratory route

Drugs that are lipid-soluble and available as gases can be administered into the respiratory tree. The respiratory tree provides an extensive, highly perfused region for enhanced absorption. Smaller doses of potent drugs can be given by this route to minimize their adverse effects. Because this route is easily accessible, it provides a convenient alternative when other routes are unavailable.

Emergency!

In emergencies, some injectable drugs, such as atropine, lidocaine and adrenaline (epinephrine), can be given directly into the lungs via an endotracheal tube (ET tube). A drug administered into the trachea is absorbed into the bloodstream from the alveolar sacs. Surfactant, for example, is administered to premature neonates via the trachea to improve their respiratory function. Also, atropine can be administered to patients with symptomatic bradycardia and no vascular access to increase their heart rate.

Breathing easy? Not so fast!

A major disadvantage of the respiratory route is that few drugs can be given this way. Other disadvantages include:
• difficulty in administering accurate doses—or full doses, if the patient isn't cooperative
• nausea and vomiting when certain drugs are delivered into the lungs
• irritation of the tracheal or bronchial mucosa, causing coughing or bronchospasm
• possible infection from the equipment used to deliver drugs into the lungs.

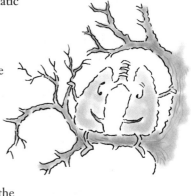

The respiratory tree provides an extensive, highly perfused region for enhanced absorption, if I do say so myself!

Buccal, sublingual and translingual routes

Certain drugs are given buccally (in the pouch between the cheek and teeth) or sublingually (under the tongue) or translingually (across the tongue) to prevent their destruction or transformation in the stomach or small intestine. Drugs given by these routes act quickly because the oral mucosa's thin epithelium and abundant vasculature allow direct absorption into the bloodstream.

Cheeky checklist

These routes can be used if the patient can take nothing by mouth, can't swallow or is intubated. What's more, the drugs have no first-pass effect in the liver and don't cause GI irritation. However, only drugs that are highly lipid-soluble may be given by these routes, and they may irritate the oral mucosa.

Oral route

Oral administration is usually the safest, most convenient and least expensive method. For that reason, most drugs are administered by this route to patients who are conscious and able to swallow.

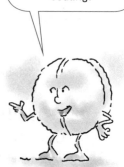

I'm designed to melt in your mouth, not in your hands! No, I take that back…that's the other little round fella with the sugar coating!

Down in the mouth

The oral route does have some disadvantages:
* It produces variable drug absorption.
* Because it moves drugs through the liver, first-pass metabolism may take place.
* Drugs can't be given orally in most emergencies because of their unpredictable and relatively slow absorption. (See *Enteral administration: Why absorption varies.*)
* Oral drugs may irritate the GI tract, discolour the patient's teeth or taste unpleasant.
* Oral drugs can be accidentally aspirated if the patient has trouble swallowing or is combative.

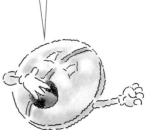

I hate to admit it, but I can be a little slow and unpredictable. So, don't count on me in an emergency.

Rectal and vaginal routes

You may instil suppositories, ointments, creams or gels into the rectum or vagina to treat local irritation or infection. Some drugs applied to the mucosa of the rectum or vagina can be absorbed systemically. Drugs may also be delivered to the rectum in a medicated enema or suppository or to the vagina in a pessary, cream or medicated douche.

The up side

Drugs administered through the rectal or vaginal routes don't irritate the upper GI tract, as some oral medications do. Also, these drugs avoid destruction by digestive enzymes in the stomach and small intestine.

The down side

However, there are some disadvantages to the rectal and vaginal routes:
* The rectal route is usually contraindicated when the patient has a disorder affecting the lower GI tract, such as rectal bleeding or diarrhoea.
* Drug absorption may be irregular or incomplete with these routes.

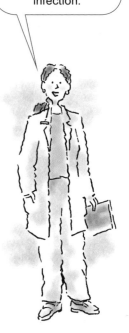

Some drugs can be administered by the rectal or vaginal route to treat local irritation or infection.

Enteral administration: Why absorption varies

A drug that's administered enterally—orally or by gastric tube—can undergo variable rates of absorption due to:

* changes in the pH of the GI tract
* changes in intestinal membrane permeability
* fluctuations in GI motility
* fluctuations in GI blood flow
* food in the GI tract
* other drugs in the GI tract.

- The rectal route usually can't be used in an emergency.
- Rectal doses of some drugs may need to be larger than oral doses.
- Because rectal administration typically stimulates the vagus nerve, this route may pose a risk for cardiac patients.
- Drugs given rectally may irritate the rectal mucosa.
- Administering a drug by the rectal or vaginal route may cause discomfort and embarrassment for the patient.

Subcutaneous route

When using the subcutaneous route, you inject small amounts of a drug beneath the dermis and into the subcutaneous tissue, usually in the patient's upper arm, thigh or abdomen. Patients with diabetes use this technique to give themselves insulin. The drug is absorbed slowly from the subcutaneous tissue, thus prolonging its effects.

Tissue issues

There are disadvantages to the subcutaneous route:
- Subcutaneous injection may damage tissue.
- The subcutaneous route can't be used when the patient has occlusive vascular disease and poor perfusion because decreased peripheral circulation delays absorption. Exceptions to this are heparin and insulin.
- The subcutaneous route can't be used when the patient's skin or underlying tissue is grossly adipose, oedematous, burned, hardened, swollen at the common injection sites, damaged by previous injections.

Intradermal route

Intradermal drug administration is used mainly for diagnostic purposes when testing for allergies or tuberculosis. To administer drugs intradermally, inject a small amount of serum or vaccine between the skin layers just below the stratum corneum. Because this route results in little systemic absorption, it produces mainly local effects.

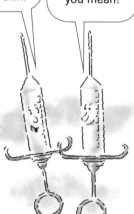

I don't know what it is about some people but sometimes they just get under my skin.

I know exactly what you mean!

Implants eliminate non-compliance

Aside from injection, another method of subcutaneous administration is to implant beneath the skin pellets or capsules that contain small amounts of a drug. From the dermis, the medication seeps slowly into the tissues. Goserelin, one such implant, is inserted into the upper abdominal wall to manage advanced prostate cancer.

Because subcutaneous implants require no patient action after they're in place, they eliminate the problem of non-compliance. Their major drawback is the need for minor surgery to insert or remove them.

Intramuscular route

The intramuscular (I.M.) route allows you to inject drugs directly into various muscle groups at varying tissue depths. You'll use this route to give aqueous suspensions and solutions in oil and to give medications that aren't available in oral form. The effect of a drug administered by the I.M. route is relatively rapid, and aqueous I.M. medications can be given to adults in doses of up to 5 ml in some sites. The I.M. route also eliminates the need for an intravenous (I.V.) site.

Intramuscular miscues

Despite the advantages, there are many disadvantages to the I.M. route:
• A drug delivered I.M. may precipitate in the muscle, thereby reducing absorption.
• The drug may not absorb properly if the patient is hypotensive or has a poor blood supply to the muscle.
• Improper technique can cause accidental injection of the drug into the patient's bloodstream, possibly causing an overdose or an adverse reaction.
• The I.M. route may cause pain and local tissue irritation, damage bone, puncture blood vessels, injure nerves or breakdown muscle tissue, thus interfering with myoglobin—a marker for acute myocardial infarction.

Intravenous route

The I.V. route allows injection of substances directly into the bloodstream through a vein. Appropriate substances include drugs, fluids, diagnostic contrast agents and blood or blood products. Administration can range from a single dose to an ongoing infusion delivered with great precision.

In the I.V. league

Because the drug or solution is absorbed immediately and completely, the patient's response is rapid. Instant bioavailability (the drug's availability for target tissues) makes the I.V. route the first choice for giving drugs during an emergency. This route has no first-pass effect in the liver and avoids damage to muscle tissue caused by irritating drugs. Because absorption into the bloodstream is complete and reliable, large drug doses can be delivered at a continuous rate.

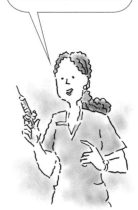

I.M. injections are helpful in a lot of situations, but they require proper technique to prevent pain, tissue breakdown, nerve injury and even accidental overdose.

This road can be bumpy

Life-threatening adverse reactions may arise if I.V. drugs are administered too quickly, if the flow rate isn't monitored carefully enough or if incompatible drugs are mixed together. Also, the I.V. route increases the risk of complications, such as extravasation, vein irritation, systemic infection and air embolism.

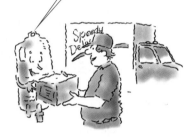

No, next-day delivery isn't good enough…I need this delivered immediately to the bloodstream.

Specialised infusions

Under certain circumstances, drug infusion may take place directly at the site of intended activity. Using specialised catheters and devices, drugs and solutions can be delivered to an organ or its blood vessels to manage emergencies, treat disease, infuse tumours or relieve pain. These infusions may be given by the epidural, intrapleural, intraperitoneal, intra-articular or intraosseous routes. (See *Reviewing specialised infusions*.)

Caution! Only registered nurses and medical staff, who have received additional theoretical and competence-based training, can administer I.V. medication.

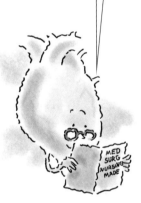

Let's see, what kind of specialised infusions do they have today? I could use a little pick-me-up.

Reviewing specialised infusions

If drug therapy needs to take a direct route to a specific site in the patient's body, you may use one of the specialised routes of drug administration as shown in this chart.

Route	Characteristics
Epidural infusion	• The drug is injected into the epidural space, outside or above the dura mater. • The drug is absorbed into cerebrospinal fluid and works directly on the central nervous system. • Epidural anaesthesia or analgesia is given through a special catheter and is considered safe and versatile. It may be tailored to affect a specific area of the body from the legs up to the upper abdomen. • The drug infused through an epidural catheter must be preservative-free to prevent serious reactions to the preservative. • Epidural catheters should be labelled 'for epidural use only' to prevent the accidental injection of other drugs into the epidural space.

(continued)

Route	Characteristics
Reviewing specialised infusions (continued)	
Intrapleural infusion	• The drug is injected into the pleural cavity. • The drug crosses the pleural membrane and enters the pleural space, where it works locally at the disease site. • Chemotherapy is an example of a drug given by this type of infusion to minimise systemic effects and increase drug effects on the tumour.
Intraperitoneal infusion	• The drug is injected into the peritoneal cavity. • The drug or solution crosses the peritoneal membrane and enters the peritoneal space, where it works locally. • This administration route is used for peritoneal dialysis, in which the peritoneum functions as a diffusible semi-permeable membrane. • Fluid or electrolyte imbalances can be corrected, toxins removed and normal renal excretion facilitated using this route.
Intra-articular infusion	• The drug is injected into the synovial cavity of a joint to suppress inflammation, prevent contractures and delay muscle atrophy. • This route is most commonly used to treat rheumatoid arthritis, gout, systemic lupus erythematosus (SLE), osteoarthritis and other joint disorders. • Corticosteroids, anaesthetics and lubricants are most commonly administered into the shoulder, elbow, wrist, finger, knee, ankle or toe joints. • This route is used sparingly because of the risk of infection.
Intraosseous infusion	• The drug is injected into the rich vascular network of a long bone for rapid absorption. • Drugs and solutions administered through bone marrow are absorbed as rapidly as those administered I.V. • With a special intraosseous access needle, this route has been used successfully in children and adults for emergency infusions when normal vascular access isn't possible.

Pharmacokinetics

A solid understanding of pharmacokinetics—the movement of a drug through the body—can help you predict your patient's response to a prescribed drug regimen and anticipate potential problems. Anytime you give a drug, a series of physiochemical events takes place in the patient's body and includes four basic processes:

 absorption

 distribution

 metabolism

 excretion. (See *What happens after drug administration*, page 126.)

What happens after drug administration

Drug disposition begins as soon as a drug is administered. The drug proceeds through pharmacokinetic, pharmacodynamic and pharmacotherapeutic phases. This chart shows the various phases, the activities that occur during them and the factors that influence those activities.

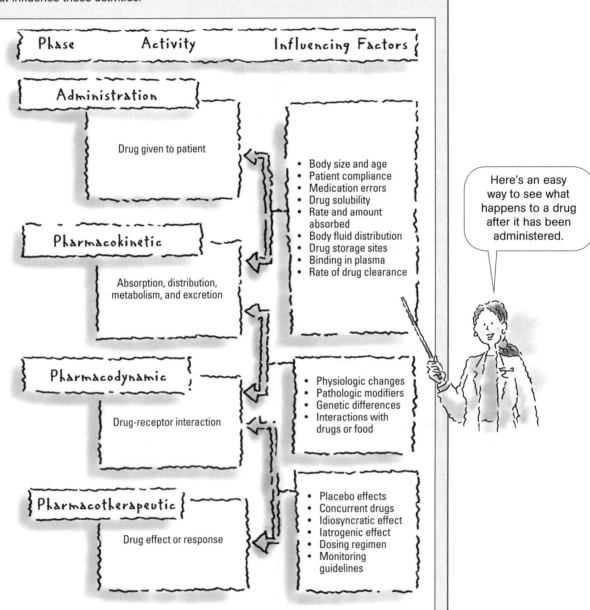

Phase	Activity	Influencing Factors
Administration	Drug given to patient	• Body size and age • Patient compliance • Medication errors • Drug solubility • Rate and amount absorbed • Body fluid distribution • Drug storage sites • Binding in plasma • Rate of drug clearance
Pharmacokinetic	Absorption, distribution, metabolism, and excretion	
Pharmacodynamic	Drug-receptor interaction	• Physiologic changes • Pathologic modifiers • Genetic differences • Interactions with drugs or food
Pharmacotherapeutic	Drug effect or response	• Placebo effects • Concurrent drugs • Idiosyncratic effect • Iatrogenic effect • Dosing regimen • Monitoring guidelines

Here's an easy way to see what happens to a drug after it has been administered.

Absorption

Before a drug can act on the body, it must be absorbed into the bloodstream. How well a patient's body absorbs a drug depends on several factors. These include:
- the drug's physiochemical properties
- the drug's form
- the route of administration
- the drug's interactions with other substances in the GI tract
- various patient characteristics, especially the site and the condition of the absorbing surface.

These factors can also determine the speed and amount of drug absorption.

Becoming bioavailable

When taken orally, some drug forms, such as tablets and capsules, may have to disintegrate before free particles are available to dissolve in the gastric juices. Only after dissolving in these juices can the drug be absorbed, circulate in the bloodstream and thus become bioavailable. A bioavailable drug is one that's ready to produce a physiologic effect.

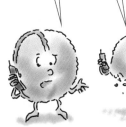

Say again? I can't hear you... you seem to be breaking up.

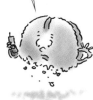

Sorry... have got to... losing signal...

Timing is everything

Some tablets have enteric coatings, which delay disintegration until after the tablets leave the acidic environment of the stomach. Oral solutions and elixirs, which don't have to disintegrate and dissolve to take effect, are usually absorbed more rapidly.

If the patient has had a bowel resection, anticipate slow absorption of any oral drug you administer. And remember that a drug given I.M. must first be absorbed through the muscle before it can enter the bloodstream. Rectal suppositories must first dissolve to be absorbed through the rectal mucosa. Drugs administered I.V.—thereby placed directly into the bloodstream—are completely and immediately bioavailable.

"Now circle to the left, and a do-si-do..."

I don't get it. If we're in a circle, why do they call this square dancing?

Distribution

When a drug enters the bloodstream, it's distributed to body tissues and fluids through the circulatory system. To better understand drug distribution, think of the body as a system of physiologic compartments defined by blood flow. The bloodstream and highly perfused organs—such as the brain, heart, liver and kidneys—make up the central compartment. Lesser perfused areas form the peripheral compartment, which is subdivided into the

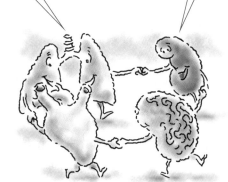

How the body stores a drug

The body can store a drug in fat, bone or skin. Knowing the characteristics of each drug storage compartment will help you understand how distribution can affect a drug's duration of action.

Fat storage

A drug that dissolves easily in lipids migrates to adipose tissue (what we commonly think of as fatty tissue). Because this tissue lacks receptors for drug action, the drug remains inactive there. Eventually, it's released by fat cells to exert its pharmacological effect. With some drugs, this slow, prolonged action is an advantage. For example, slow release of anaesthetic barbiturates provides effective anaesthesia during surgery. With other drugs, such prolonged action can be dangerous.

Bone storage

Bone acts as a storage compartment for certain drugs. Tetracycline, for example, is distributed throughout bone and may eventually crystallise there. In a growing child, this can cause tooth discolouration. Lead and some chemicals can also accumulate in bone, resulting in prolonged exposure to toxins.

Skin storage

Storage of drugs in the skin typically causes photosensitivity. Tetracycline and amiodarone are examples of drugs that are stored in the skin.

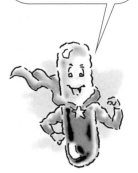

Some drugs can't cross cell membranes, but not I! I leap membranes in a single bound, for I am Super Drug!

tissue compartment (viscera, muscle and skin) and the deep compartment (fat and bone).

Highly perfused tissues receive the drug before lesser perfused areas do. Each compartment then stores portions of the drug, releasing it as plasma drug levels decline. (See *How the body stores a drug*.)

Leaping lipid barriers

Distribution also depends partly on a drug's ability to cross lipid membranes. Some drugs can't cross certain cell membranes and thus have limited distribution. For example, antibiotics have trouble permeating the prostate gland, abscesses and exudates.

It's got to be free

Distribution can also be affected if the drug binds to plasma proteins, especially albumin. Only a free, unbound drug can produce an effect at the drug receptor site, so such binding greatly influences the drug's effectiveness and duration of action.

Disease disrupts distribution

Certain diseases impede drug distribution by altering the volume of distribution—the total amount of drug in the body in relation to the

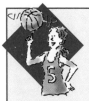

Stay on the ball

Dosing dilemma

Some drugs—such as digoxin, gentamicin and tobramycin—are poorly distributed to fatty tissue. Therefore, dosing based on actual body weight in a highly obese patient may lead to overdose and serious toxicity.

amount in plasma. Heart failure, dehydration and burns are examples of such disorders. If the patient has heart failure, expect to increase the dosage because the drug must be distributed to a larger fluid volume. On the other hand, if the patient is dehydrated, expect to decrease the dosage because the drug will be distributed to a much smaller fluid volume. (See *Dosing dilemma*.)

Metabolism and excretion

Most drugs are metabolised in the liver and excreted by the kidneys. The rate at which a drug is metabolised varies with the individual. Some patients metabolise drugs so quickly that their blood and tissue levels prove therapeutically inadequate. Others metabolise drugs so slowly that even ordinary doses can produce toxic results.

Slow or fast? Here's some help...

Drug metabolism may be faster in smokers than in non-smokers because cigarette smoke contains substances that induce production of hepatic enzymes. Also, a diet high in fat or carbohydrates may slow the metabolism of certain drugs, whereas a diet high in protein may speed metabolism.

Hepatic diseases, or diseases that interfere with hepatic blood flow or transport of drugs to the liver, may affect one or more of the liver's metabolic functions. Thus, in patients with hepatic disease, drug metabolism may be increased or decreased. All patients with hepatic disease must be monitored closely for drug effects and toxic reactions.

The kidneys can be key

Some drugs, such as digoxin and gentamicin, are eliminated almost unchanged by the kidneys. Thus, inadequate renal function causes the drug to accumulate, producing toxic

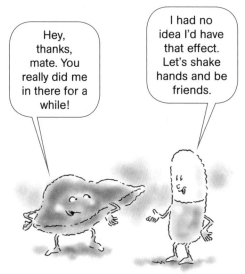

Hey, thanks, mate. You really did me in there for a while!

I had no idea I'd have that effect. Let's shake hands and be friends.

effects. Some drugs can block renal excretion of other drugs, thereby allowing them to accumulate and enhancing their effects. In contrast, some drugs can promote renal excretion of other drugs, thus diminishing their effects.

Different escape routes

Although most drugs are excreted by the kidneys, not all are. Some are excreted hepatically, via the bile and into stool. A few drugs leave the body in sweat, saliva and breast milk. Certain volatile anaesthetics—for example, halothane—are eliminated primarily by exhalation. When natural excretion mechanisms fail, as in drug overdose or renal dysfunction, many drugs can be removed through dialysis.

Underlying disease

Underlying disease can have a marked influence on drug action and effect. For example, acidosis may cause insulin resistance. Genetic diseases, such as glucose-6-phosphate dehydrogenase (G6PD) deficiency and hepatic porphyria, may turn drugs into toxins. As a result, patients with G6PD deficiency may develop haemolytic anaemia when given sulphonamides or certain other drugs.

It's in your genes

A genetically susceptible patient can develop an acute porphyria attack if given a barbiturate.

Toxic conditions

Also, patients with highly active hepatic enzyme systems (rapid acetylators, for example) can develop hepatitis when treated with isoniazid because of the rapid intrahepatic build-up of a toxic metabolite.

Sphere of influence

Other conditions that may influence a patient's response to drug therapy include infection, fever, stress, starvation, hypersensitivity, sunlight, exercise, variations in circadian rhythm, alcohol intake, pregnancy, lactation, immunisation, barometric pressure, and GI, renal, hepatic, cardiovascular and immunologic function. (See *Age-old influence*.)

Patient-specific direction

A patient-specific direction (PSD) is a prescription that remains in effect indefinitely or for a specified period. The prescriber either writes the

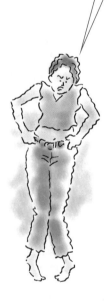

So many conditions and factors can influence a person's response to drug therapy, even genes. There's nothing worse than a pair of tightfitting genes (or jeans, in my case)!

Ages and stages

Age-old influence

The patient's age has an important influence on a drug's overall action and effect. Older adults usually have decreased hepatic function, less muscle mass and diminished renal function. Consequently, they need lower doses and, sometimes, longer dosage intervals to avoid toxicity.

Neonates have underdeveloped metabolic enzyme systems and inadequate renal function, which can also lead to toxicity. They need highly individualised dosages and careful monitoring.

medication on the medicines administration record (MAR) or enters it into a computer. (The MAR is commonly known as the drug chart)

MAR

To help ensure the safe administration of medication to the patient the MAR must specify the name of the patient, and the medication, dosage, route of administration, frequency and duration (if time limited). (See *Essential criteria of a medicines administration record*, page 132.) If a patient has more than 1 MAR they must be clearly numbered 1 of 2, 2 of 2 etc.

Stop!

If a PSD doesn't specify a stop date, the direction usually remains in effect until the prescriber writes another direction to replace or discontinue it. For some types of drugs, however, the amount of time covered by the order may be limited by local guidelines. For example, opioid orders may have a specified number of doses. Some antibiotics may have a specified time of 7 days. If the patient still needs the drug after the termination date has passed, the prescriber must write another order. The same is true for post-operative medications; the prescriber must review all medications that are to continue after surgery.

Stat orders

If a patient needs a medication right away for an urgent problem, a prescriber writes a stat order. For example, they may order an immediate single dose of an antianxiety drug to calm an acutely agitated patient. For a patient with acute chest pain, they may write a stat order for nitroglycerin (GTN) (sublingual, spray or I.V. form).

Essential criteria of medicines administration record

For inpatients, a prescriber writes a prescription on a patient's MAR on a chart or enters it into the computer system. An example of a written MAR is shown here.

Criteria

Whether written or entered into the computer, all medication must contain:

- patient's full name and date of birth
- hospital number and ward number
- date of the prescription

- name of the drug being ordered using the generic name
- dose amount
- administration route
- times for administration
- prescriber's signature or computer code
- any allergies the patient may have
- patient's weight.

Medication Administration Record

NHS Trust

Patients details

REGISTRATION DETAILS		Tick box	HOSPITAL: ROYAL
Surname SMITH	Ward 2	NHS ✓	KNOWN DRUG SENSITIVITIES– yes ☐ no ☑
			1 -------------------------------------
First Name JOHN	Consultant MR GREEN	PP	2 -------------------------------------
Registration No. 123456	Date of Birth 1/03/49	Over seas Visitor	Patient's weight: 78.5 Kgs Patient's surface area: ☐

ONCE ONLY and PREMEDICATION

DATE	TIME	DRUG	DOSE	ROUTE	PRESCRIBERS SIGNATURE	PHARM	TIME GIVEN	ADMIN. BY
4/2/10	10.00	PARACETAMOL	1g	Oral	P.A. Jones		10.15	J Brown

Date & time

Name of medication

Route of administration

Prescriber's signature

Time given

Administered by

Dosage form and amount

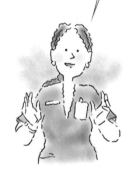

Here's a medicines administration record (MAR) with all the pertinent components.

P.R.N. orders

The term p.r.n. comes from a Latin phrase *pro re nata* that means 'as required'. A p.r.n. order allows you to give a medication when the patient needs it for a specified problem, such as pain, fever and constipation. Naturally, you should exercise sound professional judgement in determining when and how often to administer a drug p.r.n.

Record it in the record

Anytime you administer a p.r.n. medication, explain your reason for giving it in the patient's record. Also, describe its degree of effectiveness.

Patient group direction

Patient group directions (PGDs) are a specific set of written instructions derived from strict guidelines created by a doctor, pharmacist and a member of the professional group who will be administering the PGD. They are for use in *specific* settings to treat patients who fit set criteria. The health-care professional must be competent to administer the medication, but it does not require a prescription (MHRA, 2005).

> **Note!** Student nurses must not supply or administer any PGD but must have some understanding of purpose and process (NMC, 2009).

An emergency

In an emergency, a registered nurse may take a verbal message over the telephone; this must be confirmed by written instructions via e-mail, text or fax. They must make sure the prescription chart is signed by the prescriber within 24 hours (NMC, 2008). Whenever possible, avoid them because miscommunications can occur and you'll lack a written record of the direction. A bad connection, commotion on either end or the lack of non-verbal communication cues can easily result in medication errors if you fail to clarify exactly what the prescriber wants.

Many trusts require the prescriber to repeat their instuctions to two registered nurses. (See *Telephone message accuracy*, page 134.)

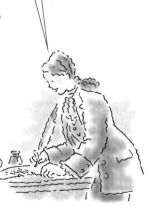

Getting a signature after a verbal message is just as important as getting it right!

Check aloud!

In urgent situations, you may not be able to avoid verbal orders. Repeat the order aloud so the prescriber can verify that you understood it. For example, your patient goes into hypoglycaemic or insulin shock and the doctor tells you to immediately prepare 50 ml of 50% glucose for I.V. administration. To verify, show the doctor the label on the empty glucose vial and say the drug's name out loud as you hand them the syringe. That way, they can confirm the accuracy of the drug and its dose.

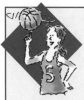

Stay on the ball

Telephone message accuracy

If you have to take a medication message over the telephone, follow these steps to help ensure its accuracy:

- Have another nurse listen in on the call to confirm that she heard the same message you did.
- Repeat the name of the ordered drug to the prescriber to verify that you heard it correctly. Have the prescriber spell the drug name, if necessary.
- Repeat the individual digits of the dose ordered to allow the prescriber to confirm the amount or correct it.
- Write on the prescription, noting that it was a verified telephone message, then sign and date it. (Students should not be involved with this!)
- Administer the medication as ordered.
- The prescriber must sign your written order within 24 hours (72 hours maximum over a weekend or bank holiday).

Please note that student nurses should not take this type of order unless they are directly supervised by a registered nurse.

It may be verbal, but still get a signature

Anytime you accept a verbal message, it's your responsibility to ensure the accuracy of the communication. This holds true even in an emergency. Ask the prescriber to spell the drug's name if you aren't sure what it is. Afterwards, write and sign the order that was given to you verbally by the prescriber. Then have the prescriber sign your written copy within 24 hours (maximum).

Administration procedures

Making sure you understand a prescription is just the start of your responsibilities when it comes to administering medications correctly. Next, you have to make your own judgement about the correctness of the prescription based on your knowledge of the medication and your understanding of the patient's condition.

The MAR looks good

If you're convinced that the MAR contains all the information you need to safely administer the medication to the patient involved, your next step is to prepare to administer the medication by following the five rights of medication administration.

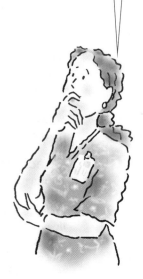

Use your good judgement before administering a medication.

The five rights

Following a tried-and-true set of safeguards known as the five rights can quickly and easily help you avoid the most basic and common sources of medication error. Each time you administer a medication, confirm that you have the:

right drug

right dose

right patient

right time

right route.

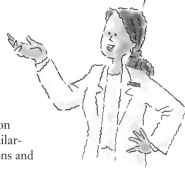

Before giving a drug, make sure you confirm the five rights of medication administration.

Right drug

Always compare the name of an ordered drug with the name printed on the container label. Take your time and do it carefully; drugs with similar-sounding and similar-looking names may have very different indications and effects.

From the mouth of the patient

Besides carefully checking the ordered medicine name against the container label, also check the patient's reaction to the medicine as you try to administer it. If they say, 'I usually take one pink pill, but you've given me two yellow pills', stop what you're doing and recheck the prescription. Perhaps you'll simply explain to the patient that the pink pill contains 10 mg of the drug and the yellow ones contain 5 mg each. Or perhaps you'll discover that you're giving the patient the wrong medication. Either way, you must carefully follow up on any comment a patient makes about changes in a medication *before* you administer it.

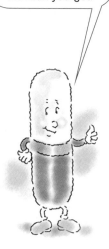

Be a namedropper… before giving me to your patient, mention my name to see what kind of reaction you get.

Right dose

Many commercially prepared medications are available in various tablet sizes, decreasing the number of calculations you have to do to determine the dosage.

Even so, you still need to know how and when to perform the appropriate dose calculations. (See *Keeping calculations correct*, page 136.)

Double up!

Whenever possible, double-check all your calculations with another nurse or with a pharmacist. Many hospitals require these double-checks when your dosage calculations involve children's medications or drugs with narrow safety margins, such as heparin and insulin.

Stay safe

Keeping calculations correct

To help keep your medication calculations correct, use these safeguards:

- Think about whether a dosage seems right, given the patient's diagnosis and the medication involved.
- If your calculation indicates that you need several dosage units to prepare a prescribed dose, double-check the calculation.
- If your calculation indicates that you need a small fraction of a dosage unit to prepare a prescribed dose, double-check the calculation.
- Be especially careful when calculating with decimal points because a mistake can increase or decrease the intended dose many times over.

- Minimise the possibility of confusion anytime you have to write down a dose that contains a decimal point by putting a zero in front of a decimal point that has no other number in front of it. In other words, write 0.25 mg rather than .25 mg, which someone could easily mistake for 25 mg. Likewise, never write a zero after a dose that includes a decimal point. In other words, don't write 0.250 mg for a dose of 0.25 mg.
- Never break an unscored tablet to prepare a calculated dose because you won't get an exact amount. Instead, ask a pharmacist for a form of the drug that you can measure accurately.

Right patient

To reduce the risk of medication errors, always check the patient's identity band before giving any medication.

Roll call

As an additional check, also call them by their full name. (Don't say something like, 'You're John, right?' because the patient could misunderstand you, could be confused or could be a different John than the one scheduled for a medication.)

Right time

The 'right time' is the time and date the medication has been prescribed for on the MAR. It may be therapeutic, practical or both. For therapeutic purposes, the right time is one that appropriately maintains the level of drug in the patient's bloodstream. For practical purposes, the right time is one that's convenient for the staff and the patient. Naturally, therapeutic goals take precedence over practical ones.

Remember that you're part of a team. Consult with the doctor and pharmacist if you think a drug isn't effective

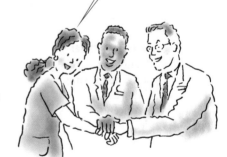

Working around the clock

To meet therapeutic goals, delivery of the medications may need to be spaced evenly around the clock. Doing so helps to maintain a consistent level of the drug in the patient's bloodstream.

For some drugs, you may need to measure the patient's therapeutic response before determining whether it's the right time to give another dose. For example, you should check the patient's pulse rate for 1 minute before giving digoxin; if it is below 60 beats per minute advice must be taken on whether the digoxin should be given. Patient's respiratory rate must be assessed before giving morphine as morphine can slow the respiration rate. Advice should be taken if the rate is 8 to 10 respirations per minute. (In both examples local policies must be followed.)

The perfect plan

Besides maximising the therapeutic effect, giving medications at specified, evenly spaced intervals provides some practical benefits. Some medicines need to be given with food to enable metabolism of the drug, while others may need to be given on an empty stomach.

Another practical benefit of standardised administration times is that they establish a habit in the patient's mind. This may make it easier for them to keep taking the medication appropriately when they get home.

If it's on the schedule, you need to be on time

Regardless of the reasons behind the administration times you establish for the patient, you'll need to follow those times carefully.

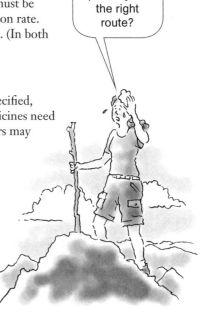

Can this possibly be the right route?

Right route

Always pay careful attention to the administration route specified on the MAR and on the product's label. Also, make sure the ordered form of the drug is appropriate for the intended route. Only drugs labelled 'for injection' should be used for injections of any kind.

Before you give the drug, consider whether the amount ordered is appropriate for the route by which you're preparing to give it. For example, 10 mg is an appropriate amount of morphine sulphate to give by the I.M. route to relieve pain in an adult. If the patient will be receiving it by the I.V. route, however, the equivalent dose would be more like 2 to 4 mg. If they are taking the drug orally, they will need more than 10 mg to achieve the same effect.

Different routes

Remember that the route by which you give a drug affects the rate at which it gets absorbed into the patient's bloodstream. Because certain forms of a drug may be intended for specific routes, be careful not to interfere with a drug's action by changing routes or circumventing the chemical preparation. For example, you wouldn't want to crush an enteric-coated tablet or open a sustained-release capsule. (See *Working with sustained-release drugs*, page 138.)

Different speeds

You can decrease the rate of absorption and effectiveness of a drug. For example, if a patient chews or swallows a sustained-release drug, absorption and effectiveness will be increased.

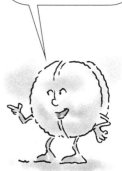

You can increase or decrease the rate of absorption of a drug, depending on the application.

Working with sustained-release drugs

A growing number of drugs are being formulated to exert an effect over many hours. The components of each drug dose dissolve at different rates, thus releasing the drug gradually but continuously into the patient's bloodstream. Convenient for staff and patients, sustained-release drugs require fewer doses per day and provide steadier control over symptoms.

Easy identification

Sustained-release drugs are supplied as plain tablets, coated tablets, and capsules filled with tiny granules. They may be identified by an SR (for sustained release) after the drug name.

Don't split, crush or chew

Never split or crush a sustained-release drug. Warn the patient not to chew the drug and to never open a sustained-release capsule to mix the granules into foods or beverages. All of these actions could alter the drug's absorption rate, put too much drug into the patient's bloodstream too quickly or reduce the drug's overall effect.

Procedural safeguards

The five rights of medication administration afford you a basic level of protection against medication errors. However, most experts consider them the minimum requirement. Here are some additional measures you should take to help avoid medication errors.

Storage and preparation

Follow these guidelines when storing and preparing drugs:
• Store and handle drugs carefully to maintain their stability and potency. Remember that some drugs can be altered by temperature, air, light and moisture; make sure you follow all drug-specific precautions. Some drugs may need to be kept in brown bottles. Some I.V. bags may need to be covered to block the light during infusion.
• Always keep drugs in the containers in which the pharmacy dispensed them. Cap all containers tightly. If you see small packets in a container, they probably serve to absorb moisture and keep the product fresh; don't remove them.
• Store drugs at room temperature unless you're instructed to refrigerate them. Refrigeration causes moisture to form and could alter some drugs through condensation.
• As required by law, all controlled drugs must be kept under double lock.

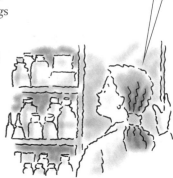

Always follow the manufacturer's recommendations and your local policies for storing and handling all medications.

Out of date? Out of the question!

- Always note a medication's expiration date—the date after which it loses some amount of potency. Never administer an outdated medication or one that looks or smells unusual.
- If the original package looks like someone may have tampered with it, don't give the drug; instead, return it in its package to the pharmacy for an investigation.
- Check the medication label three times—when you take it from the shelf or drawer, before putting it into the medication cup, and before returning the container to the shelf or drawer—to make sure you're giving the prescribed medication.
- You may need to reconstitute a medication dispensed as a powder just before you administer it. Label the container with the date, time, strength and your initials or signature.
- Never administer a medication that you did not prepare yourself.
- Discard any drug that will reach its expiration date before another dose is scheduled.
- If you find an unlabelled syringe with medication inside, discard it.
- Let a refrigerated drug reach room temperature before administering it, unless you're instructed otherwise.

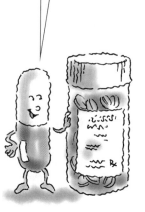

Check all medication labels and packaging carefully. Note the expiration date, too.

Administration

Follow these guidelines when administering drugs:
- Before administering a medication based on a new prescription, review the patient's medication history for known allergies or other problems.
- If you know a patient has a drug allergy, make sure their chart clearly displays the allergy.
- When you deliver drugs to a patient, stay with the drug trolley. Never leave without locking it.
- Assess the patient's physiological and psychological condition before administering any medication.
- Stay with the patient until they take the medication.
- Never leave medication doses at a patient's bedside.
- Administer only medications you've prepared personally or that the pharmacist prepared.
- When administering an oral drug, urge the patient to drink water, if appropriate. Doing so helps move the medication out of the oesophagus and into the stomach. It also dilutes the drug, thus reducing the chance of gastric irritation.

Write it down!

- Document drugs immediately after you administer them. Delayed charting, especially of p.r.n. medications, can result in repeated doses.
- Document if medication was not given and the reason why.
- Record your observations of the patient's positive and negative responses to the medication. For example, if you give an antibiotic to a patient with

pneumonia, chart such positive responses as decreased sputum, reduced fever and easier breathing to confirm the drug's effectiveness. Also, chart such adverse reactions as skin eruptions or gastric upset. Severe adverse reactions may prompt the prescriber to substitute another drug.

Controlled drugs

A 'controlled drug' is medication that a person can become dependent on (addicted). Examples of these are morphine, pethidine and diamorphine; the sale, storage and administration of controlled drugs is strictly controlled by both the law and professional requirements.

Common medication errors

In addition to following the NMC Standards for Medicines Administration (2008) and your trust's policies faithfully, you can help prevent medication errors by studying common ones and avoiding the slip-ups that allowed them to happen.

I just need to check your identification…

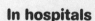

Similar names

As you read earlier, drugs with similar-sounding names can be easy to confuse. Keep in mind, however, that even different-sounding names can look similar when written out rapidly by hand on an MAR. Anytime a patient's prescription doesn't seem right for their diagnosis, call the doctor to clarify the prescription.

In hospitals

- All controlled drugs must be stored together in a locked cupboard. No other medications should be in there. The cupboard must have a separate key, not the same as any other used in the area (RPSGB, 2005).
- Only an authorised signatory can order controlled drugs from the pharmacy (NMC, 2008).
- The Registrant in Charge must enter all controlled drugs received from pharmacy into a Controlled Drug Record Book. This should be done in the presence of another registered healthcare worker (NMC, 2008).
- Controlled drugs must be administered by a registered healthcare worker in the presence of a another registered healthcare worker. Where this is not possible local policy may allow the second signatory to be someone who is assessed as competent (NMC, 2008).

A case of mistaken identity

Drug names aren't the only kinds of words you can confuse. Patient names can cause trouble as well if you fail to verify each person's identity. This problem can be especially troublesome if two patients have the same first name.

Consider this clinical scenario: Robert Brewer, age 5, was hospitalised for measles. Robert Brinson, also age 5, was admitted after a severe asthma attack. The boys were assigned to adjacent beds on a small paediatric unit. Each had a non-productive cough. When Robert Brewer's nurse came to give him an expectorant, the child's mother told her that Robert had already inhaled a medication through a mask.

The nurse quickly figured out that another nurse, new to the unit, had given Robert Brinson's medication to Robert Brewer in error. Fortunately, no harmful adverse effects ensued. Had the nurse checked her patient's identity more carefully, however, no error would have occurred in the first place.

Checking ID

Always check each patient's full name. Also, teach each patient (or parent) to offer a wristband for inspection and to state their name before taking the medication. Also, urge patients to tell you if their wristband falls off, is removed or gets lost. Replace it right away. (See *Reducing medication errors through patient teaching*.)

Teacher's lounge

Reducing medication errors through patient teaching

You aren't the only one who's at risk for making medication errors. Patients are at an even greater risk because they know so much less about medications than you do.

Clearly, patient teaching is a crucial aspect of your responsibility in minimising medication errors and their consequences—especially as more patients receive outpatient, rather than inpatient, care.

Teaching tips

You can help minimise medication errors by:

- teaching the patient about their diagnosis and the purpose of the medication

- providing the patient with their medication in writing
- asking if they take over-the-counter medications at home in addition to the prescribed drugs
- asking about herbal remedies and other nutritional supplements
- urging the patient to report anything about their medication that concerns or worries them.

Allergy alert

After you've verified your patient's full name, take time to check whether they have drug allergies—even if they are in distress. Anytime you're in a tense situation with a patient who needs or wants medication fast, resist the temptation to act first and document later. Skipping that crucial assessment step could easily lead to a medication error.

> An allergic reaction is nothing to sneeze at. Take the time to check for drug allergies before giving any medication.

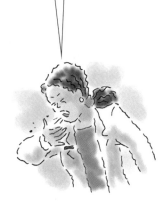

MAR errors

Many medication errors stem from compound problems, a mistake that could have been caught at any of the several steps along the way. For a medication to be administered correctly, each member of the health-care team must fulfil the appropriate role. The doctor must write the MAR correctly and legibly. The pharmacist must evaluate whether the prescription is appropriate and then fill it correctly. In addition, the nurse must evaluate whether the prescription is appropriate and then administer it correctly.

Chain reaction

A breakdown anywhere along this chain of events can lead to a medication error. That's why it's so important for members of the health-care team to act as a real team, checking each other and catching any problems that arise before those problems affect the patient's health. Do your best to foster an environment in which professionals can double-check each other.

For example, the pharmacist can help clarify the number of times a drug should be given each day, label drugs in the most appropriate way and remind you to always return unused or discontinued medications to the pharmacy.

> The health-care team—always professional and working together!

Clear the confusion

You must clarify any prescription that doesn't seem clear or correct. You must also correctly handle and store any multidose vials obtained from the pharmacist. Additionally, store drugs in their original containers to avoid errors.

Route trouble

Many medication errors stem at least in part from problems related to the route of administration. The risk of error increases when a patient has several lines running for different purposes.

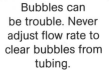

Caught in a tangle of lines

Consider this example: a nurse prepared a dose of digoxin elixir for a patient who had a central I.V. line and a jejunostomy tube—and she mistakenly administered the drug into the central I.V. line. Fortunately, the patient had no adverse reaction. To help prevent such mix-ups in administration route, prepare all oral medications in a purple oral syringe.

Bubble trouble

Here's another error that could have been avoided: to clear air bubbles from a 9-year-old patient's insulin drip, a nurse disconnected the tubing and raised the pump rate to 200 ml/hour to flush the bubbles through quickly. She then reconnected the tubing and restarted the drip, but she forgot to reset the rate back to 2 units/hour. The child received 50 units of insulin before the error was detected. To prevent this kind of error, never increase a drip rate to clear bubbles from a line. Instead, remove the tubing from the pump, disconnect it from the patient and use the flow-control clamp to establish gravity flow.

You carry a great deal of responsibility for making sure that patients get the right drugs in the right concentrations at the right times and by the right routes. By diligently applying the guidelines offered here, you can minimise your risk of medication errors and maximise the therapeutic effects of your patients' drug regimens.

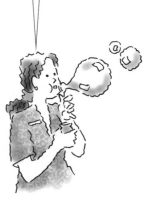

Bubbles can be trouble. Never adjust flow rate to clear bubbles from tubing.

Quick quiz

1. Which branch of pharmacology deals with the study of interactions between drugs and living tissues and serves as the basis of drug treatment?
- A. Pharmacokinetics
- B. Pharmacodynamics
- C. Steady-state dosing
- D. Bioavailability

Answer: B. Pharmacodynamics is the study of the interactions between drugs and living tissues and serves as the basis of drug treatment. It encompasses drug action and drug effect.

2. Which of the following routes of administration is a student nurse unable to use to administer medication?
- A. I.M.
- B. Oral
- C. Topical
- D. I.V.

Answer: D. Student nurses must not give I.V. medication. Only registered nurses and medical staff, who have received additional theoretical and competence-based training, can administer I.V. medication.

3.   If a verbal message is taken for medication, within what period of time must the prescription be signed by the prescriber?
  A.   Within 24 hours
  B.   Within 12 hours
  C.   Within 6 hours
  D.   It does't need to be signed

Answer: A. The NMC guidelines (2008) state that this needs to be done within 24 hours.

Scoring

★★★   If you answered all three questions correctly, excellent! You're on the route to greatness.

★★   If you answered two questions correctly, you're getting the essentials! You used the key concepts to unlock the door to understanding.

★   If you answered fewer than two questions correctly, don't worry! Go back and review this chapter, and soon you'll be pharmacodynamite.

(10) Medication administration

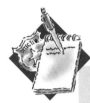

Just the facts

In this chapter, you'll learn:

♦ how to administer medication by the oral, nasogastric tube and gastric routes

♦ correct procedures for administering topical, ophthalmic, ear and nasal medication

♦ advantages and disadvantages of rectal and vaginal administration methods

♦ how to administer medication via the respiratory route

♦ principles of injecting medication

♦ methods for preparing an injection

♦ proper techniques for administering medication subcutaneously and intramuscularly.

Administering oral medication

Oral medication administration offers the safest, most convenient and least costly way to administer a host of medication. Usually, you'll give tablets, capsules or liquid medication (such as an elixir, syrup or suspension) by the oral route. However, oral medication is also available as powders, granules and oils.

> No doubt about it…these guys are the safest, most convenient and least expensive way to go.

Giving a tablet or capsule

You usually give tablets or capsules whole. However, if a tablet requires crushing this must be in the patient's best interest and

Breaking a scored tablet

To split a scored tablet, follow these steps:

- Wash your hands.
- Notice the location of the score mark.
- Using a tablet cutter, place the tablet into the device so the score mark lines up with the blade.

- Close the lid of the cutting device to force the blade through the tablet.
- Place the correct dose in a medicine container.
- Wash the tablet cutter.

advised by a pharmacist, as the therapeutic properties of the medicine may alter and the medicines are not covered by their product licence (NMC, 2007). It is much better to get the medicine prescribed in liquid form for patients that have swallowing difficulties. Where a tablet requires breaking, this should only be done with a scored tablet. Breaking of a tablet may cause an incorrect dose to be given or gastrointestinal irritation (See *Breaking a scored tablet*).

What you need

Prescribed medication in tablet or capsule form ✳ patient's *medicines administration record* (MAR) ✳ medicine pot ✳ glass of water or other liquid to help the patient swallow the medication ✳ tablet cutter (if splitting a scored tablet)

Getting ready

- Wash your hands.
- Check the patient's MAR to make sure that it is legible, clear and correct, and that the medication has not been given.
- Check the patient's allergies and gain consent.
- Before administering check: ✳ patient identity ✳ medication ✳ dosage ✳ time ✳ route.

How you do it

Keeping tabs

- If the tablet is in a bottle, open the bottle and pour the required number of tablets or capsules into the lid of the bottle. Then put them in the medicine pot without touching them. Tablets or capsules in blister packs should be pushed through the foil into the medicine pot, again without touching them.
- Assess your patient's ability to swallow before giving him an oral medication. Impaired swallowing can lead to aspiration.
- Confirm the patient's identity using the identity band and the patient's MAR as per local policy.
- Help the patient to a sitting position.

There's got to be an easier way of getting out of that drug container!

One at a time please

- Offer the tablets or capsules one at a time. Ask the patient to place it in their mouth and take enough liquid to swallow it comfortably.
- If the medication is chewable, make sure the patient chews it thoroughly before swallowing it.

Practice pointers

Look for the designer label

- Don't give tablets or capsules from a poorly labelled or an unlabelled bottle.
- Never give a tablet or capsule that has been poured by someone else.

Gotta get a witness

- If the patient questions you about the medication you're giving or the amount you're giving, double-check their MAR. If the medication and dose are correct, reassure and inform the patient about their medication and any changes in dosage. (See *Teaching about giving a tablet or a capsule*.)

Administering a liquid medication

For an infant, child or patient who has trouble swallowing pills, you may give a liquid medication. (If the patient has a nasogastric (NG), gastrostomy or jejunostomy tube, you may give the medication through the tube rather than orally.)

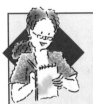

Take note!

Documenting oral medication administration

After administering a tablet or capsule, be sure to record:

- medication and dose given; date and time as per local policy
- record on the patient's MAR
- patient's ability to swallow the medication you administered (if the patient has had problems swallowing oral medication)

- patient's vital signs if you give a medication that could affect them
- adverse reactions that arise
- patient's refusal and notification of a doctor as needed (if a patient refuses a tablet or capsule)
- omission or withholding of a medication for any reason.

Teacher's lounge

Teaching about giving a tablet or a capsule

- Caution the patient not to chew tablets that aren't supposed to be chewed, especially enteric-coated ones.
- Teach the patient about the medication you're administering, including its name, purpose and possible adverse effects.
- If the patient will be taking the tablets or capsules independently at home, make sure the patient thoroughly understands and plans to follow the regimen.
- Be sure to tell them to report anything that could be an adverse reaction to the medication.

What you need

Patient's MAR ✳ graduated medicine pot ✳ prescribed medication

Getting ready

- Wash your hands.
- Complete the same checks as for administering a tablet or capsule.

How you do it

- Shake the bottle well, and then uncap it. Place the cap upside down on a clean surface to avoid contaminating the inside surface.

Graduate to the next level

- While holding a graduated medicine pot at eye level, use your thumb to mark the correct level on the cup.
- Hold the bottle so the liquid flows from the side opposite the label so that the liquid won't stain or obscure the label if it runs down the bottle.
- Pour the medication into the medicine pot to the correct dose mark.
- Set the medicine pot down and again—still at eye level—to double-check your accuracy. If you've poured too much, discard the excess rather than pour it back into the bottle.
- An *oral syringe* should be used for oral liquid medicines that are not prescribed in multiples of 5 ml (BNF, 2009).

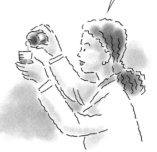

Like everything else in nursing, it's all in the technique.

Give lip service

- Remove drips from the lip of the bottle using a damp paper towel. Then clean the sides of the bottle, if necessary.
- Confirm the patient's identity checking the patient's name, date of birth and hospital number against their identity band and MAR or as per local policy.
- To administer a liquid medication to an infant, follow the steps outlined in *Administering a liquid medication to an infant*.

Practice pointers

- Don't give medication from a poorly labelled or an unlabelled container.
- Never give a medication that has been poured by someone else.

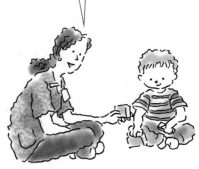

Always evaluate your patient's ability to swallow oral drugs first.

Swallow

- Assess your patient's ability to swallow before administering a liquid medication.
- If the patient or a parent questions you about the medication you're giving or the amount you're giving, double-check the patient's MAR. If the medication and dose are correct, reassure and inform the patient or parent about the medication and any changes in dosage.

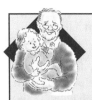

Ages and stages

Administering a liquid medication to an infant

To administer a liquid medication to an infant, be sure to follow these steps:

- Confirm the patient's identity using the identify band and the prescription as per local policy.
- Wash your hands.
- Place a bib or towel under the infant's chin if required.
- Withdraw the correct amount of liquid medication from the medication bottle using a purple oral syringe.
- Hold the infant securely in the crook of your arm and raise their head to about a 45-degree angle.

- Place the tip of the oral syringe into and towards the side of the infant's mouth so the medication will run into the pocket between their cheek and gum. Slowly discharge the liquid, allowing time for the liquid to be swallowed. This action keeps the child from spitting out the medication and also reduces the risk of aspiration.
- Dispose of syringe as per local policy.

Ages and stages

Administering oral medications to children

The oral route of medication administration is the preferred route in children because it's more comfortable and is usually safer and easier to use. When administering oral medications to children, use these guidelines:

- If the patient is a toddler, don't mix a liquid medication with food without discussing with the pharmacist to see that it is all right to do so and then discuss with the parent(s). Draw up a liquid medicine with an oral syringe first and pour into a medicine tot for an older child, unable to tolerate

tablet form. If the medication is available only in tablet form, crush it and mix it with compatible syrup after consulting the pharmacist. Check with the pharmacist first to make sure it's safe to crush the tablet.
- If the patient is an older child who can swallow a tablet or a capsule by themselves, ask them to place the tablet on the back of their tongue and swallow it with water or fruit juice. Remember, milk or milk products may interfere with medication absorption.

Gastric administration

If your patient has a nasogastric or gastrostomy tube, you can deliver medication directly to the gastric mucosa through the tube. If they have a jejunostomy tube, you can deliver medication to the intestinal lumen.

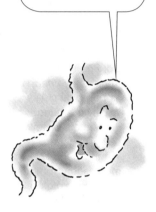

With a tube in place, my medicine is delivered wholesale, directly to me—no big-mouthed middleman needed!

Going down the tubes

An NG tube extends from the patient's nose into the stomach. Your patient may have an NG tube in place if they have trouble swallowing or have an altered level of consciousness. In either case, it may be necessary to administer their oral medication through the tube rather than through the oral route.

Crossing over

Unlike an NG tube, a gastrostomy tube crosses the abdominal wall to enter the stomach. It may be surgically inserted, or it may be placed during an endoscopic, a laparoscopic or a radiologic procedure.

A gastrostomy tube reduces the risk of aspiration and it's more comfortable for the patient than an NG tube. You'll use the tube to deliver feeding solutions and medication directly into the patient's stomach.

What you need

Patient's MAR ✳ prescribed medication (liquids or soluble tablet preferred formulation) ✳ non-sterile gloves ✳ tap or sterile water (depending on local policy and exit site of tube) ✳ 50 ml enteral syringe ✳ pH indicator strip (to confirm tube placement)

Getting ready

• All medication delivered through an NG or a gastrostomy tube must be in liquid form so they can pass easily through the tube. Administering crushed tablets or opened capsules via feeding tubes usually falls outside of a medication's product licence. The medicines should be prescribed as a liquid or a soluble tablet. The crushing of tablets or opening of capsules should only be a last resort, after discussion with the pharmacist. If your patient's medication comes in tablet form, you'll need to crush it and mix it with 10 to 15 ml of water. If the medication comes in capsule form, you'll need to empty the contents of the capsule into 10 to 15 ml of water.

• Check whether it is necessary to give medication or if an alternative route can be used.

• Check that the medication is absorbed from the site of delivery.

• Check the patient's MAR to make sure that it is legible, clear and correct and that the medication has not been given.

• Check the patient's allergies and gain consent.

- Before administering check: ✳ patient identity ✳ medication ✳ dosage ✳ time ✳ route.
- Confirm the patient's name, date of birth and hospital number against his identity band and MAR, or as per local policy.
- Explain the procedure to the patient.
- Wash your hands and put on non-sterile gloves.

How you do it

- If a feed is in progress, stop the feed and flush the tube with at least 30 ml of water, with an enteral syringe.
- Check with the pharmacist whether there needs to be a break between the feed and administering the medicines.
- Prepare the medicines for delivery. Each medication should be prepared and given separately via a 50 ml enteral syringe.
- Help the patient into a semi-upright position.
- If there is not a feed in progress always verify placement of an NG tube before administering any medication. Using a syringe aspirate a small amount of stomach contents from the NG tube.

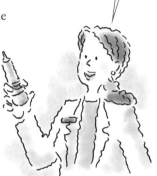

Always aspirate a small amount of stomach contents to verify correct tube placement before administering medicines through a gastric tube.

Grassy green

- Examine the aspirate and place a small amount on a pH indicator strip. Probability of gastric placement is increased if the aspirate has a typical gastric fluid appearance (grassy green, brown or clear and colourless with mucous shreds) and the pH is less than or equal to 5.5.
- If no gastric contents appear when you draw back on the syringe, the patient needs to be on their side to allow the tip of the tube to enter the gastric contents. Inject 10 to 20 ml of air down the tube to dislodge the end from the gastric mucosa.
- Where there is still no aspirate, check the external position of the tube is the same as documented when the tube was passed. The tube may have risen into the oesophagus, and you'll have to advance the tube 10–12 cm and then recheck aspirate.
- If you meet resistance when aspirating for gastric contents, stop the procedure. *Resistance may indicate a non-patent tube or improper tube placement.* (Keep in mind that some smaller tubes may collapse when aspiration is attempted.)
- After you've confirmed that the tube is in the proper position, remove the syringe from the end of the tube.
- Draw water into the syringe and use it to irrigate the tube with about 30 ml of water. Then remove the syringe from the tube.
- Administer medicine down the tube using the 50 ml enteral syringe.
- Rinse the tablet crusher equipment with a small amount of water and draw up into 50 ml syringe and flush this down the tube. This is to ensure that the whole dose is given.
- If you're giving more than one medicine, flush the tube with 10 ml of water between medication, to avoid any interaction.

Getting carried away

- When the last medication has been given, flush the tube with a minimum of 30 ml of water.
- If the patient needs to have their feed restarted, check whether a break is required.

Positioning

- Ask the patient to remain in a semi-sitting or in a side-lying position for at least 30 minutes after administration *to prevent oesophageal reflux* (backward or return flow of stomach contents into the oesophagus).
- Clean and store the equipment, or dispose it of as appropriate.

Practice pointers

- Remember that all medication instilled through the tube must be in liquid form. Check with a pharmacist if you aren't sure whether a tablet can be safely crushed or a capsule safely opened.
- Never crush an enteric-coated or a sustained-release medication, hormone preparations or cytotoxics.

Administering topical medication

Topical medication exerts its effects after being applied to a patient's skin or the mucous membrane in the patient's mouth or throat.

Most forms are local

Topical medication may take the form of a lotion, cream, ointment, paste, powder or spray that you apply to an affected skin area. Other topical medication forms include a spray, mouthwash, gargle and lozenge to treat a problem in the patient's mouth or throat.

Usually, you'll use these topical administration methods to obtain local, rather than systemic, medication effects. The medication moves through the epidermis and into the dermis, based in part on the vascularity of the region to which it's applied.

Transport

Certain types of topical medication, known as *transdermal medication*, are meant to enter the patient's bloodstream and exert a systemic effect after you apply a paste or patch to the patient's skin.

Vive la difference

Keep in mind the differences between lotions, creams, ointments, pastes and powders:

- A *lotion* contains an insoluble powder suspended in water or an emulsion. When you apply a lotion, it leaves a uniform layer of powder in the film on the patient's skin.

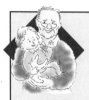

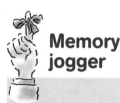

Memory jogger

Trans means 'across' or 'through'; *dermal* means 'related to the skin'. A transdermal medication moves *through the skin* and into the bloodstream.

- A *cream* is an oil-in-water emulsion in semi-solid form. It lubricates the skin and acts as a barrier.
- An *ointment* is a semi-solid substance that, when applied to the skin, helps to retain body heat and provides prolonged contact between the skin and the medication.
- A *paste* is a stiff mixture of powder and ointment. It provides a uniform coat to reduce and repel moisture.
- A *powder* is an inert chemical that may contain medication. It helps dry the skin and reduces maceration and friction. (See *Tips for tots*.)

Administering a transdermal medication

Transdermal medication delivers a constant, controlled amount of medication through the skin and into the bloodstream, thereby achieving a steady, prolonged systemic effect.

Patch him up

To give a transdermal medication, you'll either apply a measured amount of ointment to a selected area of the patient's skin, or you'll apply a transdermal patch that contains medication. (See *Understanding a transdermal patch*, page 154.)

The transdermal team

Medication that are commonly given via the transdermal route include:
- glyceryl trinitrate to control angina
- hyoscine to treat motion sickness
- estradiol to provide hormone replacement after menopause
- fentanyl to control chronic pain.

A matter of time

The appropriate form—ointment or patch—by which to give the medication depends largely on the desired delivery time; typically, a patch delivers the

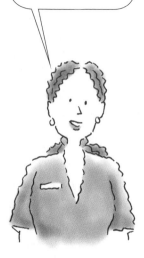

A transdermal patch delivers a constant, controlled amount of medication that achieves a steady, prolonged systemic effect.

Understanding a transdermal patch

A transdermal patch is made up of several layers. The outermost layer is an aluminised polyester barrier that holds the medication in the patch. The next layer is the medication reservoir, which contains the main dose of the medication. The next layer, a membrane, controls release of the medication from the reservoir.

Stick with it

The innermost adhesive layer keeps the patch on the patient's skin and holds a small amount of medication as it moves from the patch into the skin. The dots in this illustration show the medication moving through the skin and into the bloodstream.

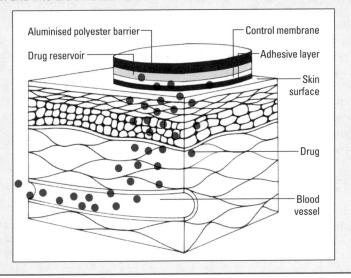

medication for a longer period. For example, transdermal glyceryl trinitrate ointment dilates coronary vessels for up to 4 hours, whereas a glyceryl trinitrate patch lasts for up to 24 hours. In patch form, hyoscine lasts up to 72 hours, estradiol up to a week and fentanyl up to 72 hours.

What you need

Transdermal ointment
Patient's MAR ✳ prescribed medicated ointment ✳ applicator strip ✳ semi-permeable dressing (if required) ✳ gloves ✳ soft wipes, soap, warm water and towel

Transdermal patch
Patient's MAR ✳ prescribed medicated patch ✳ soft wipes, soap, water and towel

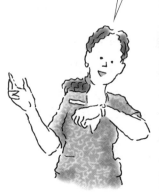

Generally, patches deliver drugs for longer periods of time than ointments do.

Getting ready
• Check the patient's MAR to make sure that it is legible, clear and correct and that the medication has not been given.
• Check the patient's allergies and gain consent.
• Before administering check: ✳ patient identity ✳ medication ✳ dosage ✳ time ✳ route.
• Confirm the patient's name, date of birth and hospital number against his identity band and MAR, or as per local policy.
• Wash your hands and put on gloves.

How you do it
Follow these steps for applying a transdermal ointment or a transdermal patch.

Applying a transdermal ointment
• Choose the application site, usually a dry, hairless spot on the patient's chest or arm.
• To promote absorption, wash the site with soap and warm water. Dry it thoroughly.
• If the patient has a previously applied medication strip at another site, remove it and wash this area to clear away medication residue.

Splitting hairs
• If you must use an area that's hairy, clip excess hair rather than shaving it; shaving causes irritation, which may be exacerbated by the medication.
• Squeeze the prescribed amount of ointment on the application strip as shown. Don't let the medication touch your skin.
• Apply the strip, medication side down, directly to the patient's skin.
• Manoeuvre the strip slightly to spread a thin layer of the ointment over a 7.5 cm area, but don't rub the ointment into the skin.
• Secure the application strip to the patient's skin by covering it with a semi-permeable dressing.

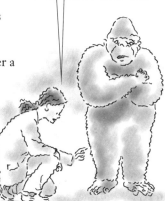

Now if I can just find that hairless spot again …I know it's here, somewhere!

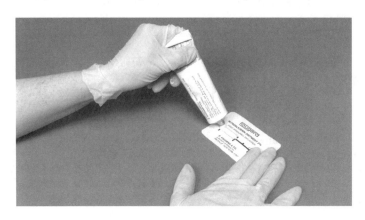

Skin tight

- Press firmly with the palm of one hand to ensure that the dressing adheres well, especially around the edges.
- Label the strip with the date, time and your initials.
- Remove your gloves and wash your hands.

Applying a transdermal patch

- Remove the old patch.
- Choose a dry, hairless application site. Be sure to rotate application sites. Don't attempt to apply the patch to an area with alterations in skin integrity.
- If necessary, clip any hair from the site, but don't shave the area. The most commonly used sites are the upper arm, the chest, the back, and behind the ear.
- Clean the application site with soap and warm water. Dry it thoroughly.
- Open the medication package and remove the patch.
- Remove the clear plastic backing, without touching the adhesive surface.
- Apply the patch to the application site, without touching the adhesive.

Practice pointers

- Apply any transdermal medication at the prescribed intervals to ensure a continuous effect.
- Don't apply the medication if the patient has skin allergies or has experienced skin reactions to the medication.

Saved by his own skin

- Avoid areas of broken or irritated skin; the medication could increase the irritation.
- Don't apply a transdermal medication to scarred or callused skin because either one may impair absorption.
- If you need to defibrillate a patient who has a transdermal patch in place, see *A shocking experience*.
- Teach the patient about taking transdermal medication. (See *Teaching about transdermal medications.*)

Here are the facts, Jack

- Also be sure to alert the patient to potential adverse reactions to the particular medication being delivered. For example:
  – glyceryl trinitrate may cause headaches and, in elderly patients, postural hypotension.

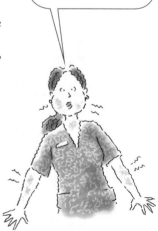

Don't apply transdermal drugs if your patient has skin allergies or has had a previous skin reaction to the drug.

Teacher's lounge

Teaching about transdermal medications

- Review medication-specific precautions the patient must know. For example, make sure they know to thoroughly remove an old application of glyceryl trinitrate ointment before applying a new dose.
- Make sure the patient knows how to choose an appropriate application site, and tell them to avoid scarred or callused areas, bony prominences and hairy surfaces.
- Warn them not to get transdermal ointment on their hands, and to wash them thoroughly after applying a transdermal medication.

Dry as a bone

- Make them aware that they need to keep the area around the application site as dry as possible.
- If the patient will be applying hyoscine, tell them not to drive or operate machinery until they know how the medication affects them.
- Warn the patient about the possible adverse reactions that can occur with transdermal medication delivery, such as skin irritation, itching and rashes.

Stay on the ball

A shocking experience

Don't place a defibrillator paddle on a transdermal patch. The aluminium on the patch can cause electrical arcing during defibrillation, resulting in smoke, thermal burns and, possibly, ineffective electrical cardioversion. If a patient's patch is on a standard paddle site, remove the patch before applying the paddle.

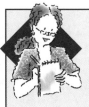

Take note!

Documenting transdermal medication administration

Be sure to record:

- date and time of a transdermal application
- medication used
- location of the ointment or patch on the patient's body
- effects of the medication
- patient teaching you provided.

– hyoscine most commonly causes a dry mouth and drowsiness.
– transdermal estradiol may increase the risk of endometrial cancer, thromboembolic disease and birth defects. (See *Documenting transdermal medication administration*.)

Administering ophthalmic medication

Typically, you'll give ophthalmic medication (diagnostic and therapeutic) in the form of drops or ointment. Sometimes, you'll need to apply a patch over a patient's eye after you instil an ophthalmic medication.

Instilling eye drops

Eye drops can be used for several diagnostic and therapeutic purposes, including:
- dilating the pupil
- staining the cornea to detect abrasions or scars
- anaesthetising the eye
- lubricating the eye
- protecting the vision of a neonate
- treating certain eye disorders, such as infections or glaucoma.

What you need
Patient's MAR ✳ prescribed eye drops ✳ gloves (as per local policy) ✳ warm sterile 0.9% sodium chloride for irrigation ✳ sterile gauze swabs ✳ facial tissues ✳ eye dressing (if necessary)

Getting ready
- Check the patient's MAR to make sure that it is legible, clear and correct and that the medication has not been given.
- Check the patient's allergies and gain consent.
- Before administering check: ✳ patient identity ✳ medication ✳ dosage ✳ time ✳ route.
- Confirm the patient's name, date of birth and hospital number against their identity band and MAR, or as per local policy.
- Read the label to make sure the medication is intended for ophthalmic use.

Seeing is believing
- Check the expiration date on the eye drop container and inspect the drops for cloudiness, discolouration and precipitates. If the solution appears abnormal in any way, don't use it.
- Keep in mind that some ophthalmic medication are in suspension form and normally appear cloudy. When in doubt, check with a pharmacist.

Not the same eye-dea
- Take extra care when checking a patient's MAR for eye drops because different medication or dosages may be ordered for each eye.

- Explain the procedure to the patient.
- Wash your hands and put on gloves (as per local policy).

How you do it
- If the patient has an eye dressing in place, remove it by gently pulling it down and away from the patient's forehead.

Careful clean up

- If the patient has discharge around the eye, moisten sterile gauze swabs with warm sterile 0.9% sodium chloride for irrigation.
- Wipe the eye gently to clean away debris, moving from the inner canthus to the outer canthus as shown. Use a fresh sterile gauze swab for each stroke.
- If the patient has crusted secretions around their eye, moisten a sterile gauze swab with warm 0.9% sodium chloride for irrigation. Then ask the patient to close their eye, and place the moist swab over their closed eye for 1 or 2 minutes.
- Remove the swab and reapply new moist sterile gauze swabs, as needed, until the secretions become soft enough that you can remove them without injuring the tender ocular tissues.

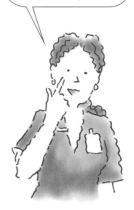

When removing discharge from around the eye, remember to wipe from the inner canthus to the outer canthus using a fresh, sterile gauze swab with each wipe.

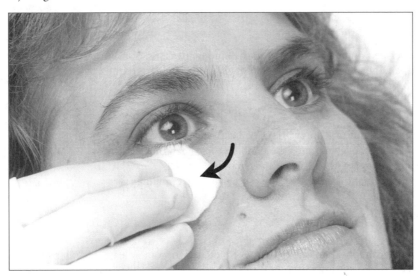

Full tilt

- To help minimise systemic reactions to eye drops, see *Minimising systemic reactions to eye drops*, page 160.
- Remove the dropper cap from the bottle (unless the bottle has a built-in dropper) and draw the eye drops into the dropper, taking care not to contaminate the dropper.
- Ask the patient to look up and away *to move the cornea away from the lower lid and minimise the risk of touching the cornea with the dropper if the patient blinks*.

• Steady the hand holding the dropper or eye drop bottle by resting it against the patient's forehead. Use your other hand to gently pull down the patient's lower eyelid as shown.

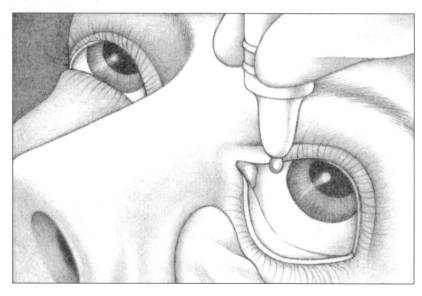

• Instil the prescribed number of drops into the conjunctival sac, not onto the patient's eyeball. Then release the patient's eyelid and ask them to blink to distribute the drops throughout their eye.

Practice pointers

• If you're opening a multiple-application medication container for the first time, write the date on the label. Once the container has been opened, the medication should be used within 1 week and then discarded.
• To prevent contamination, never use the same eye drop container for more than one patient.

Worth the wait

• If the patient needs more than one type of eye medication, wait at least 5 minutes between administering different doses.
• Teach the patient the correct procedure for instilling eye drops at home, if prescribed. (See *Teaching about eye drops*.)
• For tips on teaching an older patient, see *Managing eye drop non-sense*.

Administering ophthalmic ointment

An ointment formulation helps keep an ophthalmic medication in contact with the treatment area for as long as possible—an especially useful tactic for children. Usually, you'll use an antibiotic ointment to treat eye infections.

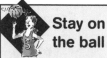

Stay on the ball

Minimising systemic reactions to eye drops

Systemic reactions to eye drops, such as tachycardia, palpitations, flushing, dry skin, ataxia and confusion, can be minimised by asking the patient to press a finger over their tear duct at the inner canthus as you instil the drops. This action compresses the nasolacrimal tear ducts, thus preventing the drops from draining out of their eye.

In addition, ask your patient to tilt their head back and towards the side of the affected eye to ensure that the drops will flow away from the tear duct at the inner canthus. If you'll be placing drops in their left eye, ask your patient to tilt to the left, to the right if you'll be placing drops in their right eye. By tilting their head, the patient will reduce the chance that the drops will drain into the tear duct and cause systemic effects.

Teacher's lounge

Teaching about eye drops

- Explain why the doctor prescribed the eye drops.
- Stress the importance of proper hand-washing technique.
- Teach the patient to make sure they have the right medication, the correct number of drops and the correct eye.
- Tell them that they can warm the drops to room temperature by holding the bottle between their hands for about 2 minutes.
- If the patient is using more than one kind of drop, tell them to wait 5 minutes between administering them.
- Teach them to protect the container from light and heat.

- Teach them the potential adverse effects of the medication and when they should notify the doctor.
- Stress the importance of never placing any medication in their eyes unless the label reads 'For Ophthalmic Use' or 'For Use in Eyes'.
- If your patient can see through the eye drop container, teach them to hold it up to the light and look at it. If the liquid is discoloured or if it contains sediment, tell them not to use it but to take the container back to the pharmacy and have it checked.
- Provide the patient with written instructions so they can review the proper administration steps after they get home.

Memory jogger

When instilling eye drops, remember *up, up and away*—ask the patient to look up and away from you.

What you need

Patient's MAR ✳ prescribed eye ointment ✳ gloves (as per local policy) ✳ warm 0.9% sodium chloride for irrigation ✳ sterile gauze swabs ✳ facial tissues ✳ eye dressing (if necessary)

Getting ready

- Check the patient's MAR to make sure that it is legible, clear and correct and that the medication has not been given.
- Check the patient's allergies and gain consent.
- Before administering check: ✳ patient identity ✳ medication ✳ dosage ✳ time ✳ route.
- Read the label to make sure the medication is intended for ophthalmic use.
- Double-check the patient's MAR when administering ophthalmic ointment because different medication or dosages may be ordered for each eye.
- Confirm the patient's name, date of birth and hospital number against their identity band and MAR, or as per local policy.
- Explain the procedure to the patient.
- Wash your hands and put on gloves (as per local policy).

Ages and stages

Managing eye drop non-sense

If your patient is an older adult, they may have trouble sensing whether a drop has gone into their eye. If so, suggest that they chill their eye drops before using them. Most people find it easier to feel a drop entering the eye when the drop is cold.

How you do it

- If the patient has an eye dressing in place, remove it by gently pulling it down and away from their forehead.
- If they have discharge around their eye, moisten sterile gauze swabs with warm 0.9% sodium chloride for irrigation.
- Gently wipe the eye to clean away debris, moving from the inner canthus to the outer canthus. Use a fresh sterile gauze swab for each stroke.
- If the patient has crusted secretions around their eye, moisten a sterile gauze swab with 0.9% sodium chloride for irrigation. Ask the patient to close their eye, then place the moist swab over it for 1 or 2 minutes.
- Remove the pad and reapply new moist sterile gauze swabs, as needed, until the secretions are soft enough to be removed without injuring the tissue.

Conquering crust

- If the tip of the ointment tube has crusted, wipe it with a sterile gauze swab to remove the crust.
- Ask the patient to look up and away *to move the cornea away from the lower lid and minimise the risk of touching the cornea with the tip of the ointment tube if the patient blinks.*
- Steady the hand holding the ointment tube against the patient's forehead. Use your other hand to gently pull down their lower eyelid.

Avoiding eye contact

- Squeeze a small ribbon of ointment along the edge of the conjunctival sac from the inner to the outer canthus as shown. Don't let the tip of the tube touch the patient's eye. (If it does, discard the tube.)

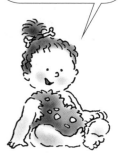

You might want to consider an ophthalmic ointment for someone young like me—chances are, it will stay in place a little longer than eye drops will.

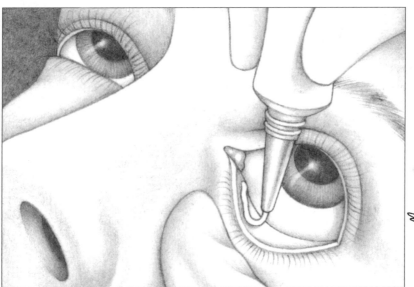

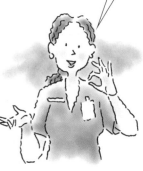

Remember, a little dab will do...but avoid touching the tube against the patient's eye.

• Cut off the ribbon of ointment by turning the tube. Then release the patient's eyelid and ask the patient to roll their eyes behind closed lids *to help distribute the medication.*

• Use a clean tissue to remove excess ointment that leaks from the patient's eye. Use a fresh tissue for each eye *to prevent cross-contamination.*

• Lastly, apply a new eye dressing, if indicated.

Practice pointers

• If you're opening the medication container for the first time, write the date on the label. When the container has been opened, the medication should be used within 1 week and discarded.

An ounce of prevention

• To prevent contamination, never use the same medication container for more than one patient.

• Systemic reactions are unlikely with ophthalmic ointments because they don't empty quickly into the lacrimal duct, as eye drops do.

• Carefully document the procedure. (See *Documenting ophthalmic medication administration.*)

• Teach the patient how to apply ophthalmic ointment for home use, if prescribed. (See *Teaching about ophthalmic ointment.*)

Take note!

Documenting ophthalmic medication administration

After administering an ophthalmic medication, be sure to record:

• eye treated
• date and time
• prescribed medication
• dose administered
• patient's response to the instillation procedure (Note the appearance of the patient's eye before and after they receive eye drops.)
• patient or family teaching you provided.

Teacher's lounge

Teaching about ophthalmic ointment

• Explain why the doctor prescribed the ointment, and review the proper steps for using the ointment at home.
• Tell the patient to wash their hands before and after applying eye ointment. Be sure to warn them not to contaminate the lid of the ointment tube or touch the tip of the tube to their eye or to the skin around their eye.
• Tell the patient to apply ointment from the inner to the outer corner of their eye. Let them know that their vision may be blurry for several minutes after they put the ointment in their eye.

Administering medication to the ear

Medication may be instilled to:
- treat infections and inflammation
- soften cerumen (earwax) for later removal
- produce local anaesthesia
- aid removal of a foreign object trapped in the ear.

Instilling ear drops

You probably won't administer ear drops to a patient with a perforated eardrum (although it may be permitted with certain medications and with sterile technique). Certain ear drops may be prohibited in other conditions as well, for example, hydrocortisone is contraindicated if the patient has a viral or fungal infection.

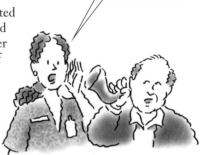

I said, the doctor thinks ear drops might help soften your earwax a little so that maybe we can loosen the horn that's attached to your ear!

What you need
Patient's MAR ✳ prescribed ear drops ✳ pen torch ✳ facial tissues (or cotton-tipped applicators) ✳ cotton balls ✳ container for warm water ✳ non-sterile gloves (as per local policy)

Getting ready
- Check the patient's MAR to make sure that it is legible, clear and correct and that the medication has not been given.
- Check the patient's allergies and gain consent.
- Before administering check: ✳ patient identity ✳ medication ✳ dosage ✳ time ✳ route.
- To avoid adverse reactions caused by the instillation of cold ear drops (such as vertigo, nausea and pain), warm the drops to body temperature by placing the container in a basin of warm water.

Now hear this

- Don't make the drops too hot; if necessary; test their temperature by placing a drop on your wrist.
- Confirm the patient's name, date of birth and hospital number against their identity band and MAR, or as per local policy.
- Wash your hands and put on gloves (as per local policy).
- Explain the procedure to the patient.

How you do it
- Ask the patient to lie on their side with their affected ear facing up.
- Straighten the patient's ear canal. (See *Positioning a patient for ear drops*.)

Ages and stages

Positioning a patient for ear drops

Before you instil ear drops, ask the patient to lie on their side. Then straighten the patient's ear canal to help the drops reach the eardrum. In an adult, gently pull the pinna *up* and *back*; in an infant or young child, gently pull *down* and *back* as shown.

Adult

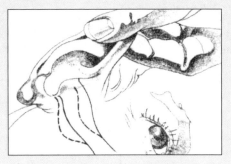

Child

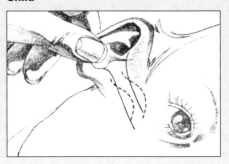

Light the way

- Using a pen torch, examine the ear canal for drainage. If you find any, clean the canal with a tissue or cotton-tipped applicator because drainage can reduce the effectiveness of the medication.
- Straighten the patient's ear canal once again and instil the prescribed number of drops. To avoid patient discomfort, aim the dropper so the drops fall against the side of the ear canal, not on the eardrum.

Disappearing act

- Hold the ear canal in position until you see the medication disappear down the canal. Then release the ear.
- Tell the patient to stay on their side for 5 to 10 minutes to allow the medication to travel down the ear canal.
- If advised by the pharmacist, tuck a cotton ball loosely into the opening of the ear canal. Don't push it too far into the ear, however, because you'll keep secretions from draining and increase pressure on the eardrum.
- Clean and dry the outer ear.
- Help the patient into a comfortable position.
- Remove your gloves (if worn) and wash your hands.

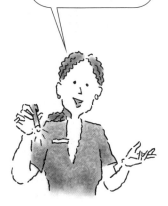

Don't know where I'd be without my trusty pentorch. (In the dark, that's for sure!)

Ages and stages

Tips for tots

When teaching parents how to administer ear drops to their child, make sure you include this helpful information:

- Warm the drops for their child's comfort by holding the bottle in their hands for about 2 minutes.
- Gently pull the earlobe down and back to straighten the child's ear canal.
- If necessary and it is safe to do so, to keep the medication from running out of the ear, place a cotton ball moistened with the medication at the very entrance to the ear canal. Remove the cotton after 1 hour. Avoid using dry cotton because it may absorb the medication.

Practice pointers

- Some conditions make the normally sensitive ear canal quite tender, so be especially gentle when instilling ear drops. (See *Tips for tots*.)
- Take special care not to injure the eardrum. Never insert any object, even a cotton-tipped applicator, so far into the ear canal that you can't see its tip.
- If the patient has vertigo, keep the side rails of his bed up and assist him as necessary. Also, move slowly to avoid aggravating his vertigo.
- Carefully document the procedure. (See *Documenting administration of ear drops*.)
- Teach the patient how to instil ear drops if they have been prescribed for home use. (See *Teaching about ear drops*.)

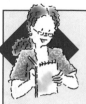

Take note!

Documenting administration of ear drops

After administering ear drops, be sure to record:

- ear treated
- name of the medication instilled
- date and time you instilled it
- dose given, and the patient's response to the instillation procedure
- appearance of the patient's ears before and after instilling ear drops
- teaching aids given to the patient or family.

Teacher's lounge

Teaching about ear drops

- Remind the patient never to insert any object into their ear.
- Review the importance of washing their hands thoroughly.
- Make sure they know how many drops to give and into which ear.
- Teach them not to use the medication and to contact their pharmacist if the liquid looks discoloured or contains sediment.
- Provide written guidelines to parents who will be administering ear drops to a child at home.

Administering nasal medication

For the most part, nasal medication produce local effects.

Instilling nose drops

You'll use drops to treat a specific nasal area and sprays and aerosols to diffuse the medication through the nasal passages.

The nose knows

The most commonly administered nasal medication are:
- vasoconstrictors, which coat and shrink swollen mucous membranes
- local anaesthetics, which promote patient comfort during such procedures as bronchoscopy
- corticosteroids, which reduce inflammation caused by allergies or nasal polyps.

What you need
Patient's MAR ✳ prescribed nasal medication ✳ gloves (as per local policy)

Getting ready
- Check the patient's MAR to make sure that it is legible, clear and correct and that the medication has not been given.
- Check the patient's allergies and gain consent.
- Before administering check: ✳ patient identity ✳ medication ✳ dosage ✳ time ✳ route.
- Confirm the patient's name, date of birth and hospital number against their identity band and MAR, or as per local policy.
- Explain the procedure to the patient and position them as needed to make sure the drops reach the intended site. This is usually done by hyper-extending the patient's neck, unless clinically contraindicated.

How you do it
- Ask the patient to blow their nose.
- Push up gently on the tip of the patient's nose to open his nostrils completely.
- Place the dropper about 1 cm inside his nostril. Angle the tip of the dropper slightly towards the inner corner of the patient's eye. Squeeze the dropper bulb to dispense the correct number of drops into each nostril.
- After you've instilled the prescribed number of drops, instruct the patient to keep their head tilted back for about 5 minutes. Encourage them to expectorate any medication that runs into their throat.

Practice pointers
- Stay with the patient after administering nose drops. Urge them to breathe through their mouth. If they cough, help them to sit up. For several minutes, observe them closely for possible respiratory problems.

Administering rectal medication

You may administer a medication rectally to a patient who's unconscious, vomiting or unable to swallow or take anything by mouth. Rectally administered medication can produce either local or systemic effects. The most commonly used forms of rectal medication include:
- suppositories
- medicated enemas.

Dodging digestion and bypassing biotransformation

Because rectal administration bypasses the upper GI tract, digestive enzymes in the stomach or small intestine don't destroy medication given by this method. Also, these medications don't irritate the upper GI tract, as some oral medication can. In addition, rectal medication bypasses the portal system, thus avoiding biotransformation in the liver. Biotransformation or medication metabolism refers to the body's ability to change a medication from its dosage form to a more water-soluble form that can be excreted. Once in the liver, enzymes metabolise medication.

Rectal medication downsides

Rectal medication does have some disadvantages, however. The administration procedure may cause discomfort or embarrassment to the patient. Also, the medication may be incompletely absorbed, especially if the patient can't retain it or if their rectum contains faeces. As a result, the patient may need a higher dose than if they had taken the same medication in oral form.

> It isn't that I have anything against you personally... it's this whole biotransformation thing we're trying to avoid.

Administering rectal suppositories

A suppository is a firm, bullet-shaped object made from a substance that melts at body temperature (such as cocoa butter). As the suppository melts, it releases the medication into the patient's rectum, where it can be absorbed across the rectal mucosa. Most suppositories are about 4 cm long (or smaller for infants and children).

Rectal suppositories commonly contain medication that reduce fever, induce relaxation, stimulate peristalsis and defecation, or relieve pain, vomiting and local irritation.

What you need

Patient's MAR ✳ prescribed rectal medication ✳ gloves ✳ absorbent pad ✳ water-soluble lubricant ✳ bedpan (if necessary)

Getting ready
- Check the patient's MAR to make sure that it is legible, clear and correct and that the medication has not been given.
- Check the patient's allergies and gain consent.
- Before administering check: ✳ patient identity ✳ medication ✳ dosage ✳ time ✳ route.
- Confirm the patient's name, date of birth and hospital number against their identity band and MAR, or as per local policy.
- Provide privacy.
- Explain the procedure to the patient and gain consent.

How you do it
- Place the patient on their left side (semi-prone with the right knee and thigh drawn up and the left arm along the patient's back). Cover them with the bedcovers, exposing only their buttocks.
- Place an absorbent pad under their buttocks *to protect the bedding.*
- Wash your hands and put on gloves.
- Remove the suppository from its wrapper, and apply a water-soluble lubricant to it.
- Using your non-dominant hand, lift the patient's upper buttock to expose their anus.

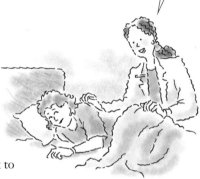

Try to have your patient lie quietly after a rectal suppository has been inserted to allow the drug time to take effect.

Take a deep breath and relax
- Tell the patient to take several deep breaths through their mouth *to relax the anal sphincter and reduce anxiety and discomfort during insertion.*

Insertion
- For information on administering a rectal suppository to a child, see *Using rectal suppositories in children.*

Ages and stages
Using rectal suppositories in children

Rectal administration via suppository may be a good alternative when the oral route can't be used, but remember that it's a less reliable method in children than in adults.

- A clear explanation needs to be given to the child and parent(s).
- Encourage the child to open their bowels first if the suppository is medicated.
- Insert the suppository fully into the rectum (using the tip of your little finger in infants).
- Infants can be laid on their back with their feet and legs held up to make insertion easier.
- Children with oncological conditions shouldn't be given medication rectally. They are prone to an increase of bacteria in the rectum and at risk of infection due to a lowered immune system.

Stay on the ball

Inserting a rectal suppository in an adult

When inserting a rectal suppository in an adult, use your index finger to direct the suppository along the rectal wall towards the patient's umbilicus, as shown, so the membrane can absorb the medication. Continue to advance it about 7.5 cm or about the length of your finger, until it passes the internal anal sphincter.

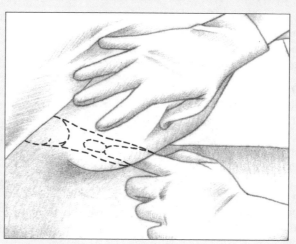

Stay on the ball

Contraindications for rectal suppositories

You'll want to avoid giving rectal suppositories to a patient who has:

- cardiac arrhythmias or has had a myocardial infarction because inserting a rectal suppository typically stimulates the vagus nerve
- undiagnosed abdominal pain because, if the pain stems from appendicitis, the peristalsis caused by rectal administration could rupture the appendix
- recently undergone colon, rectal or prostate surgery because rectal suppositories increase the risk of local trauma.

• Using your dominant hand, insert the end of the suppository into the patient's rectum. (See *Inserting a rectal suppository in an adult.*) There is conflicting information regarding which end of the suppository should be inserted first (tapered or blunt). The manufacturer's advice sheet should be followed unless your local policy indicates otherwise.

• Ensure the patient's comfort. Encourage them to lie quietly and, if applicable, to retain the suppository for an appropriate time. A suppository given to relieve constipation should be retained as long as possible (at least 20 minutes) for it to be effective.

• If the patient can't retain the suppository, place the patient on a bedpan.

Practice pointers

• Store rectal suppositories in the refrigerator, as indicated, to keep them firm and to maintain the medication's effectiveness.

• Before administering rectal medication, inspect the patient's anus. If the tissues are inflamed or if haemorrhoids are present, withhold the suppository and notify a doctor. The medication could aggravate the condition.

• To minimise the risk of local trauma, you may need to avoid this route if the patient has had recent rectal, colon or prostate surgery.

• Rectal suppositories are contraindicated in certain patients. (See *Contraindications for rectal suppositories.*)

Administering medicated enemas

When you give an enema, you instil fluid into a patient's rectum for a variable amount of time. If you're preparing the patient for a diagnostic or surgical procedure or if you're giving the enema to relieve constipation, you may perform an evacuant enema.

Cleaning crew

A evacuant enema is a procedure that involves instilling unmedicated fluid into a patient's rectum simply to clean the patient's rectum and colon. The patient expels the irrigant almost completely within about 15 minutes. (See Chapter 20 for administering evacuant enemas.) Enemas are not frequently used for children unless absolutely necessary, when other routes of medication have been tried.

Pay attention . . . the topic is retention

Enemas can also be used to deliver medication, which acidify the colon contents and lower blood ammonia levels. To deliver a medication, you'll probably give a retention enema. A retention enema is a type of enema that requires the patient to retain the fluid in his rectum and colon for 30 to 60 minutes, if possible, before expelling it. A retention enema can also be used as an emollient to soothe irritated colon tissues. *Aminosalicylates* (such as mesalazine) and *corticosteroids* (such as prednisolone) can be given as a retention enema in the treatment of inflammatory bowel disease (ulcerative colitis and crohns). They can also be administered as a foam enema via a canister with disposable applicators. You need to follow manufacturers' instructions for administering these.

Enema enemies

Enemas stimulate peristalsis by distending the colon and stimulating nerves in the rectal walls. Consequently, you shouldn't give an enema to a patient who has had:
• recent colon or rectal surgery
• myocardial infarction
• undiagnosed abdominal pain, which could be caused by appendicitis. (Giving an enema to a patient with appendicitis can irritate the inflamed area of the appendix and precipitate perforation.)

Most important, give an enema cautiously to any patient who has cardiac arrhythmias because inserting anything into the rectum stimulates the vagus nerve and could cause an increase in the cardiac arrhythmias.

Administering vaginal medication

Vaginal medication is available in many forms, including:

- suppositories
- creams
- gels
- ointments
- solutions.

These medicated preparations can be inserted to treat infection (particularly *Trichomonas vaginalis* and candidiasis), treat inflammation or prevent conception. Vaginal administration is most effective when the patient can remain lying down afterwards to retain the medication.

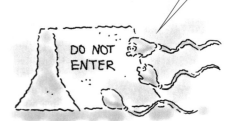

We were wrong fellas... the drug wasn't for a yeast infection this time. Maybe we should wait a week, then try again.

Giving a vaginal medication

Most vaginal medication come packaged in or with an applicator that you or the patient can use to insert the medication into the anterior and posterior fornices. When in contact with the vaginal mucosa, suppositories melt, diffusing the medication as effectively as creams, gels, and ointments.

What you need

Patient's MAR ✳ prescribed vaginal medication (with an applicator, if necessary) ✳ gloves ✳ water-soluble lubricant ✳ small sanitary pad ✳ absorbent towel ✳ absorbent pad ✳ cotton balls ✳ gauze pad ✳ paper towel ✳ soap and water (if necessary)

Getting ready

- Check the patient's MAR to make sure that it is legible, clear and correct and that the medication has not been given.
- Check the patient's allergies.
- Before administering check: ✳ patient identity ✳ medication ✳ dosage ✳ time ✳ route.
- Provide privacy.
- Explain the procedure to the patient and gain consent.
- If possible, plan to give the medication at bedtime, when the patient is recumbent.
- Confirm the patient's name, date of birth and hospital number against their identity band and MAR, or as per local policy.
- Ask the patient to empty her bladder.

Self-administration is an option

- Ask the patient whether she would rather insert the medication herself. If so, provide appropriate instructions.

How you do it

- If the patient decides not to self-administer, help her into the lithotomy position (knees drawn up and legs parted).
- Place an absorbent pad under her buttocks and cover her legs. Expose only her perineum.
- Wash your hands and put on gloves.
- Squeeze a small portion of water-soluble lubricant onto a gauze pad.

Package deal

- Unwrap the pessary, and coat it with the lubricant. If the medication is a small pessary in a pre-packaged applicator, lubricate the tip of the suppository with water-soluble lubricant. If the medication is a foam or gel, fill the applicator as prescribed, and lubricate the tip of the applicator with the water-soluble lubricant.
- Separate the patient's labia.

Examination before administration

- Examine the patient's perineum. If you find that it's excoriated, withhold the medication and notify a doctor. The patient may need a different type of medication.
- If you see discharge, wash the area.
- To wash the area, soak several cotton balls in warm, soapy water.
- While holding the labia open with one hand, wipe once down the left side of the patient's perineum with a cotton ball.
- Discard the cotton ball, pick up another one, and use the new cotton ball to wipe once down the right side of the perineum.
- Discard the cotton ball, pick up another one, and use it to wipe once down the middle of the patient's perineum.

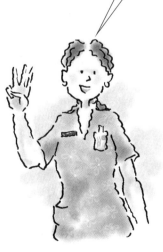

You'll need at least three cotton balls to clean your patient's perineum, so you'd better have a supply on hand.

Rounded tip first

- With the patient's labia still separated, insert the rounded tip of a pessary into her vagina, advancing it 7.5 to 10 cm along the posterior wall of the vagina, or as far as it will go.
- If you're using an applicator, insert it into the patient's vagina. (See *How to administer a vaginal medication using an applicator*, page 174.)

Time to lie down

- Tell the patient to lie down for 5 to 10 minutes with her knees flexed *to help promote absorption and allow the medication to flow into the posterior fornix.* If you inserted a pessary, tell her to remain recumbent for at least 30 minutes *to allow time for it to melt.*
- Place a small sanitary pad in the patient's underwear *to keep her clothes or bedding from becoming soiled.*

How to administer a vaginal medication using an applicator

If you're using an applicator to administer a vaginal medication to your patient, follow these steps:

- Use your dominant hand to insert the applicator about 5 cm into the patient's vagina. Direct the applicator down initially, towards the patient's spine, and then back up towards the cervix, as shown.
- Press the plunger until you empty all of the medication from the applicator.
- Remove the applicator, and place it on a paper towel to prevent the spread of micro-organisms.
- Discard the applicator as appropriate.

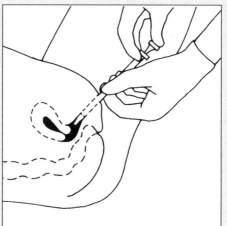

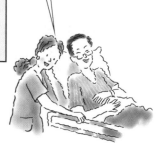

Ladies, take it from me, vaginally inserted medications are best absorbed lying down.

Practice pointers
- Refrigerate vaginal gels, foams and suppositories that melt at room temperature.

Administering respiratory medication

Several devices and procedures can be used to produce a fine, medication-carrying mist that a patient can inhale deep into his lungs.

Quick route to the capillaries

When the medication enters the lungs, it moves almost immediately into the lining of the patient's bronchi or alveoli and then into the adjacent capillaries. Medication is administered in this way because the inhaled route is the most effective method to get the medicine where it's supposed to go, directly to the airways. In addition, the total dose is low and there's little chance for systemic effect.

A breath of fresh air

To deliver medication to the respiratory tract, you'll typically use some type of handheld inhaler (sometimes with special attachments that are holding chambers called *spacers*) or a nebuliser.

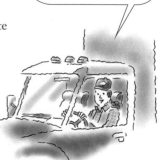

I always travel the quick and easy respiratory route to deliver drugs directly to the lungs.

Using a metered-dose inhaler

Many inhalant medication, such as bronchodilators (which help to open the bronchial airways of the lungs) and corticosteroids (used as effective anti-inflammatory agents), are available in small canisters that are inserted into a metered-dose inhaler, also known as a *puffer*. A metered-dose inhaler is a device that can be used to trigger the release of measured doses of aerosol medication from a canister. The patient can then inhale the fine mist deep into their lungs.

What you need

Patient's MAR ✳ metered-dose inhaler device ✳ prescribed medication

Getting ready

• Check the patient's MAR to make sure that it is legible, clear and correct and that the medication has not been given.
• Check the patient's allergies.
• Before administering check: ✳ patient identity ✳ medication ✳ dosage ✳ time ✳ route.
• Explain the procedure to the patient and gain consent.
• Confirm the patient's name, date of birth and hospital number against their identity band and MAR, or as per local policy.
• Place the patient in a comfortable sitting position.

How you do it

• Shake the inhaler canister well.
• Remove the cap from the canister, turn the canister upside down and insert the stem of the canister into the small hole in the flattened portion of the mouthpiece as shown.

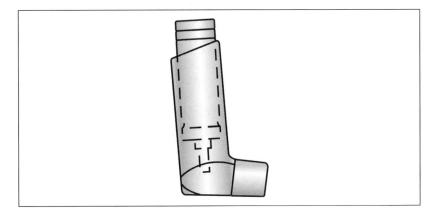

• Ask the patient to exhale, then hold the inhaler about 2.5 cm in front of their open mouth (two to three finger-widths from their mouth).
• Tell the patient to inhale slowly through their mouth and to continue inhaling until their lungs feel full.

Once is enough

• As they begin to inhale, compress the medication canister into the plastic housing of the inhaler to release a metered dose of the medication. Do this only once.

Whistle while you work

• Tell the patient to hold their breath for 10 seconds or as long as they can. Then instruct them to exhale slowly through pursed lips, as though whistling. Doing so produces backpressure, which helps to keep his bronchioles open, thus increasing absorption and diffusion of the medication.

Practice pointers

• If the patient can't co-ordinate well enough to inhale the medication as soon as you discharge it, you may need to put a spacer device on the inhaler.
• Some inhaled bronchodilators may cause restlessness, palpitations, nervousness and hypersensitivity reactions, such as rash, urticaria and bronchospasm.

Horse sense

• If the patient takes an inhaled corticosteroid, watch for evidence of hoarseness or fungal infection in his mouth or throat.
• To give inhaled medication to children, see *Giving inhaled medication to children*.
• Ask the patient to rinse their mouth and gargle with water to remove the medication from their mouth and the back of their throat. This step helps to prevent oral fungal infections. Warn them not to swallow after gargling, but rather to spit out the liquid.
• Instruct the patient to call their doctor (if the patient is at home) if their shortness of breath worsens, the medication becomes less effective or they develop palpitations, nervousness or hypersensitivity reactions such as a rash.
• If the patient takes a bronchodilator and a corticosteroid by inhaler, administer the bronchodilator 5 minutes before the corticosteroid. That way, their bronchial tubes will be as open as possible when they take the corticosteroid.
• Have the patient wait at least 1 minute between doses of a single inhaled medication.

Identification, please!

• If the patient takes an inhaled corticosteroid, urge them to carry medical identification announcing that they may need supplemental corticosteroids during stress or a severe asthma attack.

Ages and stages

Giving inhaled medication to children

When giving inhaled medication to children, remember these tips:

• If you need to give an inhaled medication to an infant or young child, have a parent or assistant hold the child to gain his co-operation.
• Children under 5 years with chronic stable asthma and bronchodilator therapy should be given corticosteroids and bronchodilator therapy via a pressurised metered dose inhaler (pMDI) and spacer system (NICE, 2000).

Preparing an injection

The ability to inject medication into a patient's subcutaneous tissue or muscle is a key nursing skill that you must exercise with great accuracy and care.

Quick and potent

These routes of administration promote a rapid onset of medication action and high medication levels in a patient's blood, in part because they sidestep the breakdown that can take place in the GI tract and liver.

It calls for preparation

To prepare for an injection, you need to know how to correctly choose a needle and withdraw liquid medication from a vial or ampoule. Then you'll need to administer the injection to the appropriate site using proper techniques.

After administering the injection, don't resheath the needle. Dispose of the syringe in the nearest sharps container.

Start at the very beginning

Typically, unless you're using one of the special needleless injection systems described later in this chapter, the first step in preparing for an injection is to choose the proper syringe and needle. Consider the route of administration, the size of the patient and the most likely injection site when you select a syringe and needle. (See *Selecting syringes and needles*, page 178.) Next, you'll need to withdraw the medication from its vial or ampoule into a syringe.

Withdrawing a medication from a vial

Withdrawing a medication from a vial may require you to perform two steps:

 reconstitution

 withdrawal.

What you need
Patient's MAR ✳ medication vial ✳ ampoule of an appropriate diluent ✳ alcohol wipes ✳ syringe ✳ two needles of appropriate size ✳ filter needle (if indicated, to screen particles that may be created during reconstitution) ✳ clean reusable plastic tray ✳ disposable gloves ✳ sharps container ✳ ampoule snapper

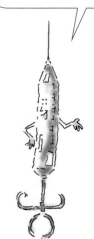

Being able to inject drugs into a patient's skin is a test of your nursing skill. It requires a great deal of accuracy and care—get my point?

Selecting syringes and needles

Success at giving injections greatly improves with your ability to choose the proper syringe and needle for the task.

Syringes

Illustrated here are four types of commonly used syringes, shown without the protection devices to prevent needle-stick injuries.

Standard syringe

The standard syringe is available in 1, 2, 3, 5, 10, 20, 30 and 50 ml sizes. It's used to administer numerous medication in various settings. It consists of a plunger, barrel, hub and needle. The dead space is the volume of fluid remaining in the syringe and needle when the plunger is depressed completely.

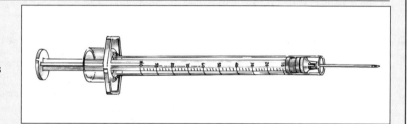

Plunger · Barrel · Hub · Needle · Dead space

Insulin syringe

The insulin syringe has an attached 25G needle and no dead space. It's divided into units rather than millilitres and should be used only for insulin administration.

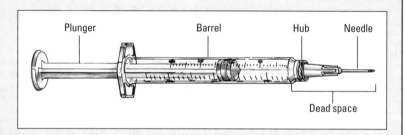

Pre-prepared syringe

The pre-prepared syringe is pre-filled with a measured medication dose in a ready-to-dispense syringe with a needle already attached. An example of this is a low molecular weight heparin.

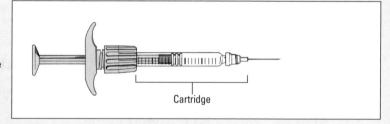

Cartridge

Needles

You'll choose different types of needles based on whether you're giving a subcutaneous or intramuscular (I.M.) injection. Needles come in various lengths and gauges (G); the higher the gauge the narrower the lumen of the needle. In the UK the needles are colour coded, depending upon the gauge.

Subcutaneous needle

For a subcutaneous injection, select a needle that's 10, 16 or 25 mm in length and 25G (orange needle).

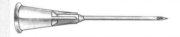

Selecting Syringes and needles (continued)

Intramuscular needle

For an I.M. injection, select a needle 38 mm in length and 21G (green needle), unless the patient doesn't have a large amount of body adipose, in which a needle 25 mm in length and 23G (blue needle) can be used.

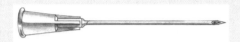

Shielded needle

To reduce the risk of needle-stick injury and the disease transmission that could result, a safety device built onto the syringe can be used to cover the needle when you're finished giving an injection, thus eliminating the temptation to resheath a used needle.

After you've completed an injection, simply grasp the syringe flanges with one hand and push the shield forward with the other hand until it clicks, as shown below. The shield is now locked firmly in place over the needle.

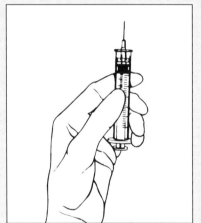
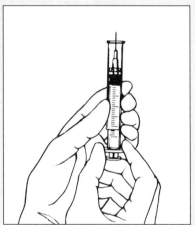
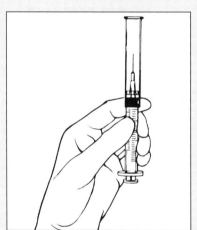

Getting ready
- Check the patient's MAR to make sure that it is legible, clear and correct, and that the medication has not been given and relates to the patient to be treated.
- Collect equipment.
- Check expiry dates, damage to vials and packaging.
- Calculate volume of medicine for injection to be given.
- Wash your hands.
- Put on disposable gloves.
- Clean tray with 70% alcohol wipe or spray.
- Using a 'non-touch' technique, assemble the syringe(s) and needle(s).

How you do it
• Tap the ampoule to dislodge diluent from neck (if glass).
• Snap open the top with an ampoule snapper (if glass) or twist the top off a plastic ampoule.
• Attach a needle to a syringe and draw up the volume required, tilting the ampoule to make it easier.
• Invert the syringe and tap gently to move bubbles to the needle end and then expel any air from the syringe.

Give it some space
• Inject the diluent into the powder-filled vial. Keep the tip of the needle above the solution and release the plunger on the syringe. The syringe will fill with air, which has been displaced by the solution.

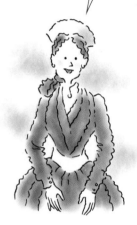

Knowing how to withdraw a drug from a vial is a fundamental procedure that every nurse must learn… it's as basic—and old a skill—as rolling bandages. Oh my, I'm dating myself, aren't I?

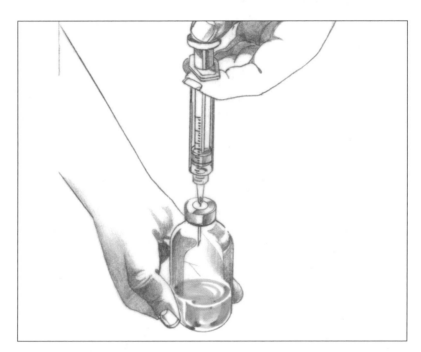

Shake and roll
• Keep the needle and syringe in the vial and gently swirl the vial until the powder has dissolved.

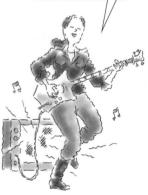

'I said shake, rattle, and roll'… your vial, that is.

Pump up the volume

- Keep the needle in the solution; depress the plunger, pushing the air from the syringe back into the vial.
- Release the plunger and the fluid will flow back into the syringe.

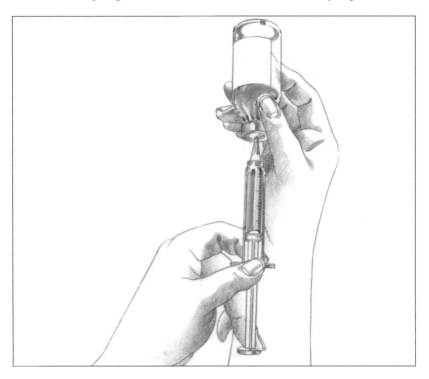

New needle needed

- Remove the needle from the syringe, and replace it with a new sterile needle. *You should do so because puncturing a rubber diaphragm can blunt a needle and increase the pain of injection, and also because medication stuck to the outside of the used needle could irritate the patient's tissues.*
- If more than one injection is to be given at the same time, label the medication-filled syringes to finish preparing it for administration (NPSA, 2007).

Practice pointers

- When inserting a needle through a rubber diaphragm, hold the needle bevel up and exert slight lateral pressure as the needle goes through the diaphragm. By using this technique, you'll avoid cutting a piece of rubber out of the stopper and pushing it into the medication in the vial.

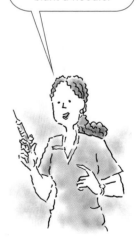

Be sure to replace the needle with a new one after withdrawing a drug from a vial. Puncturing the rubber stopper can blunt a needle.

Withdrawing a medication from an ampoule

You may be required to withdraw a medication from an ampoule.

What you need

Patient's MAR ✳ cleaned reusable plastic tray ✳ medication ampoule ✳ syringe ✳ filter needle ✳ needle for injecting the medication ✳ ampoule snapper or dry gauze pad ✳ sharps container

Getting ready

• Check the patient's MAR to make sure that it is legible, clear and correct and that the medication has not been given.
• Wash your hands.

How you do it

• Check to make sure that all of the fluid is in the bottom of the ampoule. If you see fluid in the stem or the top of the ampoule, gently flick the stem *to knock the fluid out of the stem and into the bottom of the ampoule.*
• If flicking the stem doesn't force all of the fluid to the bottom of the ampoule, try holding the ampoule by the stem, raising it to about eye level, and then quickly and carefully swinging it downward at arm's length.

Bottom of the ampoule

• If there is an ampoule snapper available, use this to break the top off the ampoule to reduce harm.
• Otherwise use a piece of gauze. When all of the fluid is in the bottom of the ampoule, wrap it in a dry gauze pad *so the pad covers the ampoule's stem.*
• Hold the body of the ampoule with one hand and the top portion of the ampoule between the thumb and first two fingers of your other hand.

It's a snap!

• While pointing the ampoule away from you and others, snap off the top.
• With a filter needle (should be used where possible) on the syringe, aspirate the correct amount of medication from the open ampoule. The filter needle strains out small pieces of glass that might have fallen into the medication.

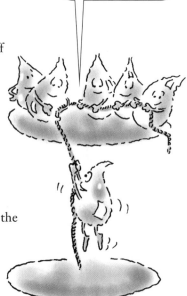

Guys, I can't hold on much longer. And watch out...if she tries that flick trick one more time, you'll all be goners, too!

New needle needed (again)

* Replace the filter needle with a fresh needle appropriate for injecting the medication. *Changing needles prevents medication on the outside of the filter needle from irritating the patient's tissues.*
* If more than one injection is being given at the same time (NPSA, 2007), label the medication-filled syringe *to finish preparing it for administration.*

Practice pointers

* An opened ampoule doesn't contain a vacuum, so you don't have to inject air as you do with a vial.

Administering intradermal medication

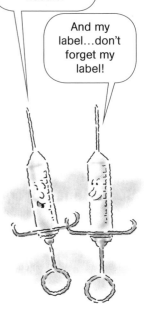

Don't forget to replace my needle.

And my label...don't forget my label!

In intradermal medication administration, a small amount of liquid (usually 0.5 ml or less) is injected into the outer layers of a patient's skin. A substance administered in this way undergoes little systemic absorption. Only registered nurses with specific training are allowed to administer intradermal injections. For this reason intradermal medication administration will not be covered in great depth in this chapter.

Identifying intradermal

The intradermal route is used to deliver substances that test for allergies and tuberculosis (TB). It may be used to deliver a local anaesthetic, before the patient undergoes an invasive procedure. Although the most common site for intradermal injection is the anterior (ventral) forearm, other sites can be used. (See *Intradermal injection sites.*)

One common use for intradermal injections is allergy testing. Now you may feel a bit itchy after this.

Intradermal injection sites

The most common intradermal injection site is the anterior (ventral) forearm. Other sites (indicated by dotted areas in these illustrations) include the upper chest, upper arm and shoulder blades. Skin in these areas is usually lightly pigmented, thinly keratinised and relatively hairless, facilitating detection of adverse reactions.

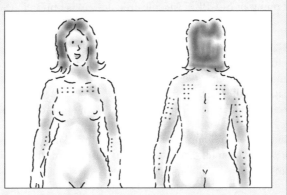

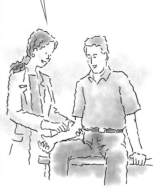

Administering subcutaneous medication

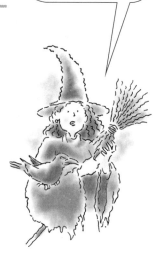

Anywhere but the wart on the tip of my nose, please!

In subcutaneous administration, you inject a small amount of liquid medication (usually 0.5 to 2 ml) into the subcutaneous tissue beneath the patient's skin. From there, the medication is absorbed slowly into nearby capillaries.

Steady and safe

As a result, a dose of concentrated medication can have a longer duration of action than it would by other injection routes. Plus, subcutaneous injection causes little tissue trauma and offers little risk of striking large blood vessels and nerves.

Subcutaneous contraindications

Typically, heparin and insulin are given by subcutaneous injection. However, a subcutaneous injection is contraindicated in areas that are inflamed, oedematous, scarred or covered by a mole, birthmark or other lesion. It may also be contraindicated in patients with impaired coagulation.

Giving a subcutaneous injection

You may be required to give a medication via the subcutaneous route, such as:
- heparin
- insulin
- ovulation-stimulating medication (or fertility medication).

What you need
Patient's MAR ✳ cleaned reusable plastic tray ✳ prepared medication (with an appropriate syringe) ✳ orange needle ✳ disposable gloves ✳ sharps container

For insulin administration
Insulin infusion pump or SQ-PEN (needle-free device) is optional. (See *Understanding insulin administration aids*)

Getting ready
- Check the patient's MAR to make sure that it is legible, clear and correct and that the medication has not been given.
- Check the patient's allergies.
- Before administering check: ✳ patient identity ✳ medication ✳ dosage ✳ time ✳ route.
- Check the medication's colour, clarity and expiration date.
- Confirm the patient's name, date of birth and hospital number against their identity band and MAR, or as per local policy.
- Explain the procedure to the patient and gain consent.
- Select an appropriate injection site. (See *Subcutaneous injection sites.*)

Understanding insulin administration aids

These days, patients have insulin delivery options beyond standard subcutaneous injections, such as subcutaneous insulin pump therapy or needle-free insulin delivery.

Subcutaneous infusion

Subcutaneous insulin pump therapy is also known as continuous subcutaneous insulin infusion (CSII). The patient carries a portable infusion pump that holds fast-acting insulin and is delivered subcutaneously at a continuous pre-set rate, according to the patient's blood glucose level. Bolus doses can also be administered if required, such as at mealtimes. This is ideal for those who need to improve their diabetes control and it will also help to reduce hypoglycaemia (a 'hypo') occurring. Due to the amount of hard work that is involved in using this therapy and the amount of motivation that is required, suitability for using this needs to be assessed on an individual basis. The National Institute for Health and Clinical Excellence (NICE) (2008) published guidance, which includes recommended criteria that an individual should meet

prior to using this form of insulin administration. This guidance is due to be reviewed by 2011.

To deliver the infusion, the patient will need either a 25G winged infusion set, a 24G cannula or as per local policy, inserted at a 45-degree angle into the abdomen, thigh or arm. The insertion site should be rotated every 2 to 3 days as you would with standard insulin injections. After needle insertion, cover the site with a transparent adhesive dressing. Teach the patient how to recognise and when to report possible problems with the device insertion site.

Needle-free insulin delivery (SQ-PEN)

The SQ-PEN is a device that delivers insulin without a needle. A spring inside the device triggers a plunger that expels a prescribed dose of insulin through a precision nozzle. When the patient holds the device against the skin surface and discharges it, a thin column of insulin penetrates the skin and disperses within the subcutaneous tissue. This device is popular for home use, especially by patients (including children) who are afraid of needles.

Subcutaneous injection sites

Potential subcutaneous injection sites (as indicated by the dotted areas in these illustrations) include the fat pads on the abdomen, upper hips, upper back and lateral upper arms and thighs.

Preferred injection sites for insulin are the arms, abdomen, thighs and buttocks. The preferred injection site for heparin is the lower abdominal fat pad, just below the umbilicus.

When you repeat, rotate

For subcutaneous injections administered repeatedly, such as insulin, rotate the injection sites. Choose one injection site in one area, move to a corresponding injection site in the next area and so on. When returning to an area, choose a new site in that area.

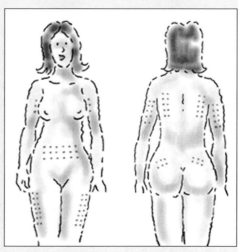

Give your patient the cold shoulder

- Before giving the injection, you may apply a cold compress to the injection site to minimise pain. (See *Ages and stages* for injecting children.)
- Wash your hands and put on disposable gloves.

How you do it
- Position and cover the patient, if necessary.

Bubble trouble

- If you're giving insulin, gently invert and roll the vial *to mix the medication*. Don't shake the vial *because air bubbles could get into the syringe and reduce the dose given*.
- Check your local policy regarding cleaning the skin with an alcohol swab. Alcohol swabs are used infrequently now unless the patient is immunocompromised. They harden the skin and can interfere with the action of subcutaneous insulin and heparin.
- Remove the protective needle sheath.

Hold the fat

- With your non-dominant hand, grasp the skin around the injection site and firmly elevate the subcutaneous tissue away from the underlying muscle. If the patient is large, you may be able to spread the skin taut rather than forming a fold. (See *Technique for subcutaneous injections*.)
- Position the needle with the bevel up, and tell the patient that they'll feel a prick as you insert it quickly—in one motion—at a 45-degree angle (90 degrees for pre-prepared low molecular heparin and insulin pens due to the shorter needle).

Try not to be irritating

- After injection, remove the needle gently but quickly at the same angle used for injection. However, when injecting heparin, leave the needle in place for 10 seconds; then withdraw it.
- Cover the injection site with a cotton ball or small piece of gauze.

Just checking

- Check the injection site for bleeding or bruising. If bleeding continues, apply pressure. If a bruise develops, apply ice. Watch for adverse reactions at the injection site for 30 minutes.
- Dispose of the equipment according to standard precautions. To avoid needle-stick injuries, don't recap the needle.

Technique for subcutaneous injections

Before giving a subcutaneous injection, elevate the subcutaneous tissue at the site by grasping it firmly, as shown. Insert the needle at a 45- or 90-degree angle to the skin surface, depending on needle length and the amount of subcutaneous tissue at the site. Some medications, such as heparin, should always be injected at a 90-degree angle.

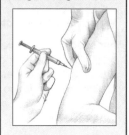

Ages and stages

Giving a child a subcutaneous injection

You may give certain medication to children by the subcutaneous route, for example insulin, heparin (post-operatively) or growth hormone injections. The procedure for subcutaneous injection differs little from that used for an adult patient. It is important that you explain the procedure to the child and parent to gain the co-operation of the child. It might be helpful to use a topical anaesthetic to reduce discomfort, especially if the injection is given regularly. Use the parent(s) or a play therapist to distract the child while the injection is being administered.

Practice pointers

Do a double take

- If you're giving insulin, double-check that you have the correct type, unit dose and syringe. Before mixing insulins in a syringe, make sure they're compatible and that it has been checked with the pharmacist. Follow your local policy about which insulin to draw up first. Don't mix insulins of different purities or origins.

Remember to rotate

- If you'll be giving repeated subcutaneous injections, as with insulin, rotate the injection sites.
- Don't administer heparin injections within 5 cm of a scar, a bruise or the umbilicus.
- Teach your patient the correct way to give a subcutaneous injection if they're on insulin or require other injections at home. (See *Teaching about subcutaneous injections*.)

Administering intramuscular medication

An I.M. injection deposits a medication deep into muscle tissue that's richly supplied with blood. As a result, the injected medication moves rapidly into the systemic circulation. Other advantages include:
- bypassing damaging digestive enzymes
- relatively little pain (because muscle tissue contains few sensory nerves)

Teacher's lounge

Teaching about subcutaneous injections

- If the patient will be giving themselves subcutaneous injections at home, teach them the correct way to perform the procedure. Send them home with written instructions to support your teaching.
- Inform the patient that different brands of syringes have differing amounts of space between the bottom line and the needle. Suggest that they tell the doctor or pharmacist if they change the brand of syringe they use.

- delivery of a relatively large volume of medication (the usual dose is 3 ml or less, but you may give up to 5 ml into a large muscle).

Be able to intradermal the candidate for I.M.

Children, elderly patients or thin people may tolerate less than 2 ml. For some medication, you may give I.M. injections using a Z-track technique or a needle-free injection system.

Giving an intramuscular injection

You may be required to inject medication intramuscularly, such as pain medications (opioids) or gold injections for arthritis.

Reflection before injection

Some situations will prevent I.M. administration of medication. (See *Precautions for intramuscular injections*.)

What you need

Patient's MAR ✳ prescribed medication ✳ cleaned reusable plastic tray ✳ 2 to 5 ml syringe ✳ 21G or 23G needle (lower gauge for a thicker medication) ✳ disposable gloves ✳ sharps container

Getting ready

- Check the patient's MAR to make sure that it is legible, clear and correct and that the medication has not been given.
- Check the patient's allergies.
- Before administering check: ✳ patient identity ✳ medication ✳ dosage ✳ time ✳ route.
- Wash your hands.
- Reconstitute the medication, if necessary; then check the medication's colour, clarity and expiration date.

Precautions for intramuscular injections

Before you give your patient an I.M. injection, remember these precautions:

- Don't give I.M. injections into inflamed, oedematous or irritated sites or sites with moles, birthmarks, scar tissue or other lesions.
- I.M. injections may be contraindicated in patients who have impaired coagulation or conditions that hinder peripheral absorption, such as peripheral vascular disease, oedema and hypo-perfusion, and during an acute myocardial infarction.
- Never give an I.M. injection into an immobile limb because the medication will absorb poorly and a sterile abscess could develop.

- Draw the correct amount into the syringe.
- Confirm the patient's name, date of birth and hospital number against their identity band and MAR, or as per local policy.
- Explain the procedure to the patient and gain consent.

Muscling up

- If your patient is an adult, consider using the dorsogluteal, ventrogluteal, vastus lateralis or deltoid muscle. (See *Locating intramuscular injection sites*.)
- If your patient is an infant or a child, consider using the vastus lateralis muscle. (See *intramuscular injection sites in infants and children*, page 191.)
- If your patient is elderly, additional points need to be considered. (See *Intramuscular injections in elderly patients*, page 192.)

How you do it

- Position and cover the patient so you have easy access to the chosen site. Locate the specific insertion site, and choose the proper needle angle.
- Check the injection site to make sure it has no lumps, depressions, redness, warmth or bruising.
- Put on disposable gloves.
- Remove the needle cover, and expel all air bubbles from the syringe.
- Urge the patient to relax the muscle that will receive the injection. A tense muscle increases pain and bleeding.
- With the thumb and index finger of your non-dominant hand, gently stretch the skin taut at the injection site.
- Position the syringe at a 90-degree angle to the skin surface, with the needle a few inches away from the skin.
- Tell the patient that they'll feel a prick, and then quickly thrust the needle into the muscle.

Seeing red? Stop!

There is limited evidence-based literature relating to injection technique. The Vaccination Administration Taskforce (VAT) (2001) reviewed the injection administration literature in depth and Malkin (2008) reviewed I.M. injection technique and discussed whether it is necessary to aspirate for blood before administering an I.M. injection.

Aspirating for blood

You should follow local policy regarding aspiration for blood before administering an intramuscular injection.
- While supporting the syringe with your non-dominant hand, use your dominant hand to aspirate for blood. If blood appears in the syringe, the needle is in a blood vessel. Withdraw it, discard it and prepare another injection with a new syringe and fresh medication.
- If you aspirate no blood, then inject the medication slowly and steadily into the muscle, allowing it to distend and accept the medication gradually. You should feel little or no resistance.

Locating intramuscular injection sites

The most common I.M. injection sites used in adults are discussed below.

Deltoid

Find the lower edge of the acromial process and the point on the lateral arm in line with the axilla. Insert the needle 2.5 to 5 cm below the acromial process, usually two or three finger-widths, at a 90-degree angle. A typical injection is 0.5 ml with a range of 0.5 to 2 ml.

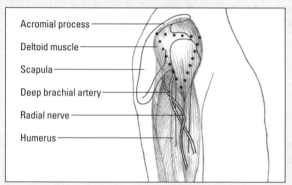

- Acromial process
- Deltoid muscle
- Scapula
- Deep brachial artery
- Radial nerve
- Humerus

Dorsogluteal

Inject above and outside a line drawn from the posterior superior iliac spine to the greater trochanter of the femur. Or, divide the buttock into quadrants, and inject in the upper outer quadrant, about 5 to 7.5 cm below the iliac crest. Insert the needle at a 90-degree angle. A typical injection is 1 to 4 ml with a range of 1 to 5 ml.

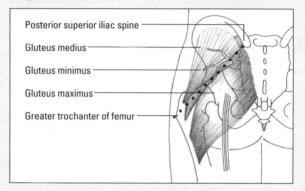

- Posterior superior iliac spine
- Gluteus medius
- Gluteus minimus
- Gluteus maximus
- Greater trochanter of femur

Ventrogluteal

Locate the greater trochanter of the femur with the heel of your hand. Then spread your index and middle fingers from the anterior superior iliac spine to as far along the iliac crest as you can reach. Insert the needle between the two fingers at a 90-degree angle to the muscle. (Remove your fingers before inserting the needle.) A typical injection is 1 to 4 ml with a range of 1 to 5 ml.

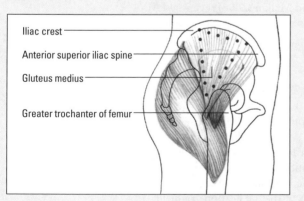

- Iliac crest
- Anterior superior iliac spine
- Gluteus medius
- Greater trochanter of femur

Vastus lateralis

Use the lateral muscle of the quadriceps group, from a handbreadth below the greater trochanter to a handbreadth above the knee. Insert the needle into the middle third of the muscle parallel to the surface on which the patient is lying. A typical injection is 1 to 4 ml with a range of 1 to 5 ml (1 to 3 ml for infants).

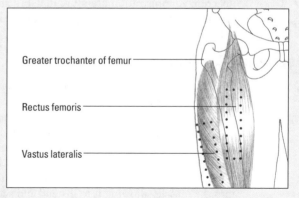

- Greater trochanter of femur
- Rectus femoris
- Vastus lateralis

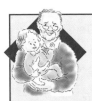

Ages and stages

I.M. injection sites in infants and children

When selecting the best site for a child's I.M. injection, consider the child's age, weight and muscular development; the amount of subcutaneous fat over the injection site; the type of medication you're administering and the medication's absorption rate. It is important to follow local policy when deciding which site to use.

Deltoid injections

This site is frequently used for vaccinations, but is inappropriate for repeated use and for young children.

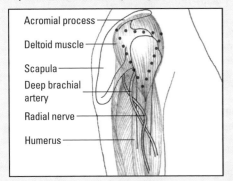

Acromial process
Deltoid muscle
Scapula
Deep brachial artery
Radial nerve
Humerus

Vastus lateralis injections

This site is commonly used for infants.

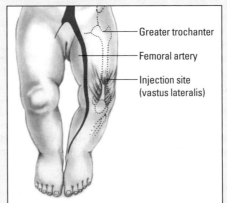

Greater trochanter
Femoral artery
Injection site (vastus lateralis)

Ventrogluteal injections

The ventrogluteal is appropriate for use in children and infants over 7 months, but is not a site commonly used.

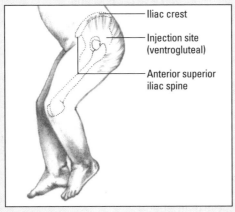

Iliac crest
Injection site (ventrogluteal)
Anterior superior iliac spine

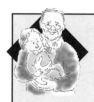

Ages and stages

Intramuscular injections in elderly patients

If your patient is elderly, consider using a shorter needle for I.M. injections. Also, because elderly people have less subcutaneous tissue and more fat around the hips, abdomen and thighs, consider using the vastus lateralis or ventrogluteal area.

Quickly yet gently

- After you've injected the medication, remove the needle quickly but gently, at a 90-degree angle.
- Apply gentle pressure and if necessary press with a cotton ball or small piece of gauze. Unless contraindicated, massage the relaxed muscle to help distribute the medication and promote absorption.

Inspection of injection

- Inspect the site for bleeding or bruising. If bleeding continues, apply pressure. If a bruise develops, apply ice. Watch for adverse reactions at the site for 30 minutes after the time of injection.
- Discard all equipment according to local policy.

Practice pointers

Continuous subcutaneous insulin infusion

- If your patient complains of pain and anxiety from repeated I.M. injections, numb the site with ice for several seconds before you give the injection.
- If you need to inject more than 5 ml of medication, split it between two different sites.

A pinch of gentleness

- If the patient is extremely thin, pinch the muscle gently to elevate it, so you won't push the needle completely through the muscle.
- Elderly patients have a higher risk of haematoma and may need direct pressure over the puncture site for a longer time than usual.

Rubbing it in

- Unless contraindicated, gently massage the injection site to aid medication absorption and distribution.
- Rotate sites if your patient needs repeated injections.
- Prevent complications associated with I.M. injections. (See *intramuscular injection complications*.)

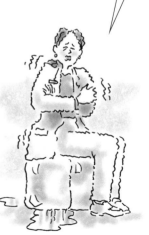

It may not be ideal, but it's one way to ice an injection site quickly.

Stay on the ball

Intramuscular injection complications

Accidentally injecting concentrated or irritating medications into subcutaneous tissue or other areas where they can't be fully absorbed can cause sterile abscesses to develop.

In addition, failing to rotate sites in patients who require repeated injections could lead to deposits of unabsorbed medications. Such deposits can reduce the desired pharmacological effect and may lead to abscess formation or tissue fibrosis.

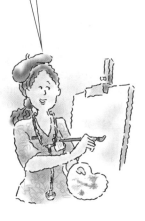

You may give zee I.M. injection another way if necessaire, n'est pas?

Giving a Z-track injection

If you need to give an irritating medication (such as iron dextran) or if you need to give an injection to an elderly patient with decreased muscle mass, use the Z-track method of I.M. administration. A Z-track injection is a method of displacing the tissues before you insert the needle for an I.M. injection. Afterward, restoring the tissues to their normal positions traps the medication inside the muscle.

How you do it
• Select an injection site appropriate for the medication to be administered.

Here's the skinny

• Place the index finger of your non-dominant hand on the injection site, and drag the skin about 1.5 cm to one side.
• Insert the needle at a 90-degree angle into the site on which you originally placed your finger.
• Inject the medication, and withdraw the needle.
• Then release the skin, allowing the displaced layers to return to their original positions. (See *Displacing the skin for Z-track injection*, page 194.)

Practice pointers
• Never inject more than 5 ml into a single site using the Z-track method.

Here's a new message: Don't massage!

• Never massage a Z-track injection site because you could cause irritation or force the medication into subcutaneous tissue.
• To increase the rate of absorption, encourage such physical activity as walking.
• For subsequent injections, alternate buttocks.

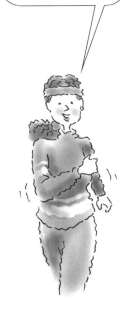

Walking is a good way to increase the rate of absorption after receiving a Z-track injection.

Displacing the skin for Z-track injection

Discomfort and tissue irritation may result from medication leakage into subcutaneous tissue. Displacing the skin helps prevent these problems.

By blocking the needle pathway after an injection, the Z-track technique allows I.M. injection while minimising the risk of subcutaneous irritation and staining from such medication as iron dextran.

How to do it

To begin, place your finger on the skin surface, and pull the skin and subcutaneous layers out of alignment with the underlying muscle, as shown below. You should move the skin about 1.5 cm.

Insert the needle at a 90-degree angle at the site where you initially placed your finger, as shown below. Inject the medication, and withdraw the needle.

Lastly, remove your finger from the skin surface, allowing the layers to return to their normal positions. The needle track (shown by the dotted line below) is now broken at the junction of each tissue layer, trapping the medication in the muscle.

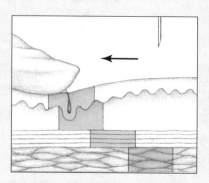
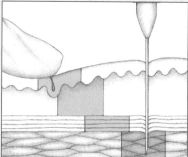
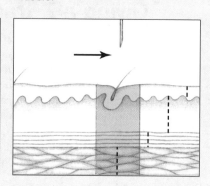

Quick quiz

1. When administering tablets or capsules by the oral route, you would:
    A. assess the patient's ability to swallow before administering the medication.
    B. give a medication that had been poured by someone else to save time.
    C. return any unused opened or unwrapped medication to the medicines trolley to avoid unnecessary waste.
    D. give a medication from a poorly labelled or an unlabeled bottle.

    Answer: A. Before administering tablets or capsules by the oral route, assess the patient's ability to swallow to prevent aspiration.

2. When instilling eye drops, instruct your patient to:
    A. look down and away.
    B. look up and away.

C. look straight ahead.
D. look up and directly at the dropper.

Answer: B. When instilling eye drops, ask your patient to look up and away. Doing so moves the cornea away from the lower lid and minimises the risk of touching the cornea with the dropper.

3. What position should your patient be in to administer an enema?
   A. on his left side with the right knee drawn up
   B. on his right side with the left knee drawn up
   C. on his left side with both legs straight
   D. on his right side with both legs straight

Answer: A. on his left side with right knee drawn up, to allow the fluid to flow easily into the rectum, following the patient's anatomy.

4. Which muscle would you choose to administer a maximum of 2 ml of medicine for injection?
   A. Deltoid
   B. Vastus lateralis
   C. Ventrogluteal
   D. Dorsogluteal

Answer: A. A typical injection into the deltoid muscle is 0.5 ml with a range of 0.5 to 2 ml.

5. Which statement *best* describes a Z-track injection?
   A. It's a method of depositing a medication deep into muscle tissue that's richly supplied with blood.
   B. It's a method of injecting a small amount of liquid medication (usually 0.5 to 2 ml) into the subcutaneous tissue beneath the patient's skin.
   C. It's a method of displacing the tissues before you insert the needle for an intramuscular injection.
   D. It's a method of aligning the tissues before you insert the needle for a subcutaneous injection.

Answer: C. A Z-track injection is a method of displacing the tissues before you insert the needle for an I.M. injection. Afterward, restoring the tissues to their normal positions traps the medication inside the muscle.

Scoring

★★★ If you answered all five questions correctly, sensational! Needle-less to say, you're in the top of your class!

★★ If you answered three or four questions correctly, great! You absorbed the material well.

★ If you answered fewer than three questions correctly, it looks like you might need a shot in the arm. Review the chapter, and you'll soon feel sharp!

11 I.V. therapy

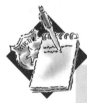

Just the facts

In this chapter, you'll learn:

♦ uses of I.V. therapy

♦ I.V. delivery methods

♦ I.V. infusion rates

♦ legal and professional standards governing the use of I.V. therapy

♦ patient teaching regarding I.V. therapy

♦ proper procedures for documenting I.V. therapy.

A look at I.V. therapy

One of your most important nursing responsibilities is to administer fluids, medications and blood products to patients. In I.V. therapy, liquid solutions are introduced directly into the bloodstream.

> Take care! Students must never administer or supply medicinal products without the direct supervision of a registered nurse (NMC, 2008).

I.V. therapy is used to:

- restore and maintain fluid and electrolyte balance
- provide medications and chemotherapeutic agents
- transfuse blood and blood products
- deliver parenteral nutrients and nutritional supplements.

Benefits of I.V. therapy

I.V. therapy has great benefits. For example, it can be used to administer fluids, drugs, nutrients and other solutions when a patient can't take oral substances.

On target and fast

I.V. drug delivery also allows more accurate dosing. Because the entire amount of a drug given I.V. reaches the bloodstream immediately, the drug begins to act almost instantaneously.

Risks of I.V. therapy

Like other invasive procedures, I.V. therapy has its downside. Risks include:
- bleeding
- blood vessel damage
- infiltration (infusion of the I.V. solution into surrounding tissue rather than the blood vessel)
- infection
- overdose (because response to I.V. drugs is more rapid)
- incompatibility when drugs and I.V. solutions are mixed
- adverse or allergic responses to infused substances.

Strings attached

Patient activity can also be problematic. Simple tasks, such as transferring to a chair, ambulating and washing oneself, can become complicated when the patient must cope with drip stands, I.V. lines and dressings.

No such thing as a free lunch

Finally, I.V. therapy is more costly than oral, subcutaneous or I.M. methods of delivering medications.

Fluids, electrolytes and I.V. therapy

One of the primary objectives of I.V. therapy is to restore and maintain fluid and electrolyte balance. To understand how I.V. therapy works to restore fluid and electrolyte balance, let's first review some basics of fluids and electrolytes.

We're all wet (well mostly!)

The human body is composed largely of liquid. These fluids account for about 60% of total body weight in an adult who weighs 70.3 kg and about 80% of total body weight in an infant.

Of solvents and solutes

Body fluids are composed of water (a solvent) and dissolved substances (solutes). The solutes in body fluids include electrolytes (such as sodium) and non-electrolytes (such as proteins).

Fluid functions

What functions do body fluids provide? They:
- help regulate body temperature
- help transport nutrients throughout the body
- carry cellular waste products to excretion sites.

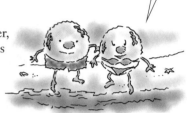

I'm feeling great…ready to take a dip?

Aim for the optimum

When fluid levels are optimal, the body performs swimmingly; however, when fluid levels deviate from the acceptable range, organs and systems can quickly become congested.

Inside and outside

Body fluids exist in two major compartments: inside the cells and outside the cells. Normally, the distribution of fluids between the two compartments is constant. Fluid is classified by whether it's inside or outside:
- intracellular fluid (ICF)—the fluid inside the cells, which is about 55% of the total body fluid
- extracellular fluid (ECF)—accounts for the rest of the body fluid.

The ABCs of ECF

ECF occurs in two forms: interstitial fluid (ISF) and intravascular fluid. ISF surrounds each cell of the body; even bone cells are bathed in it. Intravascular fluid is blood plasma, the liquid component of blood. It surrounds red blood cells and accounts for most of the blood volume.

In an adult, about 5% of body fluid is intravascular ECF; about 15% is interstitial ECF. Part of that interstitial ECF is transcellular fluid, which includes cerebrospinal fluid and lymph. Transcellular fluid contains secretions from the salivary glands, pancreas, liver and sweat glands.

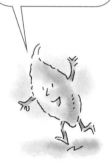

I have a very busy job. Inside, outside, and forever in-between—I'm always on the go!

It's a balancing act

Maintaining fluid balance in the body involves the kidneys, heart, liver, adrenal and pituitary glands and nervous system. This balancing act is affected by:
- fluid volume
- distribution of fluids in the body
- concentration of solutes in the fluid.

You gain some, you lose some

Every day, the body gains and loses fluid. To maintain fluid balance, the gains must equal the losses. (See *Daily fluid gains and losses*.)

Daily fluid gains and losses

Each day the body gains and loses fluid through several different processes. This illustration shows the main sites involved. The amounts shown apply to adults; infants exchange a greater amount of fluid than adults.

Note: Gastric, intestinal, pancreatic and biliary secretions total about 8,200 ml. However, because they're almost completely reabsorbed, they aren't usually counted in daily fluid gains and losses.

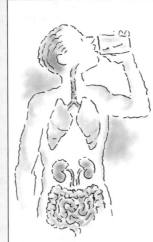

Daily total intake—2,400 to 3,200 ml
- Liquids—1,400 to 1,800 ml
- Water in foods (solid)—700 to 1,000 ml
- Water of oxidation (combined water and oxygen in the respiratory system)—1,400 to 1,800 ml

Daily total output—2,400 to 3,200 ml
- Lungs (respiration)—600 to 800 ml
- Skin (perspiration)—300 to 500 ml
- Kidneys (urine)—1,400 to 1,800 ml
- Intestines (faeces)—100 ml

Memory jogger

Remember, when it comes to body fluids, two i's make an **e**. The two i's (intravascular and interstitial fluid) are part of the **e** (**e**xtracellular fluid), not the i (intracellular fluid).

Hormones at work

Fluid volume and concentration are regulated by the interaction of two hormones: antidiuretic hormone (ADH) and aldosterone. ADH, sometimes referred to as the water-conserving hormone, affects fluid volume and concentration by regulating water retention. It's secreted when plasma osmolarity increases or circulating blood volume decreases and blood pressure drops. Aldosterone acts to retain sodium and water. It's secreted when the serum sodium level is low, the potassium level is high or the circulating volume of fluid decreases.

Water, I need water!!

The thirst mechanism (awareness of the desire to drink) also regulates water volume and participates with hormones in maintaining fluid balance. Thirst is experienced when water loss equals 2% of body weight or when osmolarity (solute concentration) increases. Drinking water restores plasma volume and dilutes ECF osmolarity.

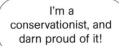

I'm a conservationist, and darn proud of it!

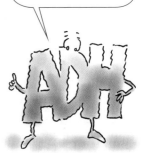

Picking out the baseline

Nurses must anticipate changes in fluid balance that may take place during I.V. therapy. Therefore, it's important to establish the patient's baseline fluid status before starting fluid replacement therapy. During I.V. therapy, changes in fluid status alert the nurse to impending fluid imbalances. (See *Identifying fluid imbalances*, page 200.)

Identifying fluid imbalances

By carefully assessing a patient before and during I.V. therapy, you can identify fluid imbalances early—before serious complications develop. The following assessment findings and test results indicate fluid deficit or excess.

Fluid deficit

- Weight loss
- Increased, thready pulse rate
- Diminished blood pressure, commonly with post-ural hypotension
- Decreased central venous pressure
- Sunken eyes, dry conjunctivae, decreased tearing
- Poor skin turgor (not a reliable sign in elderly patients)
- Pale, cool skin
- Poor capillary refill (more than 2 seconds)
- Lack of moisture in groin and axillae
- Thirst
- Decreased salivation
- Dry mouth
- Dry, cracked lips
- Furrows in tongue
- Difficulty forming words (patient needs to moisten mouth first)
- Mental status changes
- Weakness
- Diminished urine output
- Increased haematocrit (volume of red cells in the blood)
- Increased serum electrolyte levels
- Increased serum osmolarity

Fluid excess

- Weight gain
- Elevated blood pressure
- Bounding pulse that isn't easily obliterated
- Jugular vein distension
- Increased respiratory rate
- Dyspnoea
- Moist crackles or rhonchi on auscultation
- Oedema of dependent body parts; sacral oedema in patients on bed rest; oedema of feet and ankles in ambulatory patients
- Generalised oedema
- Puffy eyelids
- Peri-orbital oedema
- Slow emptying of hand veins when the arm is raised
- Decreased haematocrit (volume of red cells in the blood)
- Decreased serum electrolyte levels
- Reduced serum osmolarity

Electrolytes

Electrolytes are a major component of body fluid. There are six major electrolytes:

 sodium

 potassium

 calcium

 chloride

 phosphorus

 magnesium.

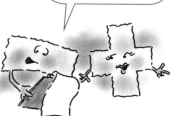

Here goes, the top 10 reasons why I'm so attracted to you…

Electric

As the name implies, electrolytes are associated with electricity. These vital substances are chemical compounds that dissociate in solution into electrically charged particles called ions. Like wiring for the body, the electrical charges of ions conduct current that's necessary for normal cell function. (See *Understanding electrolytes*.)

Understanding electrolytes

Six major electrolytes play important roles in maintaining chemical balance: sodium, potassium, calcium, chloride, phosphorus and magnesium. Electrolyte concentrations are expressed in millimols per litre (mmol/L).

Electrolyte	Principal functions	Signs and symptoms of imbalance
Calcium (Ca²⁺) • Major cation (positive ion) found in ECF of teeth and bones • Normal serum level: 2.12 to 2.62 mmol/L	• Enhances bone strength and durability (along with P) • Helps maintain cell-membrane structure, function, and permeability • Affects activation, excitation and contraction of cardiac and skeletal muscles • Participates in neurotransmitter release at synapses • Helps activate specific steps in blood coagulation • Activates serum complement in immune system function	Hypocalcaemia: muscle tremor, muscle cramps, tetany, tonic–clonic seizures, paraesthesia, bleeding, arrhythmias, hypotension, numbness or tingling in fingers, toes and area surrounding the mouth Hypercalcaemia: lethargy, headache, muscle flaccidity, nausea, vomiting, anorexia, constipation, hypertension, polyuria
Chloride (Cl⁻) • Major anion (negative ion) found in ECF • Normal serum level: 96 to 106 mmol/L	• Maintains serum osmolarity (along with Na⁻) • Combines with major cations (positive ions) to create important compounds, such as sodium chloride (NaCl), hydrogen chloride (HCl), potassium chloride (KCl) and calcium chloride (CaCl₂)	Hypochloraemia: increased muscle excitability, tetany, decreased respirations Hyperchloraemia: stupor; rapid, deep breathing; muscle weakness
Magnesium (Mg²⁺) • Major cation found in ICF (closely related to Ca²⁺ and P) • Normal serum level: 0.5 to 1 mmol/L	• Activates intracellular enzymes; active in carbohydrate and protein metabolism • Acts on myoneural vasodilation • Facilitates Na⁻ and K⁺ movement across all membranes • Influences Ca²⁺ levels	Hypomagnesaemia: dizziness, confusion, seizures, tremor, leg and foot cramps, hyperirritability, arrhythmias, vasomotor changes, anorexia, nausea Hypermagnesaemia: drowsiness, lethargy, coma, arrhythmias, hypotension, vague neuromuscular changes (such as tremor), vague GI symptoms (such as nausea), peripheral vasodilation, facial flushing, sense of warmth, slow, weak pulse

(continued)

Understanding electrolytes (continued)

Electrolyte	Principal functions	Signs and symptoms of imbalance
Phosphorus (P) • Major anion found in ICF • Normal serum phosphate level: 0.8 to 1.5 mmol/L	• Helps maintain bones and teeth • Helps maintain cell integrity • Plays a major role in acid-base balance (as a urinary buffer) • Promotes energy transfer to cells • Plays an essential role in muscle, red blood cell and neurologic function	Hypophosphataemia: paraesthesia (circumoral (around the mouth) and peripheral), lethargy, speech defects (such as stuttering or stammering), muscle pain and tenderness Hyperphosphataemia: renal failure, vague neuroexcitability to tetany and seizures, arrhythmias and muscle twitching with sudden rise in phosphate level
Potassium (K^+) • Major cation in ICF • Normal serum level: 3.5 to 5 mmol/L	• Maintains cell electroneutrality • Maintains cell osmolarity • Assists in conduction of nerve impulses • Directly affects cardiac muscle contraction • Plays a major role in acid-base balance	Hypokalaemia: decreased GI, skeletal muscle and cardiac muscle function; decreased reflexes; rapid, weak, irregular pulse; muscle weakness or irritability; fatigue; decreased blood pressure; decreased bowel motility; paralytic ileus Hyperkalaemia: muscle weakness, nausea, diarrhoea, oliguria, paraesthesia (altered sensation) of the face, tongue, hands and feet
Sodium (Na^+) • Major cation in ECF • Normal serum level: 135 to 143 mmol/L	• Maintains appropriate ECF osmolarity • Influences water distribution (with Cl^-) • Affects concentration, excretion, and absorption of potassium and chloride • Helps regulate acid-base balance • Aids nerve- and muscle-fibre impulse transmission	Hyponatraemia: muscle weakness, muscle twitching, decreased skin turgor, headache, tremor, seizures, coma Hypernatraemia: thirst, fever, flushed skin, oliguria, disorientation, dry, sticky membranes

Fluid and electrolyte balance

Fluids and electrolytes are usually discussed in tandem, especially where I.V. therapy is concerned, because fluid balance and electrolyte balance are interdependent. Any change in one alters the other, and any solution given I.V. can affect a patient's fluid and electrolyte balance.

Electrolyte balance

Not all electrolytes are distributed evenly. The major intracellular electrolytes are:
• potassium
• phosphorus.

The major extracellular electrolytes are:
- sodium
- chloride.

ICF and ECF contain different electrolytes because the cell membranes separating the two compartments have selective permeability—that is, only certain ions can cross those membranes. Although ICF and ECF contain different solutes, the concentration levels of the two fluids are about equal when balance is maintained.

Extra (cellular) credit

The two ECF components—ISF and intravascular fluid (plasma)—have identical electrolyte compositions. Pores in the capillary walls allow electrolytes to move freely between the ISF and plasma, allowing for equal distribution of electrolytes in both substances.

The protein content of ISF and plasma differs, however. ISF doesn't contain proteins because protein molecules are too large to pass through capillary walls. Plasma has a high concentration of proteins.

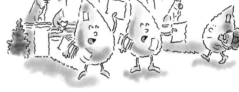

Join the Fluid Movement! Rally on library lawn at 7:00.

Fluid movement

Fluid movement is another mechanism that regulates fluid and electrolyte balance.

Ebb and flow

Body fluids are in constant motion. Although separated by membranes, they continually move between the major fluid compartments. In addition to regulating fluid and electrolyte balance, this movement is how nutrients, waste products and other substances get into and out of cells, organs and systems.

Fluid movement is influenced by membrane permeability and colloid osmotic and hydrostatic pressures. Balance is maintained when solute and fluid molecules are distributed evenly on each side of the membrane. When this scale is tipped, these molecules are able to restore balance by crossing membranes as needed.

Solute and fluid molecules have several modes for moving through membranes. Solutes move between compartments mainly by:
- diffusion (passive transport)
- active transport.
  Fluids (such as water) move between compartments by:
- osmosis
- capillary filtration and reabsorption.

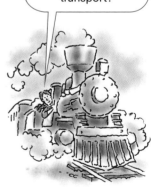

I wonder if this is what they mean by a form of active transport?

Passive is popular

Most solutes move by diffusion—that is their molecules move from areas of higher concentration to areas of lower concentration. This change is referred to as 'moving down the concentration gradient'. The result is an equal distribution of solute molecules. Because diffusion doesn't require energy, it's considered a form of passive transport.

Moving against the gradient

By contrast, in active transport, molecules move from areas of lower concentration to areas of higher concentration. This change, referred to as 'moving against the concentration gradient', requires energy in the form of adenosine triphosphate.

In active transport, molecules are moved by physiologic pumps. You're probably familiar with one active transport pump—the sodium–potassium pump. It moves sodium ions out of cells to the ECF and potassium ions into cells from the ECF. This pump balances sodium and potassium concentrations.

Osmosis

Fluids (particularly water) move by osmosis. Movement of water is caused by the existence of a concentration gradient. Water flows passively across the membrane from an area of higher water concentration to an area of lower water concentration. This dilution process stops when the solute concentrations on both sides of the membrane are equal.

Osmosis between the ECF and the ICF depends on the osmolarity (concentration) of the compartments. Normally, the osmotic (pulling) pressures of ECF and ICF are equal.

Equal, yet imbalanced

Osmosis can create a fluid imbalance between the ECF and ICF compartments, despite equal concentrations of solute, if the concentrations aren't optimal. This imbalance can cause complications such as tissue oedema.

Up against the capillary wall

Of all the vessels in the vascular system, only capillaries have walls thin enough to let solutes pass. Water and solutes move across capillary walls by two opposing processes:

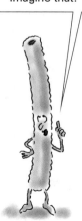 capillary filtration

capillary reabsorption.

From high to low

Filtration is the movement of substances from an area of high hydrostatic pressure to an area of lower hydrostatic pressure. (Hydrostatic pressure is the pressure at any level on water at rest due to the weight of water above it.)

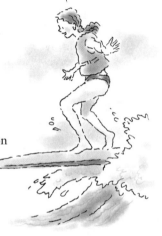

> Water moves by osmosis—flowing passively across a membrane from an area of higher concentration to one of lower concentration.

> I'm the only vessel with walls thin enough to let solutes pass. Imagine that!

Capillary filtration forces fluid and solutes through capillary wall pores and into the ISF.

Left unchecked, capillary filtration would cause plasma to move in only one direction—out of the capillaries. This movement would cause severe hypovolaemia and shock.

Reabsorption to the rescue

Fortunately, capillary reabsorption keeps capillary filtration in check. During filtration, albumin (a protein that can't pass through capillary walls) remains behind in the diminishing volume of water. As the albumin concentration inside the capillaries increases, the albumin begins to draw water back in by osmosis. Water is thus reabsorbed by capillaries.

May the force be with you

The osmotic, or pulling, force of albumin in capillary reabsorption is called colloid osmotic pressure or oncotic pressure. As long as capillary blood pressure exceeds colloid osmotic pressure, water and diffusible solutes can leave the capillaries and circulate into the ISF. When capillary blood pressure falls below colloid osmotic pressure, water and diffusible solutes return to the capillaries.

Pressure points

In any capillary, blood pressure normally exceeds colloid osmotic pressure up to the vessel's mid-point, and then falls below colloid osmotic pressure along the rest of the vessel. That's why capillary filtration takes place along the first half of a capillary and reabsorption occurs along the second half. As long as capillary blood pressure and plasma albumin levels remain normal, no net movement of water occurs. Water is lost and gained equally in this process.

Correcting imbalances

The effect an I.V. solution has on fluid compartments depends on the solution's osmolarity compared with serum osmolarity.

Osmolarity at parity?

Osmolarity is the concentration of a solution. It's expressed in milliosmols of solute per litre of solution (mOsm/L). Normally, serum has the same osmolarity as other body fluids, about 300 mOsm/L.

A lower serum osmolarity suggests fluid overload; a higher serum osmolarity suggests haemoconcentration and dehydration.

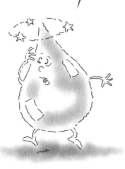

Here we go again…first I'm in, then I'm out. Somebody just point me in the right direction!

Bring back the balance

The doctor may prescribe I.V. solutions to maintain or restore fluid balance. (See *Understanding I.V. solutions.*) There are three basic types of I.V. solutions:

 isotonic

 hypotonic

 hypertonic. (See *Quick guide to I.V. solutions.*)

Isotonic solutions

An isotonic solution has the same osmolarity (or tonicity) as serum and other body fluids. Because the solution doesn't alter serum osmolarity, it stays where it's infused—inside the blood vessel (the intravascular compartment). The solution expands this compartment without pulling fluid from other compartments.

> We're the Tonic brothers. Our other brother, Gin-an', had to make a quick pit stop…but he'll be along momentarily. You'll like him…he's the life of the party.

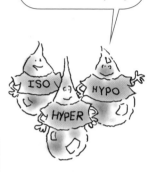

Understanding I.V. solutions

Solutions used for I.V. therapy may be isotonic, hypotonic or hypertonic. The type you give a patient depends on whether you want to change or maintain his body fluid status.

Isotonic solution

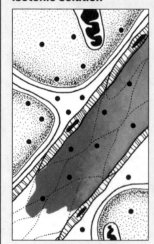

An isotonic solution has an osmolarity about equal to that of serum. Because it stays in the intravascular space, it expands the intravascular compartment.

Hypotonic solution

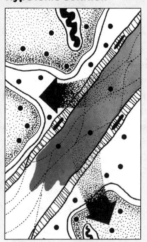

A hypotonic solution has an osmolarity lower than that of serum. It shifts fluid out of the intravascular compartment, hydrating the cells and the inter-stitial compartments.

Hypertonic solution

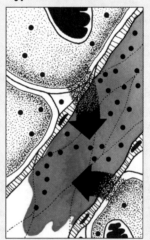

A hypertonic solution has an osmolarity higher than that of serum. It draws fluid into the intravascular compartment from the cells and the interstitial compartments.

Quick guide to I.V. solutions

A few common solutions can be used to illustrate the role of I.V. therapy in restoring and maintaining fluid and electrolyte balance. A solution is isotonic if its osmolarity falls within (or near) the normal range for serum (240 to 340 mOsm/L). A hypotonic solution has a lower osmolarity; a hypertonic solution, a higher osmolarity. This chart lists common examples of the three types of I.V. solutions and provides key considerations for administering them.

Solution	Examples	Nursing considerations
Isotonic	• 0.9% sodium chloride (normal saline) • 5% albumin • Hartmann's solution	• Because isotonic solutions expand the intravascular compartment, closely monitor the patient for signs of fluid overload, especially if he has hypertension or heart failure. • Albumin should be administered slowly if the patient has a history of cardiac or circulatory disease, to avoid a rapid rise in blood pressure and cardiac failure.
Hypotonic	• Dextrose 2.5% in water • 0.45% sodium chloride	• Administer cautiously. Hypotonic solutions cause a fluid shift from blood vessels into cells. This shift could cause cardiovascular collapse from intravascular fluid depletion and increased ICP from fluid shift into brain cells. • Don't give hypotonic solutions to patients at risk for increased ICP from stroke, head trauma or neurosurgery. • Don't give hypotonic solutions to patients at risk for third-space fluid shifts (abnormal fluid shifts into the interstitial compartment or a body cavity)—e.g. patients suffering from burns, trauma, or low serum protein levels from malnutrition or liver disease.
Hypertonic	• Gelatin (Gelofusine) • Dextrose 5% in half-normal saline • Dextrose 5% in normal saline • 25% albumin	• Because hypertonic solutions greatly expand the intravascular compartment, administer them by I.V. pump and closely monitor the patient for circulatory overload. • Hypertonic solutions pull fluid from the intracellular compartment, so don't give them to a patient with a condition that causes cellular dehydration—e.g. diabetic ketoacidosis. • Don't give hypertonic solutions to a patient with impaired heart or kidney function—his system can't handle the extra fluid.

One indication for an isotonic solution is hypotension due to hypovolaemia. Common isotonic solutions include normal saline and Hartmann's solution.

Hypertonic solutions

A hypertonic solution has an osmolarity higher than serum osmolarity. When a patient receives a hypertonic I.V. solution, serum osmolarity initially increases, causing fluid to be pulled from the interstitial and intracellular compartments into the blood vessels.

When, why and how to get hyper

Hypertonic solutions may be prescribed for patients post-operatively because the shift of fluid into the blood vessels caused by a hypertonic solution has several beneficial effects for these patients. For example, it:

- reduces the risk of oedema
- stabilises blood pressure
- regulates urine output.

Hypotonic solutions

A hypotonic solution has an osmolarity lower than serum osmolarity. When a patient receives a hypotonic solution, fluid shifts out of the blood vessels and into the cells and interstitial spaces, where osmolarity is higher. A hypotonic solution hydrates cells while reducing fluid in the circulatory system.

Hypotonic solutions may be prescribed when diuretic therapy dehydrates cells. Other indications include hyperglycaemic conditions, such as diabetic ketoacidosis and hyperosmolar hyperglycaemic non-ketotic syndrome. In these conditions, high serum glucose levels draw fluid out of cells.

Flood warning

Because hypotonic solutions flood cells, certain patients shouldn't receive them. For example patients with cerebral oedema or increased intracranial pressure shouldn't receive hypotonic solutions because the increased ECF can cause further oedema and tissue damage.

Additional uses of I.V. therapy

In addition to restoring and maintaining fluid and electrolyte balance, I.V. therapy is used to administer drugs, transfuse blood and blood products and deliver parenteral nutrition (PN).

Drug administration

The I.V. route provides a rapid, effective way of administering medications. Commonly infused drugs include antibiotics, thrombolytics, antihistamines, cytotoxic, cardiovascular and anticonvulsant drugs.

Drugs may be delivered long-term by continuous infusion, over a short period, or directly as a single dose.

Blood administration

Your nursing responsibilities may include giving blood and blood components and monitoring patients receiving transfusion therapy. Blood products can be given through a peripheral or central I.V. line. Care must be taken when administering blood products. The National Patient Safety Agency (NPSA) now requires Trusts to provide training for all personnel who deal with blood products. From those taking the initial sample to those fetching the

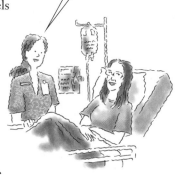

A hypertonic solution can be beneficial post-operatively because it helps reduce oedema, stabilise blood pressure and regulate urine output.

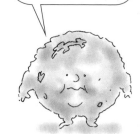

Thanks for the hypotonic solution…I needed that!

blood from the blood bank, all need to demonstrate that they have achieved competencies related to their part in the process. Various blood products are given to:
- restore and maintain adequate circulatory volume
- prevent cardiogenic shock
- increase the blood's oxygen-carrying capacity
- maintain haemostasis.

Parts of the whole

Whole blood is composed of cellular elements and plasma. Cellular elements include:
- erythrocytes (red blood cells)
- leucocytes (white blood cells)
- thrombocytes (platelets).

Each of these elements is packaged separately for transfusion. Plasma may be delivered intact or separated into several components that may be given to correct various deficiencies. Whole blood transfusions are unnecessary unless the patient has lost massive quantity of blood in a short period.

Parenteral nutrition

PN provides essential nutrients to the blood, organs and cells by the I.V. route. It isn't the same as a seven-course meal in a fine restaurant, but PN can contain the essence of a balanced diet.

It isn't gourmet, but it has all you need...

PN, although still commonly referred to as total parenteral nutrition (TPN), is customised for each patient. The ingredients in solutions developed for PN are designed to meet a patient's energy and nutrient requirements, including:
- proteins
- carbohydrates
- fats
- electrolytes
- vitamins
- trace elements
- water.

Time for PN?

PN should be used only when the GI tract is unable to absorb nutrients. A patient can receive PN indefinitely; however, long-term PN can cause liver damage.

A limited menu

Peripheral parenteral nutrition (PPN) is delivered into a peripheral vein via a peripheral line. PPN is used in limited nutritional therapy. The solution contains fewer non-protein calories and lower amino acid concentrations

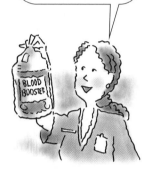

One of your responsibilities as a nurse is to administer blood and blood components and monitor transfusion therapy. So you've got to know your blood facts.

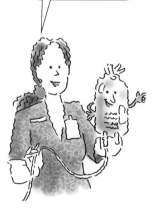

It may not be a gourmet meal, but TPN is packed with all the essential nutrients your patient needs.

than PN solutions. It may also include lipid emulsions. A patient can receive PPN for a short time. It can be used to support the nutritional status of a patient who doesn't require total nutritional support. Complications associated with PPN include the risks of vein damage and infiltration. This method should not be confused with a peripherally inserted central catheter (PICC) line.

Tracking changes

When your patient is receiving PN they are closely monitored by a nutritional support team who keep a close track of changes in their fluid and electrolyte status and glucose levels.

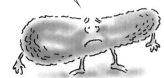

If your patient is receiving PN, please keep a close eye on my enzymes.

I.V. delivery

Depending, in part, on how concentrated an I.V. solution is, it may be delivered through a peripheral vein or a central vein. Usually, a low-concentration solution is infused through a peripheral vein in the arm or hand; a more concentrated solution must be given through a central vein. (See *Veins used in I.V. therapy.*) Medications or fluids that may be administered centrally include:
- those with a pH less than 5 or greater than 9
- those with an osmolarity greater than 500 mOsm/L
- PN formulas containing more than 10% dextrose or more than 50% protein
- continuous vesicant chemotherapy (chemotherapy that's toxic to tissues).

Delivery methods

There are three basic methods for delivering I.V. therapy:

continuous infusion

intermittent infusion

bolus injection.

Setting the terms

Continuous I.V. therapy allows you to give a carefully regulated amount of fluid over a prolonged period. In intermittent I.V. therapy, a solution (commonly a medication, e.g. antibiotics) is given for shorter periods at set intervals. A bolus injection is used to deliver a single dose of a drug, often used in emergency situations.

Veins used in I.V. therapy

This illustration shows the veins commonly used for peripheral and central venous therapy.

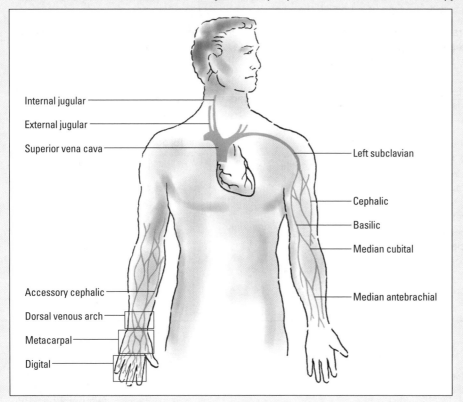

Internal jugular

External jugular

Superior vena cava

Left subclavian

Cephalic

Basilic

Median cubital

Accessory cephalic

Dorsal venous arch

Metacarpal

Digital

Median antebrachial

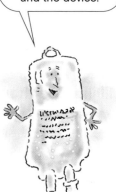

An infusion control device is an excellent way to regulate your patient's infusion rate, but you still need to monitor it and the device.

Infusion rates

A key aspect of administering I.V. therapy is maintaining accurate infusion rates for the solutions. If an infusion runs too fast or too slow, your patient may suffer complications, such as phlebitis, infiltration, circulatory overload (possibly leading to heart failure and pulmonary oedema) and adverse drug reactions.

Pumps

When a patient's condition requires you to maintain precise I.V. infusion rates, use an infusion pump. These will deliver a precise amount of fluid over an hour and, therefore, there is less chance of errors occurring.

New pumps are being developed all the time and therefore will not be discussed here as you must attend teaching sessions provided by the manufacturer to learn how to use them correctly.

It is important to note that student nurses must not set up or change the rate of delivery unless they are directly supervised by a registered nurse who is competent to do so (NMC, 2008).

Calculating infusion rates

When calculating the infusion rate (drops per minute) of I.V. solutions, remember that the number of drops required to deliver 1 ml varies with the type of administration set used and its manufacturer:

- Manufacturers may calibrate their devices differently, so be sure to look for the 'drop factor'—expressed in drops per millilitre, on the packaging that accompanies the set you're using. When you know your device's drop factor, use the following formula to calculate specific infusion rates:

$$\frac{\text{volume of infusion (in milliliters)}}{\text{time of infusion (in minutes)}} \times \text{drop factor (in drops per milliliter)} = \text{infusion rate (in drops per minute)}$$

After you calculate the infusion rate for the set you're using, remove your watch or position your wrist so you can look at your watch and the drops at the same time. Next, adjust the clamp to achieve the prescribed infusion rate and count the drops for 1 minute. Readjust the clamp as necessary and count the drops for another minute. Keep adjusting the clamp and counting the drops until you have the correct rate.

Macrodrip

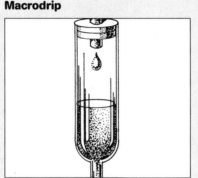

Microdrip

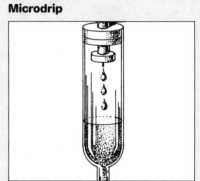

Millilitre per hour or drops per minute?

When you regulate the I.V. infusion rate with a clamp, the rate is usually measured in drops per minute. If you use a pump, the infusion rate is measured in millilitres per hour (ml/hour).

Factor these in

When you're using a roller clamp for infusion regulation, you must monitor the infusion rate closely and adjust as needed. Such factors as vein spasm, vein pressure changes, patient movement, manipulations of the clamp and bent or kinked tubing can cause the rate to vary markedly.

Other factors that affect infusion rate include the type of I.V. fluid and its viscosity, the height of the infusion container, the type of administration set and the size and position of the venous access device.

Checking infusion rates

Infusion rates can be fickle; you must check and adjust them regularly. The frequency with which you should check infusion rates depends on the patient's condition and age and the solution or medication being administered. Many nurses check the I.V. infusion rate every time they're near the patient and after each position change.

If the infusion rate slows, you can get it back on schedule by making slight adjustments. However, if the rate is off by more than 30%, consult the doctor.

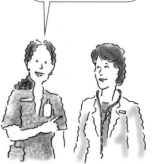

Take care!

Infusion pumps should be used for the following patients to ensure a controlled delivery of the fluids:

- critically ill patients
- patients with conditions that might be exacerbated by fluid overload
- children
- elderly patients
- patients receiving a drug that can cause tissue damage if infiltration occurs.

Minor (not major) adjustments

If the infusion rate slows significantly, you can usually get it back on schedule by adjusting the rate slightly. Don't make a major adjustment though, check with the doctor.

While you're there

The insertion site should be checked at least daily, check for signs of inflammation (erythema), swelling or pain, follow local IV cannulation policies depending on the appearance of the site.

When monitoring an I.V. line, listening to the patient is as important as monitoring the site, pump and tubing. Many clinical areas are using assessment tools to formally assess the cannula site.

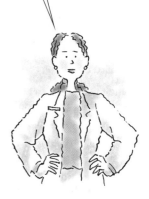

Remember! There will be local policies on I.V. administration which must be followed.

Professional and legal standards

Administering drugs and solutions to patients is one of the most important aspects of nursing, and, as a student, you must be directly supervised by a registered nurse. As a nurse, you have a legal and ethical responsibility to your patients. The good news is that if you honour these duties and meet the appropriate standards of care, you'll be safe.

By becoming aware of professional standards and laws related to administering I.V. therapy, you can provide the best care for your patients and protect yourself legally. Professional and legal standards are defined by the NMC and local policies, you must ensure you follow these. The RCN (2005), NICE (2003) and the NPSA (2008) have guidelines for I.V. administration which provide greater details and advice to follow.

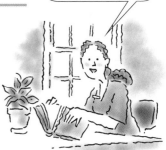

Become familiar with the scope and limitations of what you legally can and can't do regarding I.V. therapy.

Know your limits

Every nurse is expected to care for patients within defined limits. If a nurse gives care beyond those limits, they become vulnerable to charges of violating their registration.

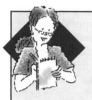

Record!

Documenting I.V. therapy

Follow these tips to document your care when you perform I.V. site care or cannula removal or when you document I.V. infusion on the fluid balance chart.

I.V. site care

When you perform I.V. site care, document the following:

- date and time of the dressing change
- condition of the insertion site, noting signs of infection (redness and pain), infiltration (coolness, blanching or oedema) or thrombophlebitis (redness, firmness, pain or oedema)
- care given and the type of dressing applied
- patient education provided. If complications are present, document:
- name of the doctor notified
- time of the notification
- specific orders given
- your interventions
- patient's response.

I.V. catheter removal

When an I.V. catheter is removed, document the following:

- date and time of removal
- condition of the site
- drainage at the puncture site
- site care given
- type of dressing applied
- patient education provided.

Fluid balance charts

- Record the type and amount of fluid infused on the fluid balance chart following local policy.
- Remember to record all oral fluids taken.
- Note output hourly or less often (but at least once each shift), depending on the patient's condition. Output includes urine, stool, vomitus and gastric drainage. For an acutely ill or unstable patient, you may need to assess urine output at least hourly.

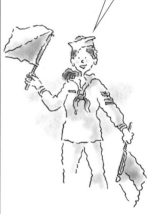

Translated, this means 'document, document, document!'

Be crystal clear when documenting how the I.V. site is maintained. I predict you will be a better nurse for doing so!

Documentation of I.V. therapy

When you initiate I.V. therapy, it's important to include specific information about when the I.V. was started, what kind of equipment was used, and what solution was infused. (See *Documenting I.V. therapy*.)

Forms, forms, forms

I.V. therapy may be documented on progress notes, a special I.V. therapy sheet, the patient's medicines administration record (MAR), a nursing care plan on the patient's chart or a fluid balance chart, so follow local policy.

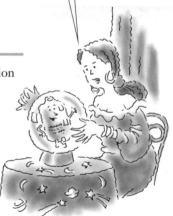

Label that dressing…

In addition to documentation in the patient's chart, you need to label the dressing on the catheter insertion site. Whenever you change the dressing, label the new one.

Teacher's lounge

Teaching about I.V. therapy

Although you may be accustomed to I.V. therapy, many patients aren't. Your patient may be apprehensive about the procedure and concerned that their condition has worsened.

Teaching the patient and, when appropriate, members of their family will help them relax and take the mystery out of I.V. therapy.

Based on past experience

Begin by determining your patient's previous infusion experience, their expectations and their knowledge of venepuncture and I.V. therapy. Then base your teaching on your findings.

Your teaching should include these steps:

- Describe the procedure. Tell the patient that I.V. means 'inside the vein' and that a plastic catheter or needle will be placed in their vein.
- Explain that fluids containing certain nutrients or medications will flow from a bag or bottle through a length of tubing, and then through the catheter or needle into their vein.
- Tell the patient how long the catheter or needle may stay in place, and explain that their doctor will decide how much and what type of fluid and medication they need.

The whole story

Give the patient as much information as possible.

- Tell the patient that although they may feel transient pain as the needle goes in, the discomfort will stop when the catheter or needle is in place.

- Explain why I.V. therapy is needed and how the patients can help by holding still and not withdrawing if they feel pain when the needle is inserted.
- Explain that the I.V. fluids may feel cold at first, but the sensation should last only a few minutes.
- Instruct the patient to report any discomfort they feel after therapy begins.
- Explain activity restrictions such as those regarding bathing and ambulating.

Easing anxiety

Give the patient time to express their concerns and fears, and take time to provide reassurance. Also, encourage the patient to use stress-reduction techniques, such as deep, slow breathing. Allow the patient and their families to participate in their care as much as possible.

But did they get it?

Make sure you evaluate how well your patient and members of the patient's family understand your instruction. Evaluate their understanding while you're teaching and when you're done. You can do this by asking frequent questions and having them explain or demonstrate what you have taught.

Don't forget the paperwork

Document all your teaching in the patient's records. Note what you taught and how well the patient understood it.

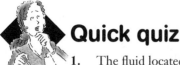

Quick quiz

1. The fluid located inside the cell is called:
A. interstitial.
B. intracellular.
C. extracellular.
D. internal.

Answer: B. The fluid inside the cells—about 55% of total body fluid—is called intracellular fluid. The rest is called extracellular fluid.

2. The major extracellular electrolytes are:
A. sodium and chloride.
B. potassium and phosphorus.
C. potassium and sodium.
D. phosphorus and chloride.

Answer: A. The major extracellular electrolytes are sodium and chloride.

3. An example of a hypertonic solution is:
A. half-normal saline.
B. 0.33% sodium chloride.
C. dextrose 2.5% in water.
D. dextrose 5% in half-normal saline.

Answer: D. Some examples of hypertonic solutions are dextrose 5% in half-normal saline, dextrose 5% in normal saline and Gelofusine.

4. When capillary blood pressure exceeds colloid osmotic pressure, which situation occurs?
A. Water and diffusible solutes leave the capillaries and circulate into the interstitial fluid.
B. Water and diffusible solutes return to the capillaries.
C. No change occurs.
D. Intake and output are affected.

Answer: A. When capillary blood pressure exceeds colloid osmotic pressure, water and diffusible solutes leave the capillaries and circulate into the interstitial fluid. When capillary blood pressure falls below colloid osmotic pressure, water and diffusible solutes return to the capillaries.

Scoring

☆☆☆   If you answered all four questions correctly, super! Your knowledge of I.V. therapy is diffuse.

☆☆   If you answered three questions correctly, bravo! You're no drip when it comes to I.V. therapy.

☆   If you answered fewer than three questions correctly, don't despair! Review the chapter for an infusion of I.V. know-how and try again.

Part III

Physiological needs

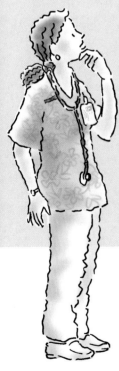

12	Oxygenation	219
13	Skin integrity and wound healing	249
14	Mobility, activity and exercise	315
15	Self-care and hygiene	339
16	Comfort, rest and sleep	365
17	Pain management	383
18	Nutrition	415
19	Urinary elimination	448
20	Bowel elimination	471

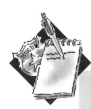

(12) Oxygenation

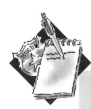

Just the facts

In this chapter, you'll learn:

♦ components that make up the respiratory system

♦ processes involved in respiration

♦ principles of acid–base balance

♦ treatments for respiratory disorders.

A look at the respiratory system

One of my main jobs is to get rid of excess carbon dioxide. Out the door with you now!

The respiratory system includes the airways, lungs, bony thorax, respiratory muscles and central nervous system. They work together to deliver oxygen to the bloodstream and remove excess carbon dioxide from the body. Knowing the basic structures and functions of the respiratory system will help you perform a comprehensive respiratory assessment and recognise any abnormalities. (See *A close look at the respiratory system*, page 220.)

Airways and lungs

The airways are divided into the upper and lower airways. The upper airways include the nasopharynx (nose), oropharynx (mouth), laryngopharynx and larynx. Their purpose is to warm, filter and humidify inhaled air. They also help make sound and send air to the lower airways.

Flapped for your protection

The epiglottis is a flap of tissue that closes over the top of the larynx when the patient swallows. The epiglottis protects the patient from aspirating food or fluid into the lower airways.

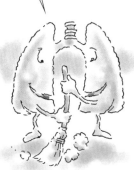

A close look at the respiratory system

The major structures of the upper and lower airways are illustrated below. The alveolus is shown in the inset.

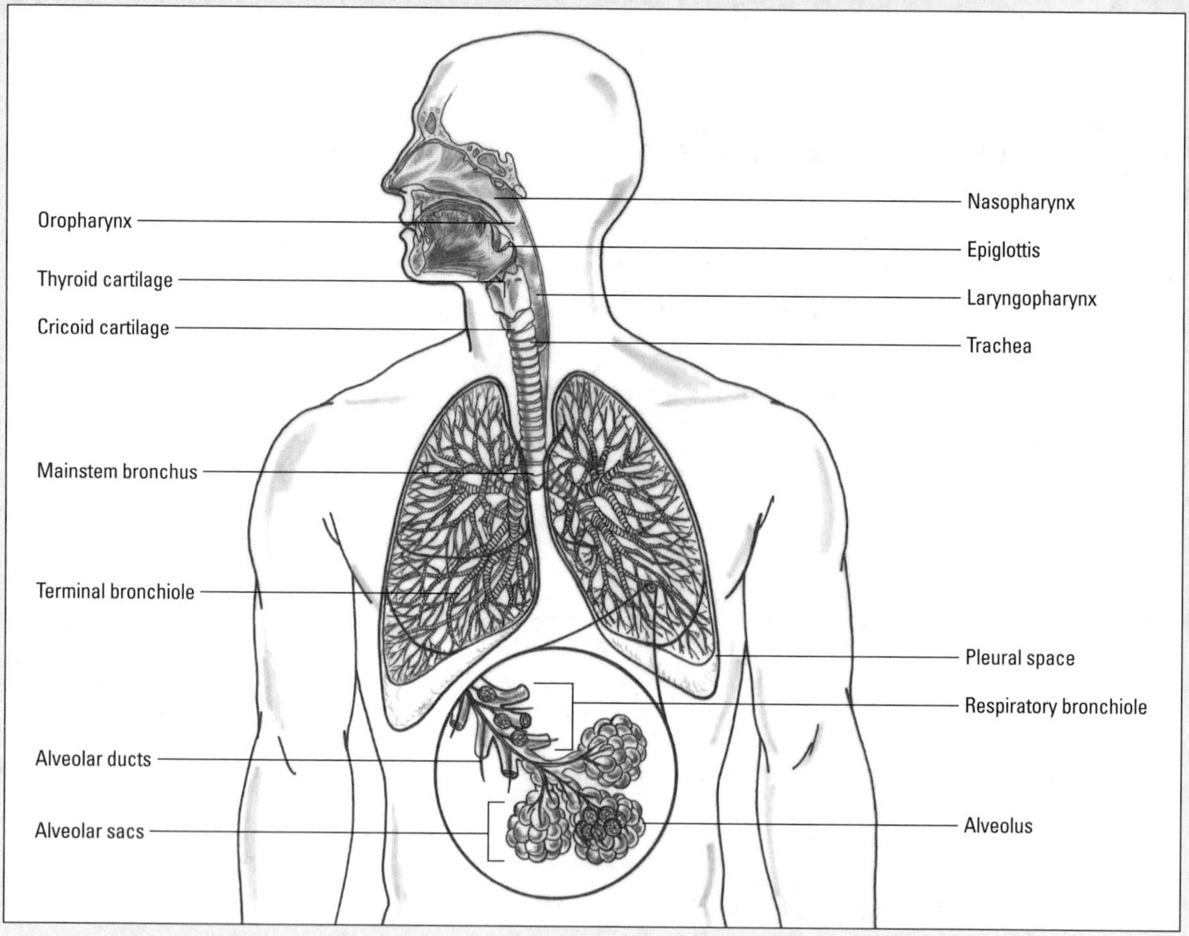

Oropharynx

Thyroid cartilage

Cricoid cartilage

Mainstem bronchus

Terminal bronchiole

Alveolar ducts

Alveolar sacs

Nasopharynx

Epiglottis

Laryngopharynx

Trachea

Pleural space

Respiratory bronchiole

Alveolus

Vocal point

The larynx is located at the top of the trachea and houses the vocal cords. It's the transition point between the upper and lower airways.

The lowdown on the lower airways

The lower airways begin with the trachea, which then divides into the right and left main stem bronchi. The main stem bronchi divide into the lobar bronchi, which are lined with mucous-producing ciliated epithelium, one of the lungs' major defence systems.

The lobar bronchi then divide into secondary bronchi, tertiary bronchi, terminal bronchioles, respiratory bronchioles, alveolar ducts and, finally, into the alveoli, the gas-exchange units of the lungs. An adult's lungs typically contain about 300 million alveoli.

Lungs and lobes

Each lung is wrapped in a lining called the *visceral pleura*. The right lung is larger and has three lobes: upper, middle and lower. The left lung is smaller and has only an upper and a lower lobe.

Smooth moves

The lungs share space in the thoracic cavity with the heart and great vessels, the trachea, the oesophagus and the bronchi. All areas of the thoracic cavity that come in contact with the lungs are lined with parietal pleura.

A small amount of fluid fills the area between the two layers of the pleura. This pleural fluid allows the layers to slide smoothly over each other as the chest expands and contracts. The parietal pleura also contain nerve endings that transmit pain signals when inflammation occurs.

Thorax

The bony thorax includes the clavicles, sternum, scapula, 12 sets of ribs and 12 thoracic vertebrae.

Rack of ribs

Ribs consist of bone and cartilage and allow the chest to expand and contract during each breath. All ribs attach to the thoracic vertebrae. The first 7 ribs also attach directly to the sternum. The 8th, 9th and 10th ribs attach to the cartilage of the preceding rib. The 11th and 12th ribs are called *floating ribs* because they don't attach to anything in the anterior thorax.

Respiratory muscles

The diaphragm and the external intercostal muscles are the primary muscles used in breathing. They contract when the patient inhales and relax when the patient exhales.

Message in a nerve

The respiratory centre in the medulla initiates each breath by sending messages to the primary respiratory muscles over the phrenic nerve. Impulses from the phrenic nerve adjust the rate and depth of breathing, depending on

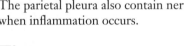

Hang tight! These lobar bronchi can get a little slippery from all that mucous in the lining.

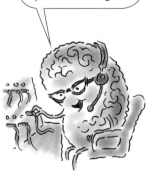

Yes, sir, it's the respiratory muscle again. He's asking whether you can slow the breathing rate just a tad... something about too much carbon dioxide in the CSF. Shall I put him through?

A close look at the mechanics of breathing

These illustrations show how mechanical forces, such as the movement of the diaphragm and intercostal muscles, produce a breath. A plus sign (+) indicates positive pressure, and a minus sign (−) indicates negative pressure.

At rest

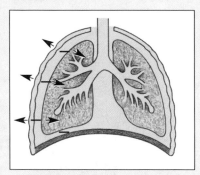

Inhalation

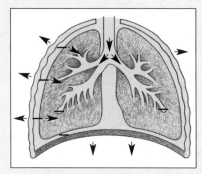

Exhalation

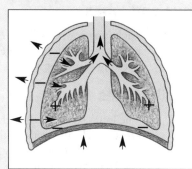

- Inspiratory muscles relax.
- Atmospheric pressure is maintained in the tracheobronchial tree.
- No air movement occurs.

- Inspiratory muscles contract.
- The diaphragm descends and flattens.
- Negative alveolar pressure is maintained.
- Air moves into the lungs.

- Inspiratory muscles relax, causing lungs to recoil to their resting size and position.
- The diaphragm ascends, returning to its resting position.
- Positive alveolar pressure is maintained.
- Air moves out of the lungs.

the carbon dioxide and pH levels in the cerebrospinal fluid (CSF). (See *A close look at the mechanics of breathing*.)

Accessory to breathing

Other muscles, called *accessory muscles*, assist in breathing. Accessory inspiratory muscles include the trapezius, the sternocleidomastoid and the scalene, which combine to elevate the scapula, clavicle, sternum and upper ribs. That elevation expands the front-to-back diameter of the chest when use of the diaphragm and intercostal muscles isn't effective.

Expiration occurs when the diaphragm and external intercostal muscles relax. If the patient has an airway obstruction, they may also use the abdominal muscles and internal intercostal muscles to exhale.

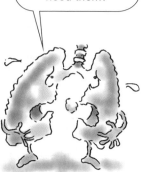

Acch. Where are those accessory muscles when you need them?

Functions of the respiratory system

The functions of the respiratory system are respiration and ventilation to help maintain acid–base balance.

Respiration

Effective respiration requires gas exchange in the tissues (internal respiration) and in the lungs (external respiration). This exchange is vital to maintain adequate oxygenation and acid–base balance. Internal respiration occurs only through diffusion. External respiration occurs through three processes:

ventilation (gas distribution into and out of the pulmonary airways)

pulmonary perfusion (blood flow from the right side of the heart, through the pulmonary circulation and into the left side of the heart)

diffusion (gas movement from an area of greater to lesser concentration through a semi-permeable membrane).

Ventilation

Adequate ventilation depends on the nervous, musculoskeletal and pulmonary systems for the requisite lung pressure changes. Any dysfunction in these systems increases the work of breathing, diminishing its effectiveness.

Nervous system influence

Although ventilation is largely involuntary, individuals can control its rate and depth. Involuntary breathing results from neurogenic stimulation of the respiratory centre in the medulla and the pons of the brain stem. The medulla controls the rate and depth of respiration; the pons moderates the rhythm of the switch from inspiration to expiration. Specialised neurovascular tissue alters these phases of the breathing process automatically and instantaneously.

A special response

When carbon dioxide in the blood diffuses into the CSF, specialised tissue in the respiratory centre of the brain stem responds. At the same time, peripheral chemoreceptors in the aortic arch and the bifurcation of the carotid arteries respond to reduced oxygen levels in the blood.

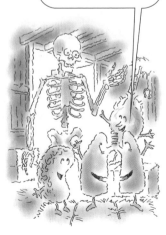

What do you say, guys? I bet with a little elbow grease and a couple more windows we could turn this into the coolest respiration clubhouse!

When the carbon dioxide level rises or the oxygen level falls noticeably, the respiratory centre of the medulla initiates respiration.

Musculoskeletal influence

The adult thorax is a flexible structure—its shape can be altered by contracting the chest muscles. The medulla controls ventilation primarily by stimulating contraction of the diaphragm and the external intercostals, the major muscles of breathing.

I'm inspired!

The diaphragm descends to expand the length of the chest cavity, while the external intercostals contract to expand the anteroposterior and lateral chest diameter. These actions produce changes in intrapulmonary pressure that cause inspiration.

Pulmonary influence

During inspiration, air flows through the right and left main stem bronchi into increasingly smaller bronchi, then into bronchioles, alveolar ducts and alveolar sacs, finally reaching the alveolar membrane. Many factors can alter airflow distribution, including airflow pattern, volume and location of the functional reserve capacity (air retained in the alveoli that prevents their collapse during respiration), amount of intrapulmonary resistance and presence of lung disease.

The path of least resistance

If disrupted, airflow distribution will follow the path of least resistance. For example, an intrapulmonary obstruction or forced inspiration will cause an uneven distribution of air.

Active, then passive

Normal breathing requires active inspiration and passive expiration. Forced breathing, as in cases of emphysema, demands active inspiration and expiration. It activates accessory muscles of respiration, which require additional oxygen to work, resulting in less efficient ventilation with an increased workload.

Non-compliance, resistance, fatigue—oh, my!

Other alterations in airflow, such as changes in compliance (distensibility of the lungs and thorax) and resistance (interference with airflow in the tracheobronchial tree), can also increase oxygen and energy demands and lead to respiratory muscle fatigue.

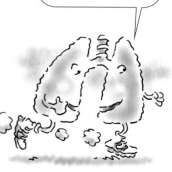

Just keep going. I'm sure we'll see the path of least resistance soon after the next bend in the road.

Pulmonary perfusion

Optimal pulmonary perfusion aids external respiration and promotes efficient alveolar gas exchange. However, factors that reduce blood flow, such as a cardiac output that's less than average (5 L/minute) and elevated pulmonary and systemic vascular resistance, can interfere with gas transport to the alveoli. Also, abnormal or insufficient haemoglobin (Hb) picks up less oxygen than is needed for efficient gas exchange.

That's heavy

Gravity can affect oxygen and carbon dioxide transport by influencing pulmonary circulation. Gravity pulls more unoxygenated blood to the lower and middle lung lobes relative to the upper lobes, where most of the tidal volume also flows.

No uniformity

As a result, neither ventilation nor perfusion is uniform throughout the lung. Areas of the lung where perfusion and ventilation are similar have good ventilation–perfusion matching. In such areas, gas exchange is most efficient. Areas of the lung that demonstrate ventilation–perfusion inequality result in less efficient gas exchange.

Diffusion

In diffusion, molecules of oxygen and carbon dioxide move between the alveoli and the capillaries. Partial pressure (the pressure exerted by one gas in a mixture of gases) dictates the direction of movement, which is always from an area of greater concentration to one of lesser concentration.

Let's move it!

During diffusion, oxygen moves across the alveolar and capillary membranes, then dissolves in the plasma, and passes through the red blood cell (RBC) membrane. Carbon dioxide moves in the opposite direction. (See *Exchanging gases*, page 226.)

Spaces in between

Successful diffusion requires an intact alveolocapillary membrane. The alveolar epithelium and the capillary endothelium are composed of a single layer of cells. Between these layers are minute interstitial spaces filled with elastin and collagen.

From the RBCs to the alveoli

Normally, oxygen and carbon dioxide move easily through all of these layers. Oxygen moves from the alveoli into the bloodstream, where it's taken up by

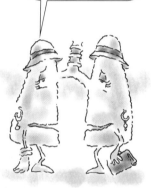

I wasn't aware of any dress code when I signed up for this job. What's all this business about ventilation and perfusion needing to match anyway?

Where do you think you're going? Diffuse yourself in the opposite direction, buddy!

Exchanging gases

Gas exchange occurs very rapidly in the millions of tiny, thin-membraned alveoli within the respiratory units. Inside these air sacs, oxygen from inhaled air diffuses into the blood while carbon dioxide diffuses from the blood into the air and is exhaled. Blood then circulates throughout the body, delivering oxygen and picking up carbon dioxide. Lastly, the blood returns to the lungs to be oxygenated again.

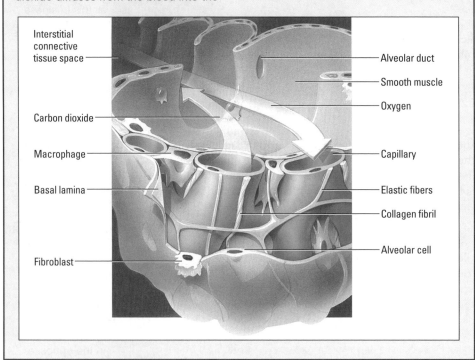

Interstitial connective tissue space

Carbon dioxide

Macrophage

Basal lamina

Fibroblast

Alveolar duct

Smooth muscle

Oxygen

Capillary

Elastic fibers

Collagen fibril

Alveolar cell

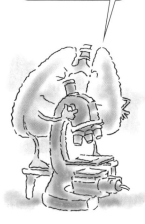

Boy, you're not kidding. Those gases whiz by so quickly. It's like, now you see it, now you don't!

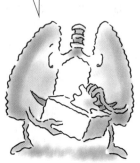

They said to look for oxygen and carbon dioxide exchange in the tissues, but I don't see anything. Think it's a prank?

Hb in the RBCs. When there, it displaces carbon dioxide (the by-product of metabolism), which diffuses from the RBCs into the blood, and then it moves to the alveoli. Most transported oxygen binds with Hb to form oxyhaemoglobin, while a small portion dissolves in the plasma (measurable as the partial pressure of oxygen in arterial blood).

Up and down

After oxygen binds to Hb, the RBCs travel to the tissues. At this point, the blood cells contain more oxygen, and the tissue cells contain more carbon dioxide. Internal respiration occurs during cellular diffusion, as RBCs release oxygen and absorb carbon dioxide. The RBCs then transport carbon dioxide back to the lungs for removal during expiration.

Acid–base balance

The lungs help maintain acid–base balance in the body by maintaining external and internal respiration. Oxygen collected in the lungs is transported to the tissues by the circulatory system, which exchanges it for the carbon dioxide produced by cellular metabolism. Because carbon dioxide is 20 times more soluble than oxygen, it dissolves in the blood, where most of it forms bicarbonate (base) and smaller amounts form carbonic acid (acid).

And back again

The lungs control bicarbonate levels by converting bicarbonate to carbon dioxide and water for excretion. In response to signals from the medulla, the lungs can change the rate and depth of ventilation.

Maintaining the balance

Such changes maintain acid–base balance by adjusting the amount of carbon dioxide that's lost. For example, in metabolic alkalosis, which results from excess bicarbonate retention, the rate and depth of ventilation decrease so that carbon dioxide is retained. This increases carbonic acid levels. In metabolic acidosis (a condition resulting from excess acid retention or excess bicarbonate loss), the lungs increase the rate and depth of ventilation to exhale excess carbon dioxide, thereby reducing carbonic acid levels.

Broken balance beam

A patient with inadequately functioning lungs can experience acid–base imbalances. For example, hypoventilation (reduced rate and depth of ventilation) of the lungs, which results in carbon dioxide retention, causes respiratory acidosis. Conversely, hyperventilation (increased rate and depth of ventilation) of the lungs leads to increased exhalation of carbon dioxide and will result in respiratory alkalosis.

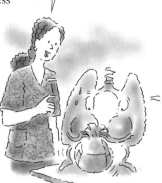

You're hyperventilating... just keep breathing slowly into the paper bag, and you'll be OK.

Therapy for altered function

When altered respiratory function occurs, such nursing interventions as coughing and deep-breathing exercises, incentive spirometry, chest physiotherapy and oxygen administration can enhance your patient's respiratory effort and improve oxygen status. Pulse oximetry allows you to monitor your patient's oxygen saturation. Surgical interventions, such as tracheostomy and chest drain insertion, can also improve oxygenation. Proper care of the patient during and after these procedures is vital.

Coughing exercises

Patients who are at risk for developing excess secretions should practise coughing exercises. However, patients who have recently had ear or eye surgery or repair of a hiatal or large abdominal hernia shouldn't do coughing exercises. Also, patients undergoing neurosurgery shouldn't practise coughing exercise post-operatively because intracranial pressure will rise.

If the patient's condition permits, instruct them to sit on the edge of his bed. Provide a small stool if their feet don't touch the floor. Tell them to bend their legs and lean slightly forward.

Slow and deep

If the patient is scheduled for or recently has had chest or abdominal surgery, teach them how to support their incision with a pillow before they cough.

In through the nose...

Instruct them to take a slow, deep breath; they should breathe in though the nose and concentrate on fully expanding their chest.

...and out through the mouth

Next, they should breathe out through the mouth and concentrate on feeling their chest sink downward and inward. Then they should take a second breath in the same manner.

Once isn't enough

Then, tell them to take a third deep breath and hold it. They should then cough two or three times in a row. (Once isn't enough.) This coughing will clear the breathing passages. Encourage them to concentrate on feeling the diaphragm force out all the air in their chest. Then they should take three to five normal breaths, exhale slowly and relax.

Say again?

Ask the patient to repeat this exercise at least once. After surgery, they'll need to perform it at least every 2 hours to help keep their lungs free from secretions. Reassure the patient that their stitches are very strong and won't split during coughing.

Deep-breathing exercises

Advise the patient that performing deep-breathing exercises several times per hour helps keep the lungs fully expanded. To deep-breathe correctly, they

Quick, grab the pillow. We have time for one good coughing session before the film begins.

must use their diaphragm and abdominal muscles—not just the chest muscles. Tell the patient to practise the following exercises two or three times per day before surgery.

Get comfortable

Ask the patient lie on their back in a comfortable position with one hand on their chest and the other over their upper abdomen. Teach them to relax and bend their knees slightly.

Inhale deeply...

Instruct them to exhale normally. The patient should then close their mouth and inhale deeply through the nose, concentrating on feeling the abdomen rise. Their chest shouldn't expand. Ask them to hold their breath and count to five.

...and then exhale.

Next, ask the patient to purse their lips as though about to whistle and then exhale completely through the mouth, without letting their checks puff out. Their ribs should sink downward and inward.

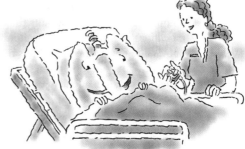

Let's go over it again one more time. Exhale normally through your nose... close your mouth and inhale deeply through your nose...

Rest and repeat

After resting several seconds, the patient should repeat the exercise 5 to 10 times. They should also do this exercise while lying on their side, sitting, standing or turning in bed.

Incentive spirometry

Incentive spirometry involves using a breathing device to help the patient achieve maximal ventilation. *This device tends to be used in specialist clinical areas.* The device measures the patient's inspiratory effort (flow rate) in cubic centimetres per second (cc/second). The device encourages the patient to take a deep breath and hold it for several seconds. This deep breath:
- increases lung volume
- boosts alveolar inflation
- promotes venous return
- loosens respiratory secretions.

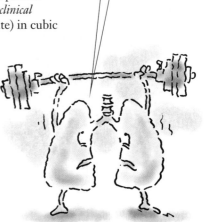

Any exercise that promises to get me back in shape is incentive enough for me.

Longer inflation, less collapse

This exercise also establishes alveolar hyperinflation for a longer time than is possible with a normal deep breath, thus preventing and reversing the alveolar collapse that causes atelectasis and pneumonitis.

What you see is what you get

Devices used for incentive spirometry provide a visual incentive to breathe deeply and encourage slow, sustained maximal inspiration. They can be divided into two types:

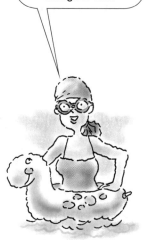

⬧ flow incentive spirometer, for patients at low risk for developing atelectasis

⬧ volume incentive spirometer, for patients at high risk for developing atelectasis. (See *Types of spirometers*.)

Let's get some incentive or float

Flow incentive spirometers contain plastic floats, which rise according to the amount of air the patient pulls through the device when he inhales. Volume incentive spirometers are activated when the patient inhales a certain volume of air. The device then estimates the amount of air inhaled. This device measures lung inflation more precisely and helps you determine whether your patient is inhaling adequately.

Benefits

Incentive spirometry benefits the patient on prolonged bed rest, especially the post-operative patient who may regain their normal respiratory pattern

> You can use a flow incentive spirometer if your patient is at low risk for developing atelectasis—or a volume incentive device, which is more precise, if he is at higher risk.

Types of spirometers

Spirometers can be volume incentive or flow incentive.

Volume incentive

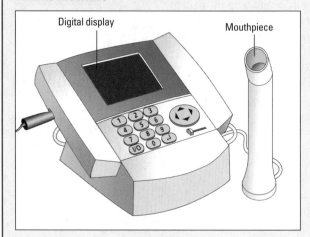

Digital display

Mouthpiece

Flow incentive

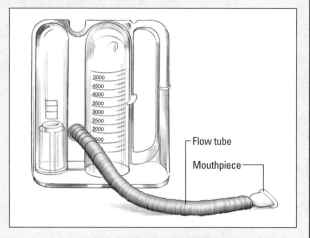

5000
4500
4000
3500
3000
2500
2000
1500

Flow tube

Mouthpiece

slowly because of such predisposing factors as abdominal or thoracic surgery, advanced age, inactivity, obesity, smoking and decreased ability to cough effectively and expel lung secretions.

What you need

Flow or volume incentive spirometer, as indicated, with sterile disposable tube and mouthpiece (The tube and mouthpiece are sterile on first use and clean on subsequent uses.) ✳ stethoscope ✳ watch

Getting ready

• Assemble the ordered equipment at the patient's bedside.
• Remove the sterile flow tube and mouthpiece from the package, and attach them to the device.
• Set the flow rate or volume goal as determined by the doctor or physiotherapist and based on the patient's pre-operative performance.
• Explain the procedure to the patient, making sure that they understand the importance of performing incentive spirometry regularly to maintain alveolar inflation.

How you do it

• Help the patient into a comfortable sitting position to promote optimal lung expansion. If you're using a flow incentive spirometer and the patient is unable to assume or maintain this position, they can perform the procedure in any position as long as the device remains upright. Tilting a flow incentive spirometer decreases the required patient effort and reduces the exercise's effectiveness.

Do you hear what I hear?

• The doctor or physiotherapist might auscultate the patient's lungs to provide a baseline for comparison with post-treatment auscultation.
• Instruct the patient to exhale normally and then tell them to insert the mouthpiece and close their lips tightly around it because a weak seal may alter flow or volume readings.

Sustained but maximal

• Then tell the patient to inhale as slowly and as deeply as possible. If they have difficulty with this step, tell them to suck as they would through a straw but more slowly. Ask the patient to retain the entire volume of air inhaled for 3 seconds or, if you're using a device with a light indicator, until the light turns off. This deep breath creates sustained transpulmonary pressure near the end of inspiration and is sometimes called a *sustained maximal inspiration*.

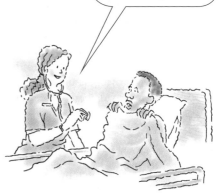

Just a quick listen before we begin with the incentive spirometry exercises. Don't worry, I remembered to warm up the stethoscope first.

• Tell the patient to remove the mouthpiece and exhale normally. Allow them to relax and take several normal breaths before attempting another breath with the spirometer. Repeat this sequence 5 to 10 times during every waking hour. Note tidal volumes.

Practice pointers

• Evaluate the patient's ability to cough effectively, and encourage them to cough after each effort because deep lung inflation may loosen secretions and facilitate their removal. Observe any expectorated secretions.

Chest physiotherapy

Chest physiotherapy is usually performed with other treatments, by a physiotherapist.

Especially important for the patient who has limited mobility, chest physiotherapy improves secretion clearance and ventilation and helps prevent or treat atelectasis and pneumonia, which can hinder recovery. Chest physiotherapy procedures include:

• percussion, which involves cupping the hands and fingers together and clapping them alternately over the patient's lung fields to loosen secretions (also achieved with the gentler technique of vibration)

• vibration, which can be used with percussion or as an alternative to it in a patient who's frail, in pain or recovering from thoracic surgery or trauma

• postural drainage, which uses gravity to promote drainage of secretions from the lungs and bronchi into the trachea

• deep-breathing exercises, which help loosen secretions and promote more effective coughing

• coughing, which helps clear the lungs, bronchi and trachea of secretions and prevents aspiration.

Doing your bit

Although you are not able to perform physiotherapy, there are things that you can do:

• Administer analgesia as prescribed to make it easier for the patient to deep-breathe and cough.

• Teach the patient to support their incision with a pillow.

• Make sure the patient is adequately hydrated to facilitate removal of secretions.

• If prescribed, administer bronchodilator and mist therapies before the treatment.

• Provide tissues and a pot for sputum.

• Provide oral hygiene after physiotherapy; secretions may taste foul or have an unpleasant odour.

Oxygen therapy

In oxygen therapy, oxygen is usually delivered by a simple oxygen mask, Venturi mask or nasal cannulae to prevent or reverse hypoxaemia and reduce

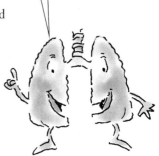

Remember to encourage your patient to cough. This helps loosen secretions.

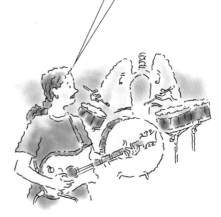

Enough with the percussion already! Let's start our next set with 'Good Vibrations.' Ready on the two… one, two…

the work of breathing. Possible causes of hypoxaemia include emphysema, pneumonia, Guillain–Barré syndrome, heart failure and myocardial infarction. (See *Oxygen delivery systems*, page 234.)

Except in an emergency situation (where oxygen should be given and documented later), oxygen therapy and concentration should always be prescribed.

The National Patient Safety Agency (NPSA) (2009) has made some recommendations in a 'Rapid Response Report' (RRR) relating to serious incidents regarding inappropriate administration and management of oxygen. Some of the actions to be completed by all hospitals include:

- minimised use of oxygen cylinders
- increased provision of piped oxygen
- reliable and adequate supplies when the use of oxygen cylinders is unavoidable
- action plans to reduce the risk of confusion over oxygen and medical compressed air
- oxygen prescribed in accordance with British Thoracic Society (BTS) guidelines
- availability of pulse oximetry where oxygen is used.

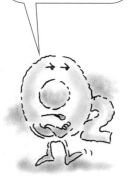

I've been waiting over an hour for the delivery truck to come and pick me up. Where is that guy?

Fire Hazard

Administrating oxygen can be a fire hazard, as oxygen is required along with heat and fuel to create a fire. It is therefore important that inflammable materials like cigarettes, grease and oil are not near oxygen supplies. Patients, relatives and visitors need to be informed of the danger of smoking when someone is receiving oxygen therapy. When oxygen is being administered in the home, the oxygen cylinder should be kept away from gas fires and naked flames.

Fully equipped

The equipment depends on the patient's age and condition as well as the required percentage of inspired oxygen. High-flow systems, such as a Venturi mask and ventilators, deliver a precisely controlled air–oxygen mixture. Low-flow systems, such as nasal cannulae or a simple mask allow variation in the oxygen percentage delivered, based on the patient's respiratory pattern. Children and infants don't tolerate masks. (See *Oxygen delivery in children*, page 235.)

Compare and contrast

Nasal cannulae deliver oxygen at flow rates ranging from 0.5 to 6 L/minute. Inexpensive and easy to use, the nasal cannulae permit talking, eating and suctioning, interfering less with the patient's activities than other devices. Even so, they may cause nasal drying and can't deliver high oxygen concentrations.

The big cover-up

Masks deliver up to 100% oxygen concentrations, but can't be used to deliver controlled oxygen concentrations. In addition, they may fit poorly, causing discomfort, and must be removed to eat.

Oxygen delivery systems

Patients may receive oxygen through nasal cannulae, a simple mask or a Venturi mask.

Nasal cannula

Oxygen is delivered in concentrations of less than 40% through a plastic cannula in the patient's nostrils.

Simple mask

Oxygen flows through an entry port at the bottom of the mask and exits through large holes on the sides of the mask. It delivers oxygen in concentrations of 40% to 60%.

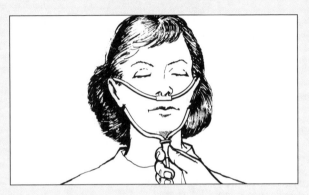

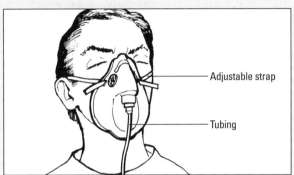

Venturi mask

The mask is connected to a Venturi device, which mixes a specific volume of air and oxygen. It delivers highly accurate oxygen concentration despite the patient's respiratory pattern.

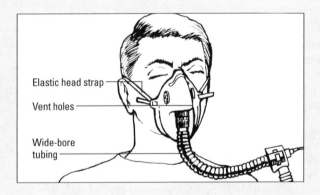

Ages and stages

Oxygen delivery in children

Oxygen delivery to children can be accomplished using a head box, a nasal cannula or prongs.

Head box

Oxygen delivery to an infant under 8 months is best tolerated by administering it through a head box, as shown below.

High as well as low concentrations of oxygen can be delivered by a head box. Remember not to allow the oxygen to flow directly on the infant's face. The oxygen is usually warmed to prevent cooling the infant, and also humidified. Older infants and children can also use a nasal cannula or nasal prongs.

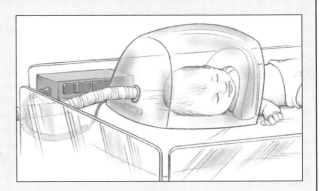

What you need

The equipment depends on the clinical need of the patient and the concentration of oxygen prescribed by the doctor. Equipment includes selections from the following list: oxygen source (wall-mounted piped oxygen unit, cylinder) ✳ flow meter ✳ adapter (if using a wall unit) or a pressure reduction gauge (if using a cylinder) ✳ sterile water for humidification and adapters ✳ appropriate oxygen delivery system small-diameter and large-diameter connection tubing ✳ jet adapter for Venturi mask (if adding humidity).

Getting ready

• Instruct the patient, other patients nearby and visitors not to use devices that can cause a spark; they shouldn't smoke or use alcohol-based sprays.
• Perform a baseline oximetry.

How you do it

• Check the oxygen concentration that has been prescribed.
• Check the patency of the patient's nostrils (may need a mask if they're blocked). Consult the doctor if a change in administration route is necessary.

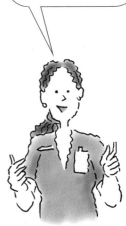

Don't forget basic position changes for patients on bed rest. Practise good skin care to prevent irritation and breakdown caused by oxygen devices.

- Assemble the equipment, check the connections and turn on the oxygen source. Make sure the humidifier bubbles and oxygen flows through the nasal cannulae or mask.
- Set the flow rate as prescribed and sign for administering the oxygen and record how it is delivered.

To everything turn, turn, turn

- If the patient is on bed rest, change their position frequently to ensure adequate ventilation and circulation.
- Provide good skin care to prevent irritation and breakdown caused by the tubing, nasal cannulae or mask.

To humidify or not to humidify

- Be sure to humidify oxygen flow exceeding 3 L/minute for over 24 hours to help prevent drying of mucous membranes. However, don't add humidity when using a Venturi mask because water can block the Venturi jets.
- Assess for signs of hypoxia, including decreased level of consciousness, tachycardia, arrhythmias, restlessness, altered blood pressure or respiratory rate, clammy skin and cyanosis. If these occur, notify the doctor, obtain a pulse oximetry reading, and check the oxygen delivery equipment to see whether it's malfunctioning. Be especially alert for changes in respiratory status when you change or discontinue oxygen therapy.

Check those symptoms

- If the patient receives high oxygen concentrations (exceeding 50%) for more than 24 hours, ask about symptoms of oxygen toxicity, such as burning, substernal chest pain, dyspnoea and dry cough. Atelectasis and pulmonary oedema may also occur.

Take a deep breath and cough

- Encourage coughing and deep breathing to help prevent atelectasis. Monitor pulse oximetry values frequently and reduce oxygen concentrations as soon as pulse oximetry values indicate it's feasible.
- Use a low flow rate if your patient has chronic pulmonary disease. However, don't use a simple facemask because low flow rates won't flush carbon dioxide from the mask and the patient will rebreathe carbon dioxide. Watch for alterations in loss of consciousness, heart rate and respiratory rate.

Go home with the flow

- If the patient needs long-term oxygen at home, this will be prescribed and then provided by the NHS. Two types of delivery systems are available: an oxygen cylinder or an oxygen concentrator. The down-side

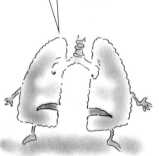

Be aware that too much oxygen can cause oxygen toxicity, with such symptoms as burning, substernal chest pain and dyspnoea.

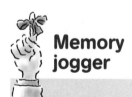

Memory jogger

If you suspect that your patient is becoming hypoxic, check for high, low, clammy and blue:

↑ heart rate, respiratory rate and restlessness

↓ level of consciousness

clammy skin

blue colouring (cyanosis).

to oxygen cylinders is that they need changing frequently, whereas the concentrator runs off electricity, taking in room air, and a filter removes the nitrogen. Make sure the patient can use the prescribed system safely and effectively. They'll need regular follow-up care to evaluate their response to therapy.

Pulse oximetry

Pulse oximetry is a non-invasive way to monitor your patient's oxygen saturation to determine how well his lungs are delivering oxygen to his blood. It can be performed continuously or intermittently.

Light reading

In pulse oximetry, two diodes send red and infrared light through a pulsating arterial vascular bed such as the one in the fingertip. A photodetector slipped over the finger measures the transmitted light as it passes through the vascular bed, detects the relative amount of colour absorbed by arterial blood and calculates the exact mix of venous oxygen saturation without interference from surrounding venous blood, skin, connective tissue or bone. (See *How oximetry works*, page 238.)

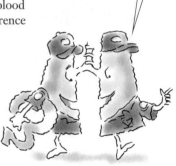

Pulse oximetry measures how well I deliver oxygen to the blood. I'd say I'm right on time, every time!

Symbolically speaking

Pulse oximeters usually denote arterial saturation values with the symbol SpO_2. Invasively measured arterial oxygen saturation values, such as from arterial blood gas analysis, on the other hand, are denoted by the symbol SaO_2.

What you need

Pulse oximeter ✳ nail polish remover, if necessary

Getting ready

• Review the manufacturer's directions for assembling the oximeter.
• Select a finger for the test. Although the index finger is commonly used, a smaller finger may be selected if the patient's fingers are too large for the equipment.
• Make sure the patient isn't wearing false fingernails, and remove any nail polish from the test finger.

How you do it

• Place the transducer (photodetector) probe over the patient's finger so that the light beam sensors oppose each other. If the patient has long fingernails, position the probe perpendicular to the finger, if possible, or clip the fingernail.

How oximetry works

The pulse oximeter allows non-invasive monitoring of a patient's arterial oxygen saturation (SaO_2) levels by measuring the absorption (amplitude) of light waves as they pass through areas of the body that are highly perfused by arterial blood. Oximetry also monitors pulse rate and amplitude.

Light-emitting diodes in a transducer (photodetector) attached to the patient's body (shown at right on the index finger) send red and infrared light beams through tissue. The photodetector records the relative amount of each colour absorbed by arterial blood and transmits the data to a monitor, which displays the information with each heartbeat. If the SaO_2 level or pulse rate varies from preset limits, the monitor triggers visual and audible alarms.

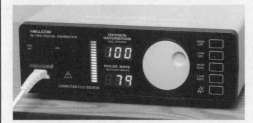
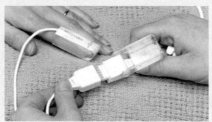

Be level with the heart

• Always position the patient's hand at heart level *to eliminate venous pulsations and promote accurate readings*. (See *Measuring pulse oximetry in infants*.)
• Turn on the power switch. If the device isn't working properly, a beep will sound, a display will light momentarily and the pulse searchlight will flash. The SpO_2 and pulse rate displays will show stationary zeros. After four to six heartbeats, the SpO_2 and the pulse rate displays will supply information with each heartbeat, and the pulse amplitude indicator will begin tracking the pulse.

Practice pointers

If oximetry has been performed properly, readings are typically accurate. However, certain factors, such as a low body temperature and low blood pressure, may interfere with accuracy.

Detour over the bridge

• If the patient has compromised circulation in their extremities, you can place a photodetector across the bridge of the nose.
• If an automatic blood pressure cuff is used on the same extremity that's used for measuring SpO_2, the cuff will interfere with SpO_2 readings during inflation.

Ages and stages

Measuring pulse oximetry in infants

If you must monitor arterial oxygen saturation in a neonate or a small infant, wrap the oximeter probe around the infant's ball of the foot so that light beams and detectors oppose each other. For a large infant, use a probe that fits around the nailbed of the big toe.

Problem-solving

- Normal SpO$_2$ levels for pulse oximetry are 95% to 100% for adults and 93.8% to 100% by 1 hour after birth for healthy, full-term neonates. Lower levels may indicate hypoxaemia, which warrants intervention. For such patients, the doctor should be notified. (See *Documenting pulse oximetry*.)

Tracheostomy care

Whether a tracheotomy is performed in an emergency situation or after careful preparation, as a permanent measure or as temporary therapy, tracheostomy care has identical goals:
- Ensure airway patency by keeping the tube free from build-up of secretions.
- Maintain mucous membrane and skin integrity.
- Prevent infection.
- Provide psychological support.

Simple, medium and complex

The patient may have one of three types of tracheostomy tube:

an uncuffed tube, which may be plastic, polyvinyl chloride or metal, comes in various sizes, lengths and styles depending on the patient's needs. It allows air to flow freely around the tracheostomy tube and through the larynx, reducing the risk of tracheal damage.

a fenestrated tube allows speech to be possible through the upper airway when the external opening is capped and the cuff is deflated. Mechanical ventilation is possible with the inner cannula in place and the cuff inflated.

a cuffed tube is made of plastic or polyvinyl chloride and is disposable. The cuff and the tube won't separate accidentally inside the trachea because the cuff is bonded to the tube. Also, it doesn't require periodic deflating to lower pressure because cuff pressure is low and evenly distributed against the tracheal wall. Although cuffed tubes may cost more than other tubes, they reduce the risk of tracheal damage.

Keepin' it clean

Whichever tube is used, tracheostomy care involving care of the stoma, changing the dressing and tapes should be performed using aseptic technique.

What you need

For changing a tracheostomy dressing and tapes
Sterile dressing pack ✳ cleaning solution such as 0.9% sodium chloride ✳ wound swab (if infection suspected) ✳ sterile 4″ × 4″ gauze pads ✳ sterile

Take note!

Document-ing pulse oximetry

In your notes, document the procedure, including the date, time, procedure type, oxygen saturation measurement and actions taken. Record the readings on appropriate charts, if indicated.

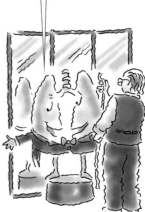

I think I like a little more cuff showing.

gloves ✳ pre-packaged sterile tracheostomy dressing ✳ equipment and supplies for suctioning and mouth care ✳ tracheostomy tapes/fixation device

Cleaning a stoma, outer cannula and changing fixation device/tapes

- Explain and discuss the procedure to the patient.
- Close the curtains around the bed area.
- Wash hands.
- Perform the procedure using an aseptic non-touch technique. Put on sterile gloves.
- Two nurses are required to change the dressing and tube fixation device/tapes. One nurse should hold the tube in place while the dressing and fixation device/tapes are changed *because of the risk of accidental tube expulsion during this procedure*. Patient movement or coughing can dislodge the tube.
- Remove the soiled dressing from around the tube. Using gauze, clean around the tube with 0.9% sodium chloride. Wipe only once with each piece of gauze and then discard it *to prevent contamination of a clean area*.
- Inspect the stoma site for colour, amount of secretions and signs of infection. Swab the site if infection is suspected.
- Dry the area thoroughly with additional sterile gauze pads; then apply a new sterile tracheostomy dressing. Wipe only once with each piece of gauze and then discard it *to prevent contamination of a clean area with a soiled pad*.
- Renew the tracheostomy fixation device/tapes, ensuring that 1 to 2 fingers can be placed between the tapes and neck.
- Remove and discard your gloves and rubbish as per local policy.
- Wash your hands and document dressing change.

What you need

For changing a tracheostomy inner tube
Disposable gloves and apron ✳ spare/new inner tube ✳ warm sterile water ✳ suction equipment ✳ alcohol hand rub

Changing a tracheostomy inner tube
- Discuss the procedure with the patient and explain that it may cause the patient to cough.
- You need to be familiar with how the inner tube is locked in place to the outer tube.
- Wash hands and put on disposable apron and gloves.
- Where oxygen is attached, temporarily disconnect.

Remove and replace

- Unlock the inner tube and remove the inner tube, following the line of the tracheostomy.

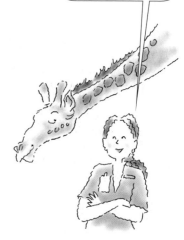

Can you imagine having to suction a patient with a trachea this long?

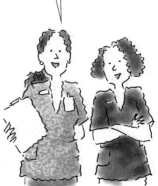

Always elicit the help of another nurse before attempting to change tracheostomy ties.

• Insert the replacement inner tube into the outer tube, following the line of the tracheostomy. Lock the inner tube in place.

Scrub a dub-dub

• If using a reusable inner tube, clean the inner tube in warm sterile water and leave to air dry before you reinsert.

Replace and record

• Reconnect oxygen if required.
• Document procedure.

Concluding tracheostomy care

• Provide oral care as needed because the oral cavity can become dry and malodorous or develop sores from encrusted secretions.

What not to do

• Refrain from changing tracheostomy ties unnecessarily during the immediate post-operative period before the stoma track is well formed (usually 4 days) *to avoid accidental dislodgment and expulsion of the tube.* Unless secretions or drainage is a problem, ties can be changed once per day.

Class time

• If the patient is being discharged with a tracheostomy, start self-care teaching as soon as they're receptive. Teach the patient how to change and clean the tube.
• Assess for complications, which can occur within the first 48 hours after tracheostomy tube insertion. Complications can include haemorrhage at the operative site, causing drowning; bleeding or oedema in tracheal tissue, causing airway obstruction; aspiration of secretions; introduction of air into the pleural cavity, causing pneumothorax; hypoxia or acidosis, triggering cardiac arrest; and introduction of air into surrounding tissues, causing subcutaneous emphysema. (See *Documenting tracheostomy care*, page 242.)

Tracheal suction

Tracheal suction involves the removal of secretions from the trachea or bronchi by means of a catheter inserted through the mouth or nose, a tracheal stoma, a tracheostomy tube or an endotracheal (ET) tube. This section will look at tracheal suction through a tracheostomy tube. *This should not be performed by a student nurse without direct supervision.*

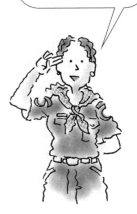

Be prepared by knowing the correct way to thread ties and secure knots. And always remember, patient safety first!

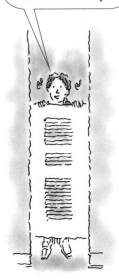

Take a lesson from teenage girls everywhere… Frequent dressing changes are, like, sooo necessary!

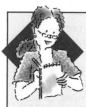

Take note!

Documenting tracheostomy care

When you've finished performing tracheostomy care, record in your notes:

- date and time of the procedure
- type of procedure
- amount, consistency, colour and odour of secretions
- stoma and skin condition
- patient's respiratory status
- tracheostomy tube changes
- complications and nursing actions taken
- patient's tolerance of the procedure
- patient or family teaching provided.

Say no to pneumonia

In addition to removing secretions, tracheal suctioning also stimulates the cough reflex. This procedure helps maintain a patent airway to promote optimal exchange of oxygen and carbon dioxide and to prevent pneumonia that results from pooling of secretions. Performed as frequently as the patient's condition warrants, tracheal suction calls for strict aseptic technique.

What you need

Wall or portable suction apparatus ✳ collection container ✳ tubing ✳ sterile suction catheters ✳ disposable plastic apron ✳ eye protection (goggles) ✳ non-sterile, clean boxed gloves ✳ sterile disposable gloves (if new surgically formed tracheostomy) ✳ bottle of sterile water (labelled 'suction' with date of opening ✳ alcohol hand rub

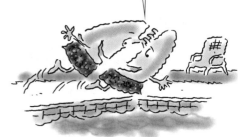

Sometimes a pool can be fun—but not when it's a pool of secretions. Yuck!

Getting ready

- Choose the correct suction catheter. The diameter should be no larger than half the inside diameter of the tracheostomy or ET tube *to minimise hypoxia during suctioning*. Use the following formula to ensure the correct size: multiply the internal diameter of the tracheostomy tube by two, and then subtract four to calculate the french gauge (Fg) size.
- Check the suction pressure is set to the appropriate level.
- Attach the collection container to the suction unit and the connecting tube to the collection container. Label and date sterile water. Put on disposable apron and goggles.

How you do it

- Assess the patient's vital signs, breath sounds and general appearance *to establish a baseline for comparison after suctioning*. Review the patient's arterial blood gas (ABG) values and oxygen saturation levels, if they're available. If you'll be performing nasotracheal suctioning, check the patient's history for a deviated septum, nasal polyps, nasal obstruction, nasal trauma, epistaxis or mucosal swelling.

• Wash your hands. Explain the procedure to the patient even if he's unresponsive.

Positioned to cough

• Unless contraindicated, place the patient in an upright position *to promote lung expansion and productive coughing*.
• If the patient is oxygen-dependent, hyper-oxygenate for 3 minutes and encourage the patient to deep-breathe before suctioning.
• Using your non-dominant hand, set the suction pressure according to local policy. Typically, pressure may be set between 80 and 150 mmHg or lower for paediatric patients. *Higher pressures may cause traumatic injury.* Occlude the suction port *to assess suction pressure*.

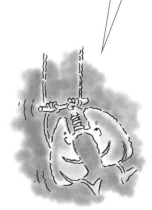

And now for my big finale...a full-twisting double front layout dismount from an upright position.

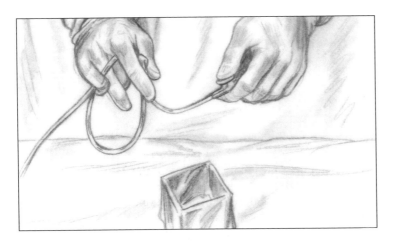

• Remove the top from the water bottle.
• Open the end of the suction catheter and use the pack to attach the catheter to the suction tubing.

For a new surgically formed tracheostomy use an individually packed sterile disposable glove on the dominant hand, and a non-sterile glove on your non-dominant hand. Non-sterile gloves on both hands can be worn for subsequent admissions.

One hand does this...

Using your dominant (sterile) hand, unwrap the catheter. Keep it coiled so it can't touch a non-sterile object.

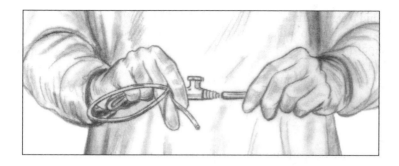

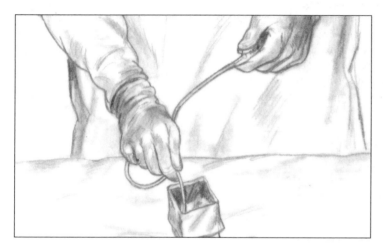

Suctioning the patient

• Introduce the catheter to about one-third of its length, until the resistance of the carina is felt or the patient coughs. If resistance is felt, withdraw the catheter approximately 1 cm before applying suction, by placing the thumb over the suction port and withdraw the remainder of the catheter gently. After inserting the catheter, apply suction intermittently by removing and replacing the thumb of your non-dominant hand over the control valve. *Monitor heart rate and oxygen saturation levels while suctioning.* Simultaneously use your dominant hand to withdraw the catheter as you roll it between your thumb and forefinger. *This rotating motion prevents the catheter from pulling tissue into the tube as it exits, avoiding tissue trauma.* Never suction more than 10 to 15 seconds (1 breath cycle) at a time *to prevent hypoxia.* Pull back glove over used catheter to contain catheter, and discard.

Oxygen

• If applicable, resume oxygen delivery by reconnecting the source of oxygen and hyperoxygenating the patient's lungs before continuing *to prevent or relieve hypoxia.*

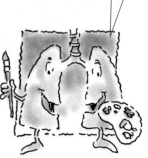

I paint a pretty good picture of the general suctioning procedure, don't I?

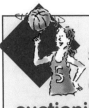

Stay on the ball

Common complications of tracheal suctioning

- hypoxaemia and dyspnoea from removal of oxygen along with secretions
- altered respiratory patterns from anxiety
- cardiac arrhythmias from hypoxia and vagus nerve stimulation
- tracheal or bronchial trauma from traumatic or prolonged suctioning
- hypoxaemia, arrhythmias, hypertension and hypotension in patients with compromised cardiovascular or pulmonary status
- bleeding in patients with those receiving anticoagulants, those who have undergone a recent tracheostomy and those with blood dyscrasias
- further rise in intracranial pressure (ICP) in patients with increased ICP.

Take note!

Documenting tracheal suctioning

In your notes, document:

- date and time of the procedure
- suctioning technique used
- reason for suctioning
- amount, colour, consistency and odour of secretions
- complications and nursing actions taken
- patient's tolerance of the procedure.

• Observe the patient, and allow him to rest for a few minutes before the next suctioning. If the patient requires further suction, repeat the above using new gloves and catheter. Repeat until the airway is clear.

After suctioning

• An assessment should be made of the type, tenacity, consistency and amount of secretions.

• Discard the gloves, apron, goggles and catheter. Clear the connecting tubing by aspirating water from the bottle of sterile water until the tubing has been rinsed through. Discard and replace suction equipment and supplies according to local policy. Wash your hands.

Practice pointers

• Don't allow the collection container on the suction machine to become more than three quarters full *to keep from damaging the machine*.

• Assess the patient for complications of tracheal suctioning. (See *Common complications of tracheal suctioning*, for details.)

• Document the procedure according to local policy. (See *Documenting tracheal suctioning*.)

Managing Chest Drains

Thoracic drainage uses gravity (and occasionally suction) to restore negative pressure, to remove material that collects in the pleural cavity or to re-expand a partially or totally collapsed lung. An underwater seal in the drainage system allows air and fluid to escape from the pleural cavity but doesn't allow air to re-enter.

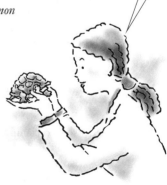

I wonder whether an aquatic turtle works as well as an underwater seal in these situations.

It is important that patients with chest drains are nursed in an environment where nurses have the relevant knowledge and experience.

Managing closed chest underwater-seal drainage

• Repeatedly note the character, consistency and amount of drainage in the drainage collection chamber.
• Mark the drainage level in the drainage collection chamber by noting the time and date at the drainage level on the chamber. Frequency of recordings will depend upon the condition of the patient and expected fluid loss. Local policy should be followed.

Look for the level

• Check the water level in the water-seal chamber every 8 hours. If necessary, carefully add sterile distilled water until the level reaches the 2 cm mark indicated on the water-seal chamber of the commercial system.
• Check for fluctuation in the water-seal chamber as the patient breathes. Normal fluctuations of 5 to 10 cm reflect pressure changes in the pleural space during respiration. To check for fluctuation when a suction system is being used, momentarily disconnect the suction system so the air vent is opened, and observe for fluctuation.

Bubbles, bubbles everywhere

• Check for intermittent bubbling/swinging in the water-seal chamber. Bubbling occurs normally when the system is removing air from the pleural cavity. If bubbling isn't readily apparent during quiet breathing, have the patient take a deep breath or cough. Absence of bubbling indicates that the pleural space has sealed.
• Check the water level in the suction-control chamber. Detach the chamber from the suction source; when bubbling ceases, observe the water level. If necessary, add sterile distilled water to bring the level to the 20 cm line or as ordered.
• Check for gentle bubbling in the suction-control chamber *because it indicates that the proper suction level has been reached.* Vigorous bubbling in this chamber increases the rate of water evaporation.
• Periodically check that the air vent in the system is working properly. Occlusion of the air vent results in a build-up of pressure in the system that could cause the patient to develop a tension pneumothorax.

Always ready to clamp down

• Be sure to keep two rubber-tipped clamps at the bedside to clamp the chest tube if the system cracks or to locate an air leak in the system. (See *Clamping alert.*)
• Encourage the patient to cough frequently and breathe deeply *to help drain the pleural space and expand the lungs.*

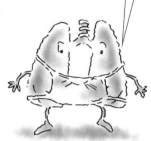

Keep it sterile to prevent pathogens from entering the pleural space.

I don't know about you but, to me, gentle bubbling indicates pure relaxation!

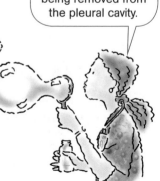

The amount of bubbling can tell you a lot about how efficiently air is being removed from the pleural cavity.

- Tell them to sit upright *for optimal lung expansion* and to splint the insertion site while coughing *to minimise pain*.
- Check the rate and quality of the patient's respirations.

Cause for alarm

- Tell the patient to report breathing difficulty immediately. Notify the doctor immediately if the patient develops cyanosis, rapid or shallow breathing, subcutaneous emphysema, chest pain or excessive bleeding.
- Check the chest tube dressing at least every 8 hours. Palpate the area surrounding the dressing for crepitus or subcutaneous emphysema, which indicates that air is leaking into the subcutaneous tissue surrounding the insertion site. Change the dressing if necessary or according to local policy.
- Give prescribed analgesia as needed for comfort and to help with deep breathing and coughing.

Practice pointers

- Avoid lifting the drainage system above the patient's chest *because fluid may flow back into the pleural space*.
- If excessive continuous bubbling is present in the water-seal chamber, especially if suction is being used, there might be a leak in the drainage system. Check for loose connections in tubing and around drainage system. Inform medical staff if no leak is found.
- If the drainage collection chamber fills, replace it. To do this, double-clamp the tube close to the insertion site (use two clamps facing in opposite directions), exchange the system, remove the clamps and retape the bottle connection.

If there's a crack

- If the commercially prepared system cracks, clamp the chest tube momentarily with the two rubber-tipped clamps at the bedside (placed there at the time of tube insertion). Place the clamps close to each other near the insertion site; they should face in opposite directions *to provide a more complete seal*. Observe the patient for altered respirations while the tube is clamped. Then replace the damaged equipment. (Prepare the new unit before clamping the tube.)
- Tension pneumothorax may result from excessive accumulation of air, drainage or both, and eventually may exert pressure on the heart and aorta, causing a precipitous fall in cardiac output.

Stay on the ball

Clamping alert

Clamping a chest drain can increase the risk of a tension pneumothorax, from pressure that builds up when air and fluid can't escape. Chest drains should only be clamped when there is accidental disconnection.

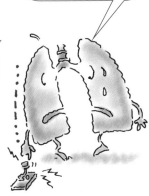

Alert the doctor immediately if the patient develops breathing difficulty or signs of complications.

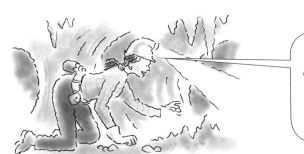

Investigate any excessive bubbling or suspected cracks promptly to rule out problems that can lead to tension pneumothorax.

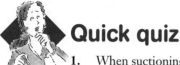

Quick quiz

1. When suctioning a patient, you should:
   A. apply suction intermittently as you insert the catheter.
   B. suction the patient for longer than 10 seconds at a time.
   C. oxygenate the patient's lungs before and after suctioning.
   D. apply suction continuously as you insert the catheter.

Answer: C. Oxygenate the patient before and after suctioning to reduce the risk of hypoxaemia, avoid suctioning for longer than 10 seconds and apply it intermittently as you withdraw the catheter.

2. To help the patient achieve maximal ventilation, use:
   A. an incentive spirometer.
   B. an MDI.
   C. a diskus.
   D. a turbo-inhaler.

Answer: A. An incentive spirometer helps achieve maximal ventilation by inducing the patient to take a deep breath and hold it.

3. Which tube permits speech through the upper airway?
   A. Uncuffed tube
   B. Cuffed tube
   C. Fenestrated tube
   D. Two-piece tube

Answer: C. A fenestrated tube permits speech through the upper airway when you cap the external opening and deflate the cuff.

4. When performing chest physiotherapy, which of the following uses gravity to promote drainage of secretions?
   A. Percussion
   B. Postural drainage
   C. Vibration
   D. Deep-breathing exercises

Answer: B. Postural drainage uses gravity to promote drainage of secretions from the lungs and bronchi into the trachea.

Scoring

✰✰✰ If you answered all four questions correctly, congrats! Your brain is saturated with knowledge of oxygenation.

✰✰ If you answered three questions correctly, good job! Your knowledge of oxygenation is perfusing nicely.

✰ If you answered fewer than three questions correctly, don't despair! Take a deep breath to re-oxygenate those tissues, and try again.

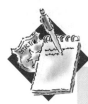

13 Skin integrity and wound healing

Just the facts

In this chapter, you'll learn:

♦ layers and functions of skin

♦ types of wounds

♦ phases of wound healing

♦ ways to classify wounds according to age, depth and colour

♦ basic wound care assessment and treatment

♦ pressure ulcer prevention, care and treatment.

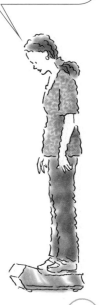

The skin accounts for about 2.5 to 3.5 kgs of a person's body weight!

A look at the skin

The skin is the largest organ in the body. It accounts for about 2.5 to 3.5 kg of a person's body weight and has a surface area of more than 20 ft^2.

The skin you're in

Skin is made up of distinct layers that function as a single unit. The outermost layer, which is actually a layer of dead cells, is completely replaced every 4 to 6 weeks by cells that migrate to the surface from the layers beneath. The living cells in the skin receive oxygen and nutrients through an extensive network of small blood vessels. In fact, every square inch of skin contains more than 158 blood vessels!

Up close and personal

Skin protects the body by acting as a barrier between internal structures and the external world. Skin also stands between each of us and the social world around us, so it's no wonder that the condition and characteristics of a person's skin influence how they feel about themself. When a person has healthy skin, unblemished skin with good tone (firmness) and colour, they feel better about themself. Skin also reflects the body's general physical health. For example if blood oxygen levels are low, skin may look bluish, (cyanosed) and skin appears flushed or red if a person has a fever.

Surgery, accidents or sun

Any damage to the skin is considered a wound. Wounds can result from planned events, such as surgery, or unplanned events, including accidents such as a fall from a bike; and exposure to the environment, such as the damage caused by ultraviolet (UV) rays in sunlight.

Functions

The skin carries out several important functions, including:

- protecting the tissues from trauma and bacteria
- preventing the loss of water and electrolytes from the body
- sensing temperature, pain, touch and pressure
- regulating body temperature through sweat production and evaporation
- synthesising vitamin D
- promoting wound repair by allowing cell replacement of surface wounds.

Layers of the skin

Skin has two main layers: the epidermis and the dermis, both of which function as one interrelated unit. A layer of subcutaneous fatty connective tissue, sometimes called the hypodermis, lies beneath these layers. Five structural networks, which are stabilised by hair and sweat gland ducts, exist within the epidermis and dermis:

 collagen fibres

 elastic fibres

small blood vessels

 nerve fibrils

 lymphatics.

Epidermis

The epidermis is the outermost of the skin's two main layers. It varies in thickness from about 0.1 mm thick on the eyelids to as much as 1 mm thick on the palms and soles. The epidermis is slightly acidic, with an average pH of 5.5. Covering the epidermis is the keratinised epithelium, a layer of cells that migrate up from the underlying dermis and die upon reaching the surface. These cells are continuously generated and replaced. The keratinised epithelium is supported by the dermis and underlying connective tissue.

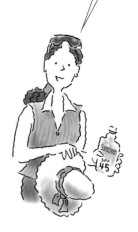

Bad burns from UV rays are wounds, too. Make sure you wear sunscreen and protect your skin!

In living colour

The epidermis also contains melanocytes, the cells that produce the brown pigment melanin, which give skin and hair their colours. The more melanin produced by melanocytes, the darker the skin. Skin colour varies not only from one person to other, but it can also vary from one area of skin on the body to another. The hypothalamus regulates melanin production by secreting melanocyte-stimulating hormone.

Layer upon layer

The epidermis is divided into five distinct layers. Each layer's name reflects its structure or its function. Here's a look at them from the outside in:

Memory jogger

You can remember the order of the skin's layers by thinking of the prefix **epi-**, which means 'upon'. Therefore, the **epi**dermis is upon, or on top of, the dermis.

The *stratum corneum* (horny layer) is the superficial layer of dead skin cells—the skin layer that's in contact with the environment. It has an acid mantle that helps protect the body from some fungi and bacteria. Cells in this layer are shed daily and replaced with cells from the layer beneath it, the stratum lucidum. In such diseases as eczema and psoriasis, the stratum corneum may become abnormally thick and irritate skin structures and peripheral nerves.

The *stratum lucidum* (clear layer) is a single layer of cells that forms a transitional boundary between the stratum corneum above and stratum granulosum below. This layer is most evident in areas where skin is thickest, as on the soles of the feet. It appears to be absent in areas where skin is especially thin, as on the eyelids. Although cells in this layer lack active nuclei, this is an area of intense enzyme activity that prepares cells for the stratum corneum.

The *stratum granulosum* (granular layer) is one to five cells thick and is characterised by flat cells with active nuclei. Experts believe this layer aids keratin formation.

The *stratum spinosum* is the area in which cells begin to flatten as they migrate towards the skin surface.

Just like this onion, your skin has a lot of layers.

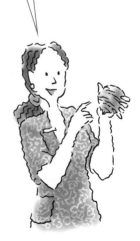

The *stratum basale*, or *stratum germinativum*, is only one cell thick and is the only layer of the epidermis in which cells undergo mitosis to form new cells. The stratum basale forms the dermoepidermal junction—the area where the epidermis and dermis are connected. Protrusions of this layer (called rete pegs or epidermal ridges) extend down into the dermis where they're surrounded by vascularised dermal papillae. This unique structure supports the epidermis and facilitates the exchange of fluids and cells between the skin layers.

Structural supports: collagen and elastin

Normally, skin returns to its original position after it's pulled on due to the actions of the connective tissues collagen and elastin—two key components of skin. Collagen and elastin work together to support the dermis and give skin its physical characteristics.

Collagen

Collagen fibres form tightly woven networks in the papillary layer of the dermis. These fibres are relatively inextensible and non-elastic and, therefore, give the dermis high tensile strength. In addition, collagen constitutes approximately 70% of the skin's dry weight and is the skin's principal structural body protein.

Elastin

Elastin is made up of wavy fibres that intertwine with collagen in horizontal arrangements at the lower dermis and vertical arrangements at the epidermal margin. Elastin makes skin pliable and is the structural protein that enables extensibility in the dermis.

Seeing the effects of age

As a person ages, collagen and elastin fibres break down and the fine lines and wrinkles that are associated with aging develop. Extensive exposure to sunlight accelerates this breakdown process. Deep wrinkles are caused by changes in facial muscles. Over time, laughing, crying, smiling and frowning cause facial muscles to thicken and eventually cause wrinkles in the overlying skin.

Memory jogger

To remember the five layers of the epidermis, think, 'Cozy Layers Generate Skin Barriers'. In other words, the epidermis consists of the stratum:

Corneum

Lucidum

Granulosum

Spinosum

Basale.

Dermis

The dermis—the thick, deeper layer of skin—is composed of collagen and elastin fibres and an extracellular matrix, which contributes to skin's strength and pliability. Collagen fibres give skin its strength, and elastin fibres provide elasticity. The meshing of collagen and elastin determines the skin's physical characteristics. (See *Structural supports: collagen and elastin*.)

In addition, the dermis contains:
• blood vessels and lymphatic vessels, which transport oxygen and nutrients to cells and remove waste products
• nerve fibres and hair follicles, which contribute to skin sensation, temperature regulation and excretion and absorption through the skin
• fibroblast cells, which are important in the production of collagen and elastin.

Laying it on thick

The dermis is composed of two layers of connective tissue:

The *papillary dermis*, the outermost layer, is composed of collagen and reticular fibres, which are important in healing wounds. Capillaries in the papillary dermis carry the nourishment needed for metabolic activity.

The *reticular dermis* is the innermost layer. It's formed by thick networks of collagen bundles that anchor it to the subcutaneous tissue and underlying support structures, such as fasciae, muscle and bone.

Sebaceous and sweat glands

Although sebaceous and sweat glands appear to originate in the dermis, they're actually appendages of the epidermis that extend downwards into the dermis.

Sebaceous glands, found primarily in the skin of the scalp, face, upper body and genital region, are part of the same structure that contains hair follicles. These sac-like glands produce sebum, a fatty substance that lubricates and softens the skin.

Sweat glands are tightly coiled tubular glands; the average person has roughly 2.6 million of them. They're present throughout the body in varying amounts. The palms and soles have many, but the external ear, lip margins, nail beds and glans penis have none.

The secreting portion of the sweat gland originates in the dermis and the outlet is on the surface of the skin. The sympathetic nervous system regulates the production of sweat, which, in turn, helps control body temperature.

There are two types of sweat glands:

Eccrine glands are active at birth and are found throughout the body. They're most dense on the palms, soles of the feet and forehead. These glands connect to the skin's surface through pores and produce sweat that lacks proteins and fatty acids. Eccrine glands are smaller than apocrine glands.

Apocrine glands begin to function at puberty. These glands open into hair follicles; therefore, most are found in areas where hair typically grows, such as the scalp, groin and axillary region. The coiled secreting portion of the gland lies deep in the dermis (deeper than eccrine glands), and a duct connects it to the upper portion of the hair follicle. The sweat produced by apocrine glands contains water, sodium, chloride, proteins and fatty acids. It's thicker than the sweat produced by eccrine glands and has a milky-white or yellowish tinge. (See *Oh no, B.O.!*)

Subcutaneous tissue

The subcutaneous tissue, or hypodermis, is a sub-dermal (below the skin) layer of loose connective tissue that contains major blood vessels, lymph vessels and nerves. Subcutaneous tissue:

* has a high proportion of fat cells and contains fewer small blood vessels than the dermis
* varies in thickness depending on body type and location
* constitutes 15% to 20% of a man's weight; 20% to 25% of a woman's weight

Oh no, B.O.!

The sweat produced by apocrine glands contains the same water, sodium and chloride found in the sweat produced by eccrine glands. However, it also contains proteins and fatty acids. The unpleasant odour associated with sweat comes from the interaction of bacteria with these proteins and fatty acids.

- insulates the body
- absorbs shocks to the skeletal system
- helps skin move easily over underlying structures.

Blood supply

The skin receives its blood supply through vessels that originate in the underlying muscle tissue. Here, arteries branch into smaller vessels, which then branch into the network of capillaries that permeate the dermis and subcutaneous tissue.

The thin and thinner of it

Within the vascular system, only capillaries have walls thin enough (typically only a single layer of endothelial cells) to let solutes pass through. These thin walls allow nutrients and oxygen to pass from the bloodstream into the interstitial space around skin cells. At the same time, waste products pass into the capillaries and are carried away. The pressure of arterial blood entering the capillaries is approximately 30 mmHg. The pressure of venous blood leaving the capillaries is approximately 10 mmHg. This 20-mmHg difference in pressure within the capillaries is quite low when compared with the pressure found in the larger arteries in the body (85 to 100 mmHg), which is known as blood pressure.

Lymphatic system

The skin's lymphatic system helps remove waste products from the dermis.

Go with the flow

Lymphatic vessels, or lymphatics for short, are similar to capillaries in that they're thin-walled, permeable vessels. However, lymphatics aren't part of the blood circulatory system. Instead, the lymphatics belong to a separate system that removes proteins, large waste products and excess fluids from the interstitial spaces in skin and transports them to the venous circulation. The lymphatics merge into two main trunks—the thoracic duct and the right lymphatic duct—which empty into the junction of the subclavian and internal jugular veins.

Functions of the skin

Skin performs or participates in a host of vital functions, including:
- protection of internal structures
- sensory perception
- thermoregulation
- excretion

- metabolism
- absorption
- social communication.

Damage to skin impairs its ability to carry out these important functions. Let's take a closer look at each.

Protection

Skin acts as a physical barrier to microorganisms and foreign matter, protecting the body against infection. It also protects underlying tissue and structures from mechanical injury. Consider the feet for a moment. As a person walks or runs, the soles of the feet withstand a tremendous amount of force, yet the underlying tissue and bone structures remain unharmed.

The skin also helps maintain a stable environment inside the body by preventing the loss of water, electrolytes, proteins and other substances. Any damage (any wound) jeopardises this protection. However, when damaged, skin goes into repair mode to restore full protection by stepping up the normal process of cell replacement.

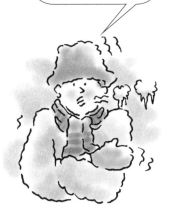

I think my nerve endings are working just fine. My sensory perception tells me I'm freezing!

Sensory perception

Nerve endings in the skin allow a person literally to touch the world around them. Sensory nerve fibres originate in the nerve roots along the spine and supply specific areas of the skin known as dermatomes. Dermatomes are used to document sensory function. This same network helps a person avoid injury by making them aware of pain, pressure, heat and cold.

Just sensational

Sensory nerves exist throughout the skin; however, some areas are more sensitive than others—for example the fingertips are more sensitive than the back. Sensation allows us to identify potential dangers and avoid injury. Any loss or reduction of sensation, local or general, increases the chance of injury.

Thermoregulation

Thermoregulation, or control of body temperature, involves the concerted effort of nerves, blood vessels and eccrine glands in the dermis.

Warming up

When skin is exposed to cold or internal body temperature falls, blood vessels constrict, reducing blood flow, and thereby conserving body heat.

Cooling down

Similarly, if skin becomes too hot or internal body temperature rises, small arteries within the skin dilate, increasing the blood flow, and sweat production increases to promote cooling.

Excretion

Unlikely as it may seem at first, the skin is an excretory organ. Excretion through the skin plays an important role in thermoregulation, electrolyte balance and hydration. In addition, sebum excretion helps maintain the skin's integrity and suppleness.

Water works

Through its more than two million pores, skin efficiently transmits trace amounts of water and body wastes to the environment. At the same time, it prevents dehydration by ensuring that the body doesn't lose too much water. Sweat carries water and salt to the skin surface, where it evaporates, aiding thermoregulation and electrolyte balance. In addition, a small amount of water evaporates directly from the skin itself each day. A normal adult loses about 500 ml of water per day this way. While the skin is busy regulating fluids that are leaving the body, it's equally busy preventing unwanted or dangerous fluids from entering the body.

Metabolism

Skin also helps maintain the mineralisation of bones and teeth. A photochemical reaction in the skin produces vitamin D, which is crucial to the metabolism of calcium and phosphate. These minerals, in turn, play a central role in the health of bones and teeth.

Let the sun shine in

When skin is exposed to sunlight—the UV spectrum in sunlight, to be specific—vitamin D is synthesised in a photochemical reaction. Keep in mind, however, that, although some sunlight works wonders, overexposure to UV light causes skin damage that reduces its ability to function properly.

Absorption

Some drugs and, unfortunately, some toxic substances—for example pesticides—can be absorbed directly through the skin and into the bloodstream. This process has been used to treat certain disorders via skin patch drug delivery systems. One of the best-known examples of this method is the patch used in some nicotine withdrawal programmes. However, today this technology is also used to administer some forms of hormone replacement therapy, nitroglycerin and some pain medications.

Social communication

A commonly overlooked but important function of the skin is its role in self-esteem development and social communication. Every time a person looks in the mirror they decide whether they like what they see. Although bone structure, body type, teeth and hair (or lack thereof!) all have an impact, the condition and characteristics of skin can have the greatest impact on a person's self-esteem. Ask any teenager with acne. If a person likes what they see, self-esteem rises; if they don't, it sags.

What you see

Virtually every interpersonal exchange includes the non-verbal languages of facial expression and body posture. Level of self-esteem and skin characteristics, which are visible at all times, have an impact on how a person communicates verbally and non-verbally and how a listener receives the person communicating.

Because the physical characteristics of skin are so closely linked to self-perception, there has been a proliferation of skin-care products and surgical techniques offered to keep skin looking young and healthy.

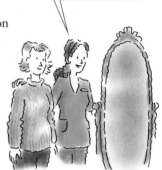

Skin is very important to self-esteem and social communication. Remember that when you're treating patients.

A look at wound healing

Any break in the skin is considered a wound. Wounds can result from a planned event, such as surgery, or from an unexpected event, such as an accident, trauma or exposure to pressure, heat, sun or chemicals. Tissue damage in wounds varies widely, from a superficial break in the epithelium to deep trauma that involves the muscle and bone.

A 'clean' wound is a wound produced by surgery. A wound is described as 'dirty' if it may contain bacteria or debris. Trauma typically produces dirty wounds. The rate of recovery is influenced by the extent and type of damage incurred as well as other intrinsic factors, such as patient circulation, nutrition, hydration and the presence of a chronic illness. However, regardless of the cause of a wound, the healing process is similar in all cases.

Types of wound healing

Wounds are classified by the way the wound closes. A wound can close by primary intention, secondary intention or tertiary intention.

Primary intention
Primary healing involves re-epithelialisation, in which the skin's outer layer grows closed. Cells grow in from the margins of the wound and out from epithelial cells lining the hair follicles and sweat glands.

Just a scratch

Wounds that heal through primary intention are, most commonly, superficial wounds that involve only the epidermis and don't involve the loss of tissue—a first-degree burn, for example. However, a wound that has well-approximated

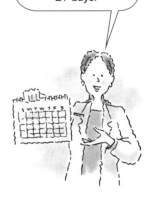

Wounds that heal by primary intention usually do so within 21 days.

edges (edges that can be pulled together to meet neatly), such as a surgical incision, also heals through primary intention. Because there's no loss of tissue and little risk of infection, the healing process is predictable. These wounds usually heal in 4 to 21 days and result in minimal scarring.

Secondary intention

A wound that involves some degree of tissue loss heals by secondary intention. The edges of these wounds can't be easily approximated, and the wound itself is described as partial-thickness or full-thickness, depending on its depth:
• Partial-thickness wounds extend through the epidermis and into, but not through, the dermis.
• Full-thickness wounds extend through the epidermis and dermis and may involve subcutaneous tissue, muscle and, possibly, bone.

Getting under the skin

During healing, wounds that heal by secondary intention fill with granulation tissue, a scar forms, and re-epithelialisation occurs, primarily from the wound edges. Pressure ulcers, burns, dehisced surgical wounds and traumatic injuries are examples of this type of wound. These wounds also take longer to heal, result in scarring, and have a higher rate of complications, such as the development of an infection, than wounds that heal by primary intention.

Tertiary intention

When a wound is intentionally kept open to allow oedema or infection to resolve or to permit removal of exudate, the wound heals by tertiary intention, or delayed primary intention. These wounds result in more scarring than the wounds that heal by primary intention but less than the wounds that heal by secondary intention.

Phases of wound healing

The healing process is the same for all wounds, irrespective of whether the cause is mechanical, chemical or thermal.

Don't let it phase you

Health-care professionals discuss the process of wound healing in four specific phases:
• haemostasis
• inflammation
• proliferation
• maturation.
    Although this categorisation is useful, it's important to remember that healing rarely occurs in this strict order. Typically, the phases of wound healing overlap. (See *How wounds heal*.)

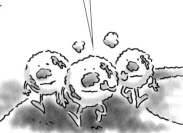

C'mon, lads! We've got to begin the process of cleaning and healing the wound!

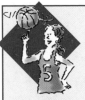

Stay on the ball

How wounds heal

The healing process begins at the instant of injury and proceeds through a repair 'cascade', as outlined here.

1. When tissue is damaged, serotonin, histamine, prostaglandins and blood from the injured vessels fill the area. Blood platelets form a clot, and fibrin in the clot binds the wound edges together.

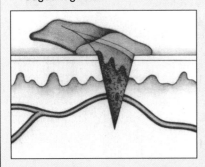

2. Lymphocytes initiate the inflammatory response, increasing capillary permeability. Wound edges swell; white blood cells from surrounding vessels move in and ingest bacteria and cellular debris, demolishing the clot. Redness, warmth, swelling, pain and loss of function may occur.

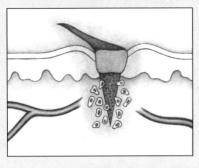

3. Adjacent healthy tissue supplies blood, nutrients, fibroblasts, proteins and other building materials needed to form soft, pink and highly vascular granulation tissue, which begins to bridge the area. Inflammation may decrease; or signs and symptoms of infection (increased swelling, increased pain, fever, and pus-filled discharge) may develop.

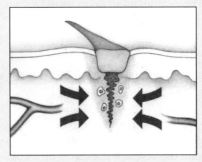

4. Fibroblasts in the granulation tissue secrete collagen, a glue-like substance. Collagen fibres crisscross the area, forming scar tissue.

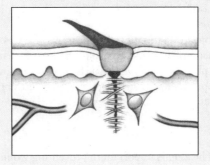

5. Meanwhile, epithelial cells at the wound edge multiply and migrate towards the wound centre. A new layer of surface cells replaces the layer that was destroyed. New, healthy tissue or granulation tissue (if the blood supply is inadequate) appears.

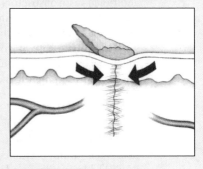

6. Damaged tissue (including lymphatics, blood vessels and stromal matrices) regenerates. Collagen fibres shorten, and the scar diminishes in size. Scar size may decrease and normal function return or the scar may hypertrophy, leading to the formation of a keloid and the development of contractures.

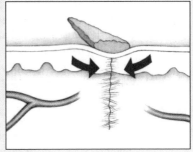

Haemostasis

Immediately after an injury, the body releases chemical mediators and intercellular messengers called growth factors that begin the process of cleaning and healing the wound.

Slow that flow!

When blood vessels are damaged, the small muscles in the walls of the vessels contract (vasoconstriction), reducing the flow of blood to the injury and minimising blood loss. Vasoconstriction can last as long as 30 minutes.

Next, blood leaking from the inflamed, dilated or broken vessels begins to coagulate. Collagen fibres in the wall of the damaged blood vessels activate the platelets in the blood in the wound. Aided by the action of prostaglandins, the platelets enlarge and stick together to form a temporary plug in the blood vessel, which helps prevent further bleeding. The platelets also release additional vasoconstrictors such as serotonin, which help prevent further blood loss. Thrombin forms in a cascade of events stimulated by the platelets, and a clot forms to close the small vessels and stop the bleeding.

This initial phase of wound healing occurs almost immediately after the injury occurs and works quickly (within minutes) in small wounds. It's less effective in stopping the bleeding in larger wounds.

Inflammation

The inflammatory phase is a defence mechanism and a crucial component of the healing process. (See *Understanding the inflammatory response*.) During this phase, the wound is cleaned and the process of rebuilding begins. This phase is marked by swelling, redness and heat at the wound site.

During the inflammatory phase, vascular permeability increases, permitting serous fluid carrying small amounts of cell and plasma protein to accumulate in the tissue around the wound (oedema). The accumulation of fluid causes the damaged tissue to appear swollen, red and warm to the touch.

Seek and destroy

During the early phase of the inflammatory process, neutrophils (one type of white blood cell [WBC]) enter the wound. The primary role of neutrophils is phagocytosis, or the removal and destruction of bacteria and other contaminants.

As neutrophil infiltration slows, monocytes appear. Monocytes are converted into activated macrophages and continue the job of cleaning the wound. The macrophages play a key role early in the process of granulation and re-epithelialisation by producing growth factors and by attracting the cells needed for the formation of new blood vessels and collagen.

Telling time

The inflammatory phase of healing is important in preventing wound infection. The process is negatively influenced if the patient has a systemic condition that

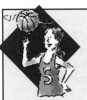

Stay on the ball

Understanding the inflammatory response

This flowchart outlines the sequence of events in the inflammatory process.

Microorganisms invade damaged tissue.

Basophils release heparin, and histamine and kinin production occurs.

Vasodilation occurs along with increased capillary permeability.

Blood flow increases to the affected tissues and fluid collects within them.

Neutrophils flock to the invasion site to engulf and destroy microorganisms from dying cells.

This repairs the tissue.

suppresses their immune system or if they're undergoing immunosuppressive therapy. In clean wounds, the inflammatory response lasts from 3 to 6 days. In dirty or infected wounds, the response can last much longer.

Proliferation

During the proliferation phase of the healing process, the body:
- fills the wound with connective tissue (granulation)
- contracts the wound edges (contraction)
- covers the wound with epithelium (epithelialisation).

All wounds go through the proliferation phase, which begins on day 3 and lasts until about day 21, but it takes much longer in wounds with extensive tissue loss. Although phases overlap, wound granulation generally starts when the inflammatory response is complete. As the inflammatory phase subsides, the wound drainage (exudate) begins to decrease.

The proliferation phase involves regeneration of blood vessels (angiogenesis) and the formation of connective or granulation tissue, which is fragile and can bleed easily. The development of granulation tissue requires an adequate supply of blood and nutrients. Endothelial cells in blood vessels in surrounding tissue reconstruct damaged or destroyed vessels by first migrating and then proliferating to form new capillary beds. As the beds form, this area of the wound takes on a red, granular appearance. This tissue is a good defence against contaminants, but it's also quite fragile and bleeds easily.

The rebuilding process

During the proliferation phase, growth factors prompt fibroblasts to migrate to the wound. Fibroblasts are the most common cell in connective tissue. They're responsible for making fibres and ground substance, also known as extracellular matrix, which provides support to cells. At first, fibroblasts populate just the margins of the wound but, later, they spread over the entire wound surface.

Fibroblasts have the important task of synthesising collagen fibres that, in turn, produce keratinocyte, a growth factor needed for re-epithelialisation. This process necessitates a delicate balance of collagen synthesis and lysis (making new and removing old). If the process yields too much collagen, increased scarring results. If the process yields too little collagen, scar tissue is weak and easily ruptured. Because fibroblasts require a supply of oxygen to perform their important role, capillary bed regeneration is crucial to the process.

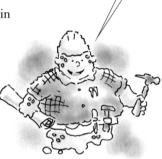

I'm your local fibroblast and I'm here to build support to these cells.

Pulling it all together

As healing progresses, myofibroblasts and the newly formed collagen fibres contract, pulling the wound edges towards each other. Contraction reduces the amount of granulation tissue needed to fill the wound, thereby speeding the healing process. (See *Contraction vs. contracture*.)

Complete healing occurs only after epithelial cells have completely covered the surface of the wound. As this occurs, keratinocytes switch from a migrating mode to a differentiating mode. The epidermis thickens and

---

Contraction vs. contracture

Contraction and contracture occur during the wound healing process. Although they have mechanisms in common, it's important to understand how contraction and contracture differ.

Contraction

Contraction, a desirable process that takes place during healing, occurs when the edges of a wound pull towards the centre of the wound to close it. Contraction continues to close the wound until tension in the surrounding skin causes it to slow and then stop.

Contracture

Contracture is an undesirable process and a common complication of burn scarring. Typically, contracture occurs after healing is complete. Contracture involves an inordinate amount of pulling or shortening of tissue, resulting in an area of tissue with only limited ability to move. It's especially problematic over joints, which may be pulled to a flexed position. Stretching is the only way to overcome contracture, and patients typically require physiotherapy.

becomes differentiated, and the wound is closed. Any remaining scab comes off and the new epidermis is toughened by the production of keratin, which also returns the skin to its original colour.

Maturation

The final phase of wound healing is maturation, which is marked by shrinking and strengthening of the scar. This is a gradual, transitional phase of healing that can continue for months or even years after the wound has closed.

During this phase, fibroblasts leave the site of the wound, vascularisation is reduced, the scar shrinks and becomes pale, and the mature scar forms. If the wound involved extensive tissue destruction, the scar won't contain hair, sweat or sebaceous glands.

The wound gradually gains tensile strength. In primary intention wounds, tissues will achieve approximately 30% to 50% of their original strength between days 1 and 14. When fully healed, tissue will achieve, at best, approximately 80% of its original strength. Scar tissue will always be less elastic than the surrounding skin.

Factors that affect wound healing

The healing process is affected by many factors. The most important influences include:

- nutrition
- oxygenation
- infection
- age
- chronic health conditions
- medications
- smoking.

Nutrition

Proper nutrition is arguably the most important factor affecting wound healing. Unfortunately, malnutrition is a common finding among patients with wounds. For older adults, the problem is more pervasive.

Poor nutrition prolongs hospitalisation and increases the risk of medical complications, with the severity of complications being directly related to the severity of the malnutrition. In older patients, malnutrition is known to increase the risk of pressure ulcers and delay in wound healing. It may also contribute to poor tensile strength in healing wounds, with an associated increase in the risk of wound dehiscence.

Good nutrition is key when it comes to getting well.

Protein is key

Protein is critical for wounds to heal properly. In fact, a person needs to double the recommended dietary allowance of protein (from 0.8 g/kg/day to 1.6 g/kg/day) before tissue even begins to heal. If a significant amount of body weight has been lost in connection with the injury, as much as 50% of the lost weight must be regained before healing will begin. A patient who lacks protein reserves heals slowly, if at all, and a patient who's borderline malnourished can easily become malnourished under this demand.

The body needs protein to form collagen during the proliferation phase. Without adequate protein, collagen formation is reduced or delayed and the healing process slows. Studies of malnourished patients indicate that they have lower levels of serum albumin, which results in slower oxygen diffusion and, in turn, a reduction in the ability of neutrophils to kill bacteria. Wound exudate alone can contain up to 100 g of protein per day.

Other necessary nutrients

Fatty acids (lipids) are used in cell structures and play a role in the inflammatory process. Also, vitamins C, B-complex, A and E and the minerals iron, copper, zinc and calcium are important in the healing process. A zinc deficiency adversely affects the proliferation phase by slowing the rate of epithelialisation and decreasing the strength of collagen produced—and, thus, the strength of the wound.

In addition to protein and zinc, collagen synthesis requires supplies of carbohydrates and fat. Collagen cross-linking requires adequate amounts of vitamins A and C, iron and copper. Vitamin C, iron and zinc are important for developing tensile strength during the maturation phase of wound healing.

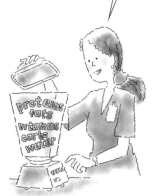

Proper wound healing depends on a blend of nutrients, including protein, fatty acids, vitamins and minerals.

Oxygenation

Healing depends on a regular supply of oxygen. For example, oxygen is critical for leucocytes to destroy bacteria and fibroblasts to stimulate collagen synthesis. If the supply is hindered by poor blood flow to the area of the wound or if the patient's ability to take in adequate oxygen is impaired, the result is the same—impaired healing.

Possible causes of inadequate blood flow to the area of the wound include pressure, arterial occlusion or prolonged vasoconstriction, possibly associated with medical conditions as peripheral vascular disease and atherosclerosis. Possible causes of a lower than necessary systemic blood oxygenation include:

- inadequate oxygen intake
- hypothermia or hyperthermia
- anaemia
- alkalaemia
- other medical conditions, such as chronic obstructive pulmonary disease.

Infection

An infection can affect wound healing or be a complication of the healing process. Infection can be systemic or localised in the wound. A systemic infection, such as pneumonia or tuberculosis, increases the patient's metabolism and thus consumes the fluids, nutrients and oxygen the body needs for healing.

Keeping it local

A localised infection in the wound itself is more common. Remember, any break in the skin allows bacteria to enter. The infection may occur as part of the injury or may develop later in the healing process. For example, when the inflammatory phase lingers, wound healing is delayed and metabolic by-products of bacterial ingestion accumulate in the wound. This build-up interferes with the formation of new blood vessels and the synthesis of collagen. Infection can also occur in a wound that has been healing normally. This situation happens especially in larger wounds involving extensive tissue damage. New or increased pain, redness, heat and drainage are signs of a new infection. In any case, healing can't progress until the cause of infection is addressed.

Age

Skin changes that occur with aging cause healing time to be prolonged in elderly patients. Although delayed healing is partially due to physiologic changes, it's also complicated by other problems associated with aging, such as poor nutrition and hydration, the presence of a chronic condition and the use of multiple medications. (See *Effects of aging on wound healing*.)

Chronic health conditions

Respiratory problems, atherosclerosis, diabetes and malignancies can increase the risk of wounds and interfere with wound healing. These conditions can interfere with systemic and peripheral oxygenation and nutrition, which affect healing.

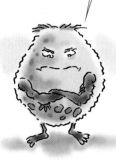

If there's a break in skin, I'll be sure to find it. Infections are my specialty.

Ages and stages

Effects of aging on wound healing

These factors impede wound healing in older adults:

- slower turnover rate in epidermal cells
- poorer oxygenation at the wound due to increasingly fragile capillaries and a reduction in skin vascularisation
- altered nutrition and fluid intake resulting from physical changes that can accompany aging, such as reduced saliva production, a declining sense of smell and taste and decreased stomach motility
- altered nutrition and fluid intake attributable to troubling personal or social issues, such as loose-fitting dentures, financial concerns, eating alone after the death of a spouse and problems preparing or obtaining food
- impaired function of the respiratory or immune systems
- reduced dermal and subcutaneous mass leading to an increased risk of chronic pressure ulcers
- healed wounds that lack tensile strength and are prone to reinjury.

Getting complicated

Impaired circulation, a common problem for patients with diabetes and other disorders, can cause tissue hypoxia (lack of oxygen). Neuropathy associated with diabetes reduces ability to sense pressure. As a result, patients with diabetes may experience trauma, especially to the feet, without realising it. Insulin dependency can impair leukocyte function, which adversely affects cell proliferation.

Hemiplegia and quadriplegia involve the breakdown of muscle tissue and reduction in the padding around the large bones of the lower body. Because a patient with one of these conditions lacks sensation, they're at risk for developing chronic pressure ulcers.

Night and day shifts

Normally, a healthy person shifts position every 15 minutes or so, even during sleep. This shifting prevents tissue damage due to ischaemia. Anything that impairs the ability to sense pressure, including spinal cord lesions, the use of pain medications and cognitive impairment, puts the patient at risk (because the patient can't feel the growing discomfort of pressure and respond to it).

Other conditions that can delay healing include dehydration, end-stage renal disease, liver disease, thyroid disease, heart failure, peripheral vascular disease and vasculitis and other collagen vascular disorders.

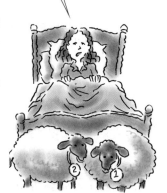

I think I've been shifting every 15 seconds! Time to try alternate measures. . .

Medications

Any medication that reduces a patient's movement, circulation or metabolic function, such as sedatives and tranquilisers, has the potential to inhibit the patient's ability to sense and respond to pressure. Also, because movement promotes adequate oxygenation, lack of motion means that peripheral blood delivers less oxygen to the extremities than it should. This decrease in oxygen is especially problematic for older adults. Remember, oxygen is important; without it, the healing process slows and the potential for complications rises.

Interruptions!

Some medications, such as steroids and chemotherapeutic agents, reduce the body's ability to mount an appropriate inflammatory response. This reduction in response interrupts the inflammatory phase of healing and can dramatically lengthen healing time, especially in a patient with a compromised immune system, such as one with acquired immunodeficiency syndrome. The use of antibiotics for long periods may place the patient at greater risk for developing an infection, which can affect wound healing.

Smoking

Carbon monoxide, a component of cigarette smoke, binds to the haemoglobin in blood in the place of oxygen. This binding significantly reduces the amount of oxygen circulating in the bloodstream, which can impede wound healing. To some extent, this reaction also occurs in people regularly exposed to second-hand smoke.

Complications of wound healing

The most common complications associated with wound healing are:
- haemorrhage
- dehiscence and evisceration
- infection
- fistula formation.

Haemorrhage

Internal haemorrhage (bleeding) can result in the formation of a haematoma— a blood clot that solidifies to form a hard lump under the skin. Haematomas are commonly found around bruises.

External haemorrhage is visible bleeding from the wound. External bleeding during healing isn't unusual because the newly developed blood vessels are fragile and rupture easily. This is one reason a wound needs to be protected by a dressing. However, each time the new blood vessels suffer damage, healing is delayed while repairs are made.

Dehiscence and evisceration

Dehiscence is a separation of skin and tissue layers. It's most likely to occur 3 to 11 days after the injury was sustained and may follow surgery. Evisceration is similar but involves protrusion of underlying visceral organs as well. (See *Recognising dehiscence and evisceration*.)

Dehiscence and evisceration may constitute a surgical emergency, especially if they involve an abdominal wound. If a wound opens without evisceration, it may need to heal by secondary intention. Poor nutrition and advanced age are two factors that increase a patient's risk of dehiscence and evisceration.

Infection

Infection is a relatively common complication of wound healing that should be addressed promptly. Infection can lead to a bacterial infection that spreads to surrounding tissue. Signs that infection may be at work include:
- redness and warmth of the margins and tissue around the wound
- fever
- oedema
- pain (or a sudden increase in pain)
- pus
- increase in exudate or a change in its colour
- odour
- discolouration of granulation tissue
- further wound breakdown or lack of progress towards healing.

Recognising dehiscence and evisceration

In wound dehiscence (top), the layers of a wound separate. In evisceration (bottom), the viscera (in this case, a bowel loop) protrude through the wound.

Wound dehiscence

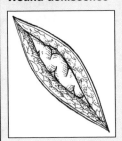

Evisceration of bowel loop

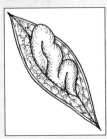

Fistula formation

A fistula is an abnormal passage between two organs or between an organ and the skin. In a wound, it may appear as undermining or a sinus tract (tunnelling) in the skin around the wound. If a sinus tract is present, it's important to determine its extent and direction.

Wound classification

The words you choose to describe your observations of a specific wound have to communicate the same meaning to other members of the health-care team, the patient's family and, ultimately, the patients themselves. This is a tall order when you consider that even wound care experts debate the descriptive phrases they use. Slough or eschar? Undermining or tunnelling? How much drainage is moderate? Is the colour green or yellow? Does the drainage have an odour?

A helpful way to classify wounds is to use the basic system described here, which focuses on three categories of fundamental characteristics:

 wound type

 wound age

 wound depth.

Wound type

There are two basic types of wounds: surgical, which is the result of a surgical procedure performed in a sterile environment, and non-surgical, which is the result of trauma or underlying health conditions, for example diabetic foot ulcers, venous leg ulcers or pressure ulcers.

Wound age

Wounds can be acute or chronic. An acute wound usually heals quickly providing nothing else alters, while chronic wounds take a long time to heal. The dilemma is—when does an acute wound become chronic if it doesn't heal?

A different way of thinking

Rather than base your determination solely on time, consider a wound an acute wound if it's new or making progress as expected and a chronic wound any wound that isn't healing in a timely fashion. The main idea is that, in a chronic wound, healing has slowed or stopped and the wound is no longer getting smaller and shallower. Even if the wound bed appears healthy, red, and moist, if healing fails to progress, consider it a chronic wound.

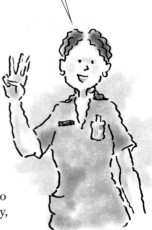

When it comes to classifying wounds, the magic number is 3—age, depth and colour.

More bad than good

Chronic wounds don't heal as easily as acute wounds. The drainage in chronic wounds contains a greater amount of destructive enzymes, and fibroblasts—the cells that function as the architects in wound healing—seem to lose their 'oomph'. They're less effective at producing collagen, divide less often, and send fewer signals to other cells telling them to divide and fill the wound. In other words, the wound changes from one that's vigorous and ready to heal, to one that's downright lazy!

Wound depth

Wound depth is another fundamental characteristic used to classify wounds. In your assessment, record wound depth as partial-thickness or full-thickness. (See *Classifying wound depth*.)

Partial-thickness

Partial-thickness wounds normally heal very quickly because they involve only the epidermal layer of the skin or extend through the epidermis into (but not through) the dermis. The dermis remains at least partially intact to generate the new epidermis needed to close the wound. Partial-thickness wounds are also less susceptible to infection because part of the body's first

---

Classifying wound depth

Wounds are classified as partial-thickness or full-thickness according to the depth of the wound. Partial-thickness wounds involve only the epidermis or extend into the dermis but not through it. Full-thickness wounds extend through the dermis into tissues beneath and may expose adipose tissue, muscle or bone. These diagrams illustrate the relative depth of both classifications.

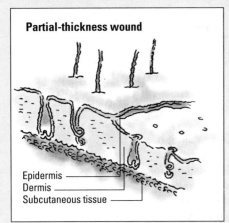

Partial-thickness wound

Epidermis
Dermis
Subcutaneous tissue

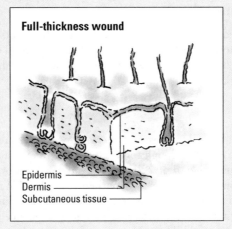

Full-thickness wound

Epidermis
Dermis
Subcutaneous tissue

level of defence (the skin) is still intact. These wounds tend to be painful, however, and need protection from the air to reduce pain and decrease the risk of infection.

Full-thickness

Full-thickness wounds penetrate completely through the skin into underlying tissues. The wound may expose adipose tissue (fat), muscle, tendon or bone. In the abdomen, you may see adipose tissue or omentum (the covering of the bowel). If the omentum is penetrated, the bowel may protrude through the wound (evisceration). Granulation tissue may be visible if the wound has started to heal.

Full-thickness wounds heal by granulation and contraction, which require more body resources and more time than the healing of partial-thickness wounds. When assessing a full-thickness wound, report the depth as well as the length, width and surface area of the wound.

The added pressure of pressure ulcers

In the case of pressure ulcers, wound depth allows you to stage the ulcer.

Wound colour

Wounds are also classified by the colour of the wound bed. Wound colour helps the wound care team determine whether debridement is appropriate. (See *Tailoring wound care to wound colour*.)

Be picky about wound bed colour! Only red will do, and the best shade is blood red—not pale pink or greyish red. There are literally thousands of words to describe colours; however, you can simplify your assessment by sticking to the red–yellow–black classification system. This system is a useful tool for developing effective wound care management plans.

Red means you're ahead

If the wound bed is red (the colour of healthy granulation tissue), the wound is healthy and normal healing is under way. When a wound begins to heal, a layer of pale pink granulation tissue covers the wound bed. As this layer thickens, it becomes beefy red.

Mellow yellow

If the wound bed is yellow, described as sloughy, beware! Yellow or sloughy wounds need to have the slough removed, so that the wound can heal. Slough is the build up of dead cells in the exudate, a part of the inflammatory stage in the healing process, but where the neutrophils die faster than they can be removed (Dealey, 2005). A yellow colour in the wound bed may be a film of fibrin on the tissue. Fibrin is a sticky substance that normally acts as glue in tissue rebuilding. However, if the wound is unhealthy or too

Tailoring wound care to wound colour

With any wound, you can promote healing by keeping the wound moist, clean and free from debris. For open wounds, using wound colour can guide the specific management approach to aid healing.

Wound colour	Management technique
Red granulation tissue	• Cover the wound, keep it moist and clean, and protect it from trauma. • Use a transparent dressing (such as Tegaderm or OpSite) over a gauze dressing moistened with normal saline solution, or use a hydrogel, foam or hydrocolloid dressing to insulate and protect the wound.
Yellow slough tissue	• Clean the wound and remove the yellow layer. • Cover the wound with a moisture-retentive dressing, such as a hydrogel or foam dressing, or a moist gauze dressing with or without a debriding enzyme.
Black necrotic tissue	• Debridement can be achieved by the use of sharp or surgical debridement, autolytic (a dressing that keeps in the moisture allowing the necrotic tissue to soften) and biosurgical methods (using maggots). • For wounds with inadequate blood supply and non-infected heel ulcers, don't debride. Keep them clean and dry.

Careful now!

A pink wound bed indicates that the wound is healing properly, epithelialisation is taking place, therefore, care must be taken not to disturb this wound bed.

Black may be best when it comes to cocktail parties, but watch out for black when it comes to the wound bed. A black wound signals necrosis.

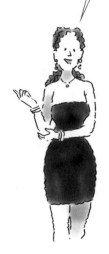

dry, fibrin builds up into a layer that can't be rinsed off and may require debridement.

Black = debridement

If the wound bed is black, be alarmed. A black wound bed signals necrosis (tissue death). Eschar (dead, avascular tissue) covers the wound, slowing the healing process and providing microorganisms with a site in which to proliferate. When eschar covers a wound, accurate assessment of wound depth is difficult and should be deferred until eschar is removed.

Ischaemia exceptions

Typically, debridement is indicated for black wounds; however, ulcers caused by ischaemia (damage due to inadequate blood supply) and uninfected heel pressure ulcers are exceptions. Ischaemic wounds won't heal until blood supply is improved, and they're less likely to become infected if kept dry. The wound can be debrided and kept moist after blood supply is re-established. The body can then fend off infection and heal the wound.

Multicoloured wounds

If you note two or even all the three colours in a wound, classify the wound according to the least healthy colour present. For example if your patient's wound appears both red and yellow, classify it as a yellow wound.

Wound assessment

Gathering information about a wound requires you to use almost all of your senses. Be sure to assess exudate, the wound bed, and patient pain. Assess the wound bed and the surrounding skin only after they've been cleaned. As you perform your assessment, remember that it doesn't matter what method you use to record your observations, it's just important to be consistent.

Assessing exudate

To begin collecting information about wound exudate, inspect the dressing as you remove it and record answers to such questions as:
- Is the drainage well contained, or is it oozing from the edges? If it's oozing, consider using a more absorbent dressing.
- In the case of an occlusive dressing, were the dressing edges well sealed? If the patient has faecal incontinence, it's even more important to note the seal status.
- Is the dressing saturated or dry?
- How much exudate is there: a scant, moderate or large amount?
- Is there an odour?
- What are the colour and consistency of the drainage? (See *Drainage descriptors*.)

Swab or not to swab?

The texture of the exudate must also be considered. If it has a thick, creamy texture, the wound contains an excessive amount of bacteria. However, this doesn't necessarily mean a clinically significant infection is present. It might be creamy because it contains WBCs that have killed bacteria. The exudate is also contaminated with surface bacteria that naturally live in moist environments on the human body, because of this, it is important to take a wound swab only when there are clinical signs of infection.

Assessing the wound bed

As you assess the wound bed, record information about:
- wound dimensions, including size and depth
- tunnelling and undermining

Drainage descriptors

This chart provides terminology that you can use to describe the colour and consistency of wound drainage.

Description	Colour and consistency
Serous	• Clear or light yellow • Thin and watery
Sanguineous	• Red (with fresh blood) • Thin
Serosanguineous	• Pink to light red • Thin • Watery
Purulent	• Creamy yellow, green, white or tan • Thick and opaque

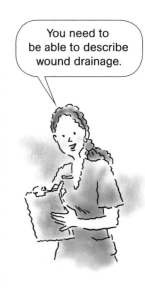

You need to be able to describe wound drainage.

- bed moisture
- wound odour
- margins and surrounding skin.

Dimensions

Get out your ruler

The most common method of measuring wound dimensions is to use a tape measure. Make sure it's a disposable device to prevent contamination and cross-contamination. Record the length of the wound as the longest overall distance across the wound (regardless of orientation), and record the width as the longest measurement perpendicular (at a right angle) to your length measurement. (See *Measuring a wound*, page 274.)

Be sure to record any observed areas of discolouration of the intact skin around the wound opening separately—not as part of the wound bed. Record all measurements in centimetres.

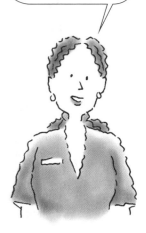

Record as much information about the wound as possible.

Trace the wound

Another way to measure the wound is to use wound tracing (in which wound margins are traced on a sheet of clear plastic). You use the tracing to calculate an approximate wound area. This method provides only a rough estimate but is simple and fairly quick.

Measuring a wound

When measuring a wound, first determine the longest distance across the open area of the wound—regardless of orientation. In this photograph, note the line used to illustrate this length.

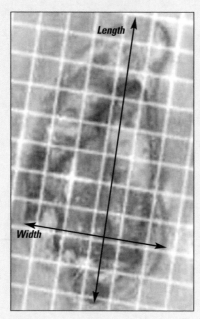

A wound's length is simply the longest distance across the wound at a right angle to the length. Note the relationship of length and width in the photograph. Also, note the area of reddened, intact skin and white macerated skin. These areas would be measured and recorded as surrounding erythaema and maceration—not as part of the wound itself. In this full-thickness ischial pressure ulcer, you would also record a depth and note areas of tunnelling or undermining.

How deep

To measure the depth of the wound, you'll need a wound swab. Gently insert the wound swab into the deepest portion of the wound and then carefully mark the probe where it meets the edge of the skin. Remove from the wound and measure the distance from your mark to the end of the wound swab to determine depth.

Tunnelling and undermining

It's also important to measure tunnelling, or sinus tracts (extensions of the wound bed into adjacent tissue), and undermining (areas of the wound bed that extend under the skin). Measure these features just as you would the depth. Carefully insert a flexible wound swab to the bottom of the tunnel or to the end of the undermined area; then mark the stick and measure the distance from your mark to the end of the swab. If a tunnel is large, palpate it with a gloved finger rather than a swab because you can sense the end of the tunnel better with your finger. Doing so also avoids damaging the tissue. (Follow local policies about measuring tunnelling and underminning, it should be done with care, by a person competent to do so.)

Smile please!

Because accurately recording wound dimensions is important, many health-care facilities use photography as a tool in wound assessment. If photography is available in your area, it should be included in your assessment of wound characteristics. Some photographic techniques produce a picture with a grid overlay that's useful for measuring. It is important to follow local policies when using photographs: gaining consent, maintaining privacy and dignity while taking the photograph, anonymity and using the pictures only for the purpose the consent was given are some of the considerations, as well as storage issues of digital photographs. Remember, however, that there are qualities of the wound that a camera simply can't record.

Moisture

The wound bed should be moist but not overly moist. Moisture allows the cells and chemicals needed for healing to move about the wound surface.

Fish out of water

In dry wound beds, cells involved in healing, which normally exist in a fluid environment, are a bit like fish in a desert—they can't move. WBCs can't fight infection, enzymes like collagenase can't break down dead material, and macrophages can't carry away debris. The wound edges curl up to preserve moisture remaining in the edge and epithelial cells (new skin cells) fail to grow over and cover the wound. Healing grinds to a halt and necrotic tissue builds up.

Flood watch

Too much moisture poses a different problem. It floods the wound and spills out onto the skin, where the constant moisture causes maceration and can result in the death of skin cells.

Odour

If kept clean, a non-infected wound usually produces little, if any, odour. (One exception is the odour normally present under a hydrocolloid dressing that develops as a by-product of the degradation process.) A newly detected odour might be a sign of infection; record it in your findings and report it to the doctor. When documenting wound odour, it's important to include when the odour was noted and whether it went away with wound cleaning.

Odour eaters

If an odour develops, it can present an embarrassing or otherwise uncomfortable situation for the patient as well as their family, guests and roommate. If you notice an odour, or if your patient says they notice one, use an odour eliminator. Odour eliminators differ from air fresheners in that they aren't scents that mask odours but rather compounds that bind with, and neutralise, the molecules responsible for the odour.

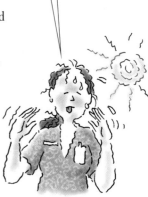

I'm no fish, but I can't go very far without moisture and neither can proper wound healing.

Margins and surrounding skin

When assessing wound margins, you'll want to see skin that's smooth—not rolled—and tightly adherent to the wound bed. Margins that are rolled under may indicate that the wound bed is too dry. Loose skin at the edges may indicate additional shearing injury (separation of skin layers), possibly due to a rough transfer or repositioning. Improving transfer and repositioning techniques and increased moisture levels may prevent recurrence. Margins that roll out may indicate malignancy and need to be referred to a specialist nurse.

Rainbow connections

In the past, sailors used the colour of the sky to predict danger at sea. In a similar fashion, the colour of the skin around the wound can alert you to impending problems that can impede healing:

• White skin indicates maceration, or too much moisture, and signals the need for a protective barrier around the wound and a more absorbent dressing.

• Red skin can indicate inflammation, injury (for example tape burn, excessive pressure or chemical exposure) or infection. Remember that inflammation is healthy only during the inflammatory phase of healing—not after! Feel for warmth!

• Purple skin can indicate bruising, one sign of trauma. Remember, abuse or non-accidental injury may result in bruising; therefore, careful history taking is needed here.

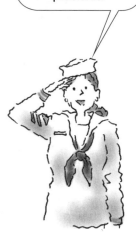

Just like sailors use the colour of the sky to predict weather, you can use wound and skin colour to alert you to potential problems.

Let your fingers do the talking

Your fingers are invaluable tools you may be taking for granted. During your assessment of the area around the wound, your fingers will tell you much. For example gently probe the tissue around the wound bed to determine if it's soft or hard (indurated). Indurated tissue, even in the absence of erythaema (redness), is one indication of infection.

Similarly, if your patient has dark skin, it may be impossible to see colour cues. Again, your fingers can help. Probe the area around the wound bed and compare the feel with surrounding healthy skin. A tender area of skin that appears shiny and feels hard may indicate inflammation in such a patient. Use the back of your hand to assess the temperature of the skin, hot skin may suggest infection present, cold skin may indicate loss of blood supply to the area.

Assessing pain

Assessing patient pain is an important part of wound assessment. You'll want to note not only the pain associated with the injury itself, but also the pain associated with healing and therapies employed to promote healing. To fully understand your patient's pain, talk to them and ask about the level of pain on

Memory jogger

Use the mnemonic **WOUND PICTURE** to help you recall and organise all of the key facts that should be included in your documentation:

Wound or ulcer location

Odour (In room or just when wound is uncovered.)

Ulcer category, stage (for pressure ulcer), or classification (for diabetic ulcer) and depth (partial-thickness or full-thickness)

Necrotic tissue

Dimension and drainage—dimension of wound (shape, length, width, depth); drainage colour, consistency and amount (scant, moderate, large)

Pain (When it occurs, what relieves it, patient's description, patient's rating on scale of 0 to 10?)

Induration (Surrounding tissue hard or soft.)

Colour of wound bed (red–yellow–black or combination)

Tunnelling (Record length and direction—towards patient's right, left, head, feet.)

Undermining (Record length and direction, using clock references to describe.)

Redness or other discolouration in surrounding skin

Edges of skin loose or tightly adhered, flat or rolled under?

a scale of 0 to 10, with 10 being the worst pain they have ever experienced. Then watch how they respond to pain and the therapies provided. As always, remember to record your findings.

Listen and learn

If your patient is conscious and can communicate, have them rate their pain before and during each dressing change. If your notes reveal that their pain is higher before the dressing change, it may indicate an impending infection, even before any other signs appear.

If your patient says the dressing change itself is painful, ensure pain medication is administered before the dressing change.

Useful tips for removal

In general, when removing adherent dressings, it's less painful if you soak the dressing or, over intact skin, use an adhesive remover. Also, keep the skin taut. Press down on the skin to release the dressing, rather than just pulling the dressing off. If the patient still says that dressing removal is painful, the team may wish to choose a less adherent dressing type.

Treatment for wounds

Treating impaired skin integrity involves a range of procedures, from basic wound care and wound irrigation to surgical wound management and closed wound drain management.

Basic wound care

Basic wound care centres on cleaning and dressing the wound. The goal of wound cleaning is to remove debris and contaminants from the wound without damaging healthy tissue. The wound should be cleaned as needed before a new dressing is applied.

The basic purpose of a dressing, to provide an optimal environment in which the body can heal itself, should be considered before one is selected. Functions of a wound dressing include:
- protecting the wound from contamination and trauma
- providing compression if bleeding
- absorbing exudate
- maintaining the temperature of the wound
- debriding necrotic tissue
- filling or packing the wound
- protecting the skin surrounding the wound.

The golden rule!
The golden rule is to keep moist tissue moist and dry tissue dry. Ideally, a dressing should keep the wound moist, absorb exudate or debris, conform to the wound, and be adhesive to surrounding skin yet be easily removable. It should also be user-friendly, require minimal changes, decrease the need for a secondary dressing layer, and be cost-effective and comfortable for the patient.

What you need
Dressing trolley or suitable clean area ✳ sterile dressing pack ✳ sterile gloves × 2 pair ✳ 30 to 50 ml syringe ✳ filling needle or quill ✳ cleaning solution: normal saline solution 0.9% ✳ selected topical dressing ✳ hand gel ✳ hypoallergenic tape or elastic netting (if required this will depend on the type of dressing selected) ✳ protection pad ✳ clinical waste bag (if not included in the dressing pack) ✳ disposable wound-measuring device (if required) ✳ disposable apron

Getting ready
- Explain the procedure to the patient to gain consent, allay fears and promote cooperation.
- Before any dressing change, wash your hands and review the principles of standard precautions.
- Assemble the equipment on the clean dressing trolley or suitable area, after checking outer packs and expiry dates.
- Attach the clinical waste bag to the trolley or table.

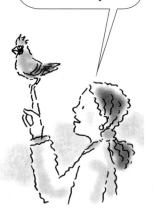

The cardinal rule of wound care is to keep moist tissue moist and dry tissue dry.

How you do it
- Provide privacy
- Position the patient in a way that maximises their comfort while allowing easy access to the wound site.
- Cover bed linen with a protection pad to prevent soiling.

Cleaning the wound
Use clean or sterile technique as appropriate.
- Open the dressing pack and spread the contents out careful not to contaminate the area.
- Pour cleaning solution into the bowl, avoid splashing.
- Open the dressing, syringe and quill, 'drop' them onto the sterile area.
- Put on gloves.
- Gently roll or lift an edge of the soiled dressing to obtain a starting point. Support adjacent skin while gently releasing the soiled dressing from the skin. When possible, remove the dressing in the direction of hair growth. (The waste bag included in the dressing pack can be used for this instead of sterile gloves).
- Assess the existing dressing for drainage, colour, amount and odour.
- Discard the soiled dressing and your contaminated gloves (if used) in the clinical waste bag to avoid contaminating the clean or sterile field.
- Wash your hands.
- Put on a clean pair of gloves.
- Inspect the wound. Note the colour, amount and odour of drainage and necrotic debris.
- Clean the wound if appropriate.

Circles on the skin

- When cleaning, be sure to move from the least-contaminated area to the most-contaminated area. For a linear shaped wound, such as an incision, gently wipe from top to bottom in one motion, along each side of the wound, moving outwards. For an open wound, such as a pressure ulcer, gently wipe around the wound or irrigate it if possible. Use a separate gauze pad each time the wound is cleaned.
- Discard the gauze pads in the clinical waste bag.
- Dry the wound with a gauze pad, using the same procedure as for cleaning. Discard the used gauze pads in the clinical waste bag.
- Next, reassess the condition of the skin and wound. Note the character of the clean wound bed and the surrounding skin.

Applying a dressing
- Prepare to apply the appropriate dressing. Instructions for applying hydrocolloid, transparent film, alginate, foam, hydrogel and hydrofibre dressings follow. (See *Choosing a wound dressing*, page 208.) For other dressings or topical agents, follow your Trust's protocol or the manufacturer's instructions.

> Remember to follow manufacturer's instructions for the individual products!

Choosing a wound dressing

The patient's needs and wound characteristics determine which type of dressing to use on a wound.

Gauze dressings

Made of absorptive cotton or synthetic fabric, gauze dressings are permeable to water, water vapour and oxygen and may be impregnated with hydrogel or another agent. When uncertain about which dressing to use or in emergency situations, you may apply a gauze dressing moistened in saline solution as a temporary measure. Gauze can stick to the wound bed and, when removed, causes pain and disturbs the healing process.

Hydrocolloid dressings

Hydrocolloid dressings are adhesive, mouldable wafers made of a carbohydrate-based material and usually have waterproof backings. They're impermeable to oxygen, water and water vapour, and most have some absorptive properties.

Transparent film dressings

Transparent film dressings are clear, adherent and non-absorptive. These polymer-based dressings are permeable to oxygen and water vapour but not to water. Their transparency allows visual inspection. Because they can't absorb drainage, they're used on partial thickness wounds with minimal exudate.

Alginate dressings

Made from seaweed, alginate dressings are non-woven, absorptive dressings available as soft white sterile pads or ropes. They absorb excessive exudate and may be used on infected wounds. As these dressings absorb exudate, they turn into a gel that keeps the wound bed moist and promotes healing. When exudate is no longer excessive, switch to another type of dressing.

Foam dressings

Foam dressings are sponge-like polymer dressings that may be impregnated or coated with other materials. Somewhat absorptive, they may be adherent. These dressings promote moist wound healing and are useful when a non-adherent surface is desired.

Hydrogel dressings

Water-based and non-adherent, hydrogel dressings are polymer-based dressings that have some absorptive properties. They're available as a gel in a tube, as flexible sheets, and as saturated gauze packing strips. They may have a cooling effect, which eases pain, and are used when the wound needs moisture.

Hydrocolloid dressing
(For wounds with moderate to low exudate)
• Choose a clean, dry, pre-sized dressing, or cut one to overlap the wound by about 2.5 cm. Remove the dressing from its package, pull the release paper from the adherent side of the dressing, and apply the dressing to the wound. Hold the dressing in place with your hand, the warmth will mould the dressing to the skin.

Smooth operator

• As you apply the dressing, carefully smooth out wrinkles and avoid stretching the dressing.
• If the dressing's edges need to be secured with tape, apply a skin sealant to the intact skin around the wound. After the area dries, tape the dressing to the skin. The sealant protects the skin from tape burns and skin stripping and

promotes tape adherence. Avoid using tension or pressure when applying the tape.
• Remove your gloves and discard them in the clinical waste bag. Dispose off refuse according to your local infection control policy.
• Before any dressing change, wash your hands, put on a disposable apron and review.
• Change a hydrocolloid dressing every 3 to 7 days, follow manufacturer's recommendations. Change it immediately if the patient complains of pain, the dressing no longer adheres, or leakage occurs.

Transparent film dressing
(For wounds with no or minimal exudate)
• Select a dressing to overlap the wound by 2.5 to 5 cm.
• Gently lay the dressing over the wound; avoid wrinkling the dressing. To prevent shearing force, don't stretch the dressing over the wound. Press firmly on the edges of the dressing to promote adherence. Although this type of dressing is self-adhesive, you may have to tape the edges to prevent them from curling.
• Change the dressing every 3 to 5 days, depending on the amount of drainage. If the seal is no longer secure or if accumulated tissue fluid extends beyond the edges of the wound and onto the surrounding skin, change the dressing.

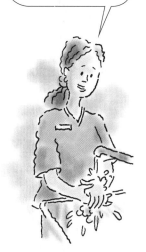

Make sure you wash your hands before and after each dressing change.

Alginate dressing
(For wounds with moderate or heavy exudate)
• Apply the alginate dressing to the wound surface. Cover the area with a secondary dressing (such as absorbent pads or foam adhesive dressing).
• If the wound is draining heavily, change the dressing once or twice daily until the drainage decreases, then change the dressing less frequently—every 2 to 4 days. When the drainage stops or the wound bed looks dry, stop using alginate dressing.

Foam dressing
(For wounds with some exudate)
• Gently lay the foam dressing over the wound.
• Use tape or elastic netting to hold the dressing in place, if foam is not adhesive.
• Change the dressing when the foam no longer absorbs the exudate.

Hydrogel dressing
(For wounds with moderate to low exudate)
• Apply a moderate amount of gel to the wound bed.
• Cover the area with a secondary dressing (transparent film or foam).
• Change the dressing every 2 to 3 days or as needed to keep the wound bed moist.
• Hydrogel dressings also come in pre-packaged, saturated gauze for wounds with cavities that require 'dead space' to be filled. Follow the manufacturer's directions.

Practice pointers
- Be aware that infection may cause foul-smelling drainage, persistent pain, severe erythema, induration and elevated skin and body temperatures. Advancing infection or cellulitis can lead to septicaemia and must, therefore, be reported immediately.
- Severe erythema may signal worsening cellulitis, which means the offending organisms have invaded the tissue and are no longer localised.

Wound irrigation

Gentle irrigation cleans tissues and flushes cell debris and drainage from an open wound. It also helps prevent premature surface healing over an abscess pocket or infected tract.

How you do it
- Explain the procedure to the patient, provide privacy and position the patient correctly for the procedure. Place the absorbent pad under the patient and place the disposable bowl below the wound so that the irrigating solution flows from the wound into the basin. (See *Irrigating a wound*.)

From clean to dirty

- Fill the syringe with the irrigating solution and connect the catheter to the syringe. Gently instil a slow, steady stream of solution into the wound until the syringe empties. Make sure the solution flows from the clean to the dirty area of the wound to prevent contamination of clean tissue by exudate. Also make sure the solution reaches all areas of the wound.
- Refill the syringe, reconnect it to the catheter, and repeat the irrigation. Continue to irrigate the wound until the solution returns clear. Note the amount of solution administered. Then remove and discard the catheter and syringe in the clinical waste bag. (See *Wound irrigation tips*, page 284.)

Positioned for success

- Keep the patient positioned to allow further wound drainage into the basin.
- Clean the area around the wound with normal saline solution and pat dry with gauze; wipe intact surrounding skin with a skin protectant wipe and allow it to dry.
- Apply a dressing.
- Remove and discard your gloves.
- Make sure the patient is comfortable.
- Dispose of drainage, soiled equipment and supplies according to your local infection prevention and control policy.
- Remove apron and wash hands.

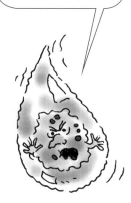

I'm a victim! I mean, there I was in my cozy wound with all my friends and then, the next thing I know, I'm floating in this bowl. Oh, the humanity!

Irrigating a wound

When preparing to irrigate a wound, attach a sterile quill or soft catheter to a 50 ml catheter tipped syringe. Use warmed 0.9% normal saline solution to irrigate the wound. To prevent tissue damage, avoid forcing the quill or soft catheter into the wound.

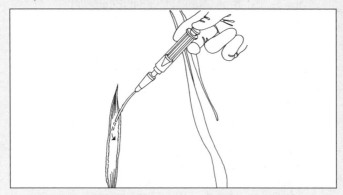

Irrigate the wound with gentle pressure until the solution returns clear. Allow the disposable bowl to remain under the wound to collect any remaining drainage.

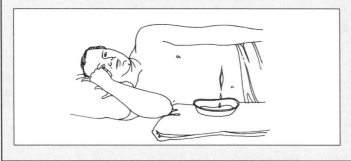

Practice pointers

• Never use a needle to irrigate a wound as this may result in a needle stick injury to you or your patient.
• Solutions used for cleaning should be at body temperature (37° C) to prevent the wound from cooling, which can delay wound healing.

Surgical wound management

When caring for a surgical wound, you carry out procedures that help prevent infection by stopping pathogens from entering the wound. In addition to promoting patient comfort, such procedures protect the skin's

Wound irrigation tips

How can you avoid mess or spillage when irrigating a wound in a hard-to-reach location? Here are some tips you can follow.

Limb wounds

An arm or leg wound can be soaked in a large vessel of warm irrigating fluid, such as tap water or normal saline solution, remember to use a disposable liner.

If possible, rinse the wound several times and carefully dispose off the contaminated liquid. Dry and store it after cleaning, follow local infection prevention and control policy. Reserve the equipment used for that particular patient.

Trunk or thigh wounds

Because they're difficult to irrigate, trunk or thigh wounds require some ingenuity. One device uses Stomahesive and a plastic irrigating chamber applied over the wound. (Run warm solution through an infusion set and collect it in a drainage bag.)

Another alternative is to use a syringe to irrigate. Where possible, direct the flow at right angles to the wound and allow the fluid to drain by gravity. Doing so requires careful positioning of the patient, either in bed or on a chair.

If soaking or irrigation isn't possible, you'll have to gently swab clean the wound. Swab away exudate before using saline solution to clean the wound (taking care not to push loose debris into the wound). The patient may need analgesia during the treatment.

---

surface from maceration and excoriation caused by contact with irritating drainage. They also allow you to measure wound drainage to monitor fluid and electrolyte balance.

Surgical site infections (SSI's) are included in NICE (2008) guidelines; surgical site infections, prevention and treatment of surgical site infections, as one of the causes of health-care-associated infections (HCAIs). Care must be taken to follow a non-touch technique when performing the dressing change, also, to assess the wound and the patient for early signs and symptoms of infection.

Suitably dressed

The primary method used to manage a draining surgical wound is dressing. Dressing a wound calls for sterile technique and sterile supplies to prevent contamination. You may use the colour of the wound to help determine which type of dressing to apply. Choosing the appropriate dressing will promote wound healing by providing optimal conditions. Careful monitoring of the wound when changing the dressing will enable early detection of problems.

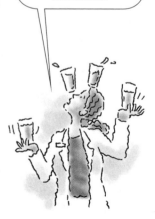

Infection-preventing procedures also allow you to monitor fluid and electrolyte imbalance.

What you need

Dressing wounds with a drain

Sterile scissors ✳ sterile 4" × 4" gauze pads without cotton lining ✳ sterile pre-cut tracheostomy pads or drain dressings

Getting ready

• Ask the patient about allergies to tapes and dressings. Assemble all equipment and check the expiration date on each sterile package, and inspect for tears.

How you do it

• Explain the procedure to the patient to allay their fears and ensure their cooperation.

Removing the old dressing

• Check the wound care plan for specific wound care instructions. Note the location of surgical drains to avoid dislodging them during the procedure.
• Assess the patient's condition.
• Provide privacy, and position the patient as necessary. To avoid chilling them, expose only the wound site.
• Put on apron and wash your hands thoroughly. Then put on clean gloves.

Go towards the wound

• Loosen the soiled dressing by holding the patient's skin and pulling the tape or dressing towards the wound to protect the newly formed tissue and prevent stress on the incision.
• Slowly remove the soiled dressing.
• Observe the dressing for the amount, type, colour and odour of drainage.
• Discard the dressing and gloves in the clinical waste bag.

Caring for the wound

• Wash your hands. Establish a sterile field with all the equipment and supplies you'll need for suture-line care and the dressing change. Pour the normal saline solution into the sterile container. Then put on sterile gloves.

No cotton balls, please!

• Saturate the sterile gauze pads with the normal saline solution. Avoid using cotton balls because they may shed fibres in the wound, causing irritation, infection, or adhesion.
• If clinically indicated, obtain a wound swab; then proceed to clean the wound.
• Irrigate the wound, if appropriate.
• Pick up the moistened gauze pad or swab, and squeeze out the excess solution.

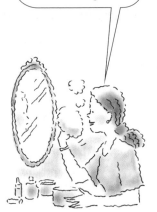

Cotton balls are great for taking off makeup but not so good for wound cleaning!

From top to bottom

- Working from the top of the incision, wipe once to the bottom and then discard the gauze pad. With a second moistened pad, wipe from top to bottom in a vertical path next to the incision (as shown below), **not** over the incision line.

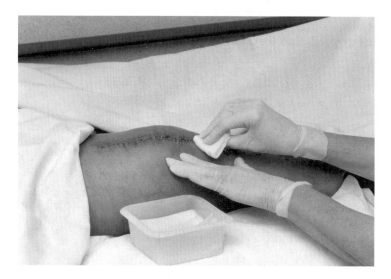

- Continue to work outwards from the incision in lines running parallel to it. Always wipe from the clean area towards the less clean area (usually from top to bottom). Use each gauze pad or swab for only one stroke to avoid tracking wound exudate and normal body flora from surrounding skin to the clean areas. Remember that the suture line is cleaner than the adjacent skin and the top of the suture line is usually cleaner than the bottom because more drainage collects at the bottom of the wound.

Watch out for the drain!

- If the patient has a surgical drain, clean the drain's surface last. Because moist drainage promotes bacterial growth, the drain is considered the most contaminated area. Clean the skin around the drain by wiping in half or full circles from the drain site outwards.
- Clean all areas of the wound to wash away debris, pus, blood, and necrotic material. Try not to disturb sutures or irritate the incision.

Line 'em up . . .

- Check to make sure the edges of the incision are lined up properly, and check for signs of infection (heat, redness, swelling, induration and odour), dehiscence and evisceration. If you observe such signs or if the patient reports pain at the wound site, notify the doctor.

Applying a fresh dressing
- Cover the wound evenly with the appropriate sterile dressing.
- Make sure the patient is comfortable.

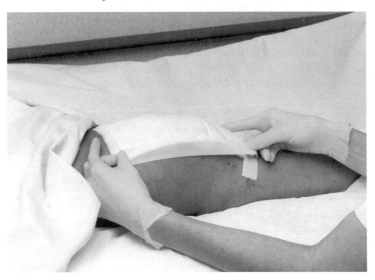

- Dispose of the soiled equipment and supplies according to your local infection prevention and control policy.
- Remove apron and wash hands.
- Document dressing change and appearance, size and amount of exudate.

Dressing a wound with a drain
- Use commercially pre-cut gauze drain dressings or prepare a drain dressing by using sterile scissors to cut a slit in a sterile 4" × 4" gauze pad. Fold the pad in half, then cut inwards from the centre of the folded edge. Don't use a cotton-lined gauze pad because cutting the gauze opens the lining and releases cotton fibres into the wound. Prepare a second pad the same way.
- Gently press one drain dressing close to the skin around the drain so that the tubing fits into the slit. Press the second drain dressing around the drain from the opposite direction so that the two dressings encircle the tubing.
- Tape the dressing in place.

Practice pointers
- If the patient has two wounds in the same area, cover each wound separately.
- Document the amount of dressing used on the wound care plan.

A time saver
- To save time when dressing a wound with a drain, use pre-cut tracheostomy pads or drain dressings instead of custom-cutting gauze pads to fit around the drain.

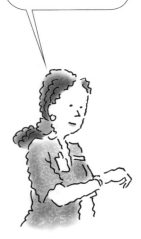

Using pre-cut tracheostomy pads or drain dressings saves time.

• Use non-allergic tape because it's less likely to cause a skin reaction and peels off more easily than adhesive tape.
• Use a skin protectant instead of a gauze dressing. This moisture- and contaminant-proof covering dries in a clear, impermeable film that leaves the wound visible for observation and avoids the friction caused by a dressing.
• Use a wound drainage bag if the wound is draining large amounts or if the surrounding skin is becoming damaged. If you use more than one collection pouch for a wound or wounds, record drainage volume separately for each pouch.
• If drainage comes through the dressing, reinforce the dressing with fresh sterile pad. A reinforced dressing shouldn't remain in place longer than 24 hours because it's an excellent medium for bacterial growth.

Check and recheck!

• For the recent post-operative patient or a patient with complications, check the dressing every 15 to 30 minutes. For the patient with a properly healing wound, check the dressing daily.
• If the dressing becomes wet, replace it as soon as possible to prevent wound contamination.

Closed-wound drain management

Typically inserted during some types of surgery in anticipation of substantial post-operative drainage, a closed-wound drain promotes healing and prevents swelling by suctioning the serosanguineous fluid that accumulates at the wound site. By removing this fluid, the closed-wound drain helps reduce the risk of infection and skin breakdown, as well as the number of dressing changes.

A closed-wound drain consists of perforated tubing connected to a vacuumed container. The distal end of the tubing lies within the wound and usually leaves the body from a site other than the primary suture line to preserve the integrity of the surgical wound. The tubing exit site is treated as an additional surgical wound; the drain is usually sutured to the skin.

If the wound produces heavy drainage, the closed-wound drain may be left in place until drainage decreases or stops. Drainage must be measured frequently and the equipment checked to maintain maximum suction and prevent strain on the suture line.

No twist and shout!

• Check the patency of the equipment. Make sure the tubing is free from twists, kinks and leaks because the drainage system must be airtight to work properly.
• Secure the drainage bottle to the patient's gown. Fasten it below wound level to promote drainage. Don't apply tension on drainage tubing when fastening the unit to avoid possible dislodgment.

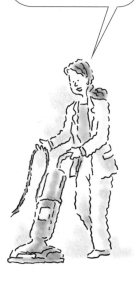

Portable vacuum units are handy in lots of places—some are even used for draining closed wounds.

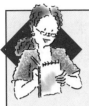

Record!

Documenting closed-wound drainage management

Follow these tips when documenting your care of a closed-wound drainage unit. On the intake and output sheet, record drainage colour, consistency, type and amount. If the patient has more than one closed-wound drain, number the drains and record the information above separately for each drainage site.

Also record:

- the date and time you empty the drain
- appearance of the drain site
- presence of swelling or signs of infection.

Be gentle

- Observe the sutures that secure the drain to the patient's skin; look for signs of pulling or tearing and for swelling or infection of surrounding skin. Gently clean the sutures with sterile gauze pads soaked in normal saline solution.

Practice pointers

- Measure and record the contents of the drain during each shift, more often if drainage is excessive.
- If the patient has more than one closed drain, number the drains so you can record drainage from each site.
- Document your care. (See *Documenting closed-wound drainage management*.)

Watch out!

- Be careful not to mistake chest tubes with water seal drainage devices for closed-wound drains because the care of these devices differs from closed-wound drainage systems, and the vacuum of a chest tube should never be released.

A look at pressure ulcers

Pressure ulcers are a serious health problem. UK-wide incidence and prevalence figures are difficult to establish; Trusts and other institutions gather their own data, and are not yet required to release their figures. Some data gathered by bed companies suggest that the prevalence of pressure ulcers

> *Note!* It is important to note that people of **any** age, including infants and neonates, are at risk of developing a pressure ulcer, not just the elderly!

remains at 10%. Although this finding is significant in itself, prevalence in some groups—such as patients with spinal cord injuries, patients in intensive care units and nursing home residents—may be higher.

At what cost?

Although there are little overall statistics, what has become starkly evident are the costs associated with pressure ulcers—the cost in terms of suffering and diminished quality of life for patients, the cost to the NHS in terms of resources consumed and manpower hours dedicated to managing the problem, and the very real monetary cost to individuals and NHS, the suggested cost was £1.4 to 2.1 billion (Bennett et al., 2004).

Pressure ulcers are chronic conditions—they take time to heal and tend to recur frequently, therefore prevention and early intervention are critical for more effective management.

The closer you get

Better disease management in pressure ulcer cases depends on closer collaboration among all health-care professionals, patients and their carers. All involved are paying closer attention to prevention and the effectiveness of interventions, and they're finding better methods of quantifying and disseminating results. NICE (2005) indicate the reporting of pressure ulcers graded 2 and above, is required via the critical incident reporting system, which highlights the importance of assessment and prevention.

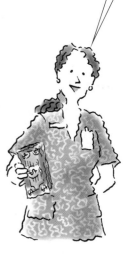

Pressure ulcers are costly—for the patient and the health-care industry.

Causes

Chronic wounds are those that fail to heal in a timely manner, resist treatment and tend to recur. Pressure ulcers are chronic wounds resulting from tissue death due to prolonged, irreversible ischaemia brought on by compression of soft tissue.

If you want to get technical

Technically speaking, pressure ulcers are the clinical manifestation of localised tissue death due to lack of blood flow in areas under pressure.

Simplify, simplify!

Now, let's back up a bit to break down and better understand this description. First of all, different tissues have different tolerances for compression. Muscle and fat have comparatively low tolerances for pressure, whereas skin has a somewhat higher tolerance. All cells, regardless of tissue type, depend on blood circulation for the oxygen and nutrients they need. Tissue compression interferes with circulation, reducing or completely cutting off blood flow. The result, known as ischaemia, is that cells fail to receive adequate supplies of oxygen and nutrients. Unless the pressure relents, cells eventually die. By the time inflammation signals impending necrosis on the surface of the skin, it's likely that necrosis has occurred in deeper tissues.

Location, location, location

Pressure ulcers are most common in areas where pressure compresses soft tissue over a bony prominence in the body; the tissue is pinched between the outer pressure and the hard underlying surface. Other factors that contribute to the problem include shear, friction and moisture. Planning effective interventions for prevention and treatment requires a sound understanding of the causes of pressure ulcers.

Pressure

Capillaries are connected to arteries and veins through intermediary vessels called arterioles and venules. In healthy individuals, capillary filling pressure is approximately 32 mmHg where arterioles connect to capillaries and 12 mmHg where capillaries connect to venules. Therefore, external pressure greater than capillary filling pressure can cause problems. In frail or ill people, capillary-filling pressures may be much lower. External pressure that exceeds capillary perfusion pressure compresses blood vessels and causes ischaemia in the tissues supplied by those vessels.

Tip of the iceberg

If the pressure continues long enough, capillaries collapse and thrombose, toxic metabolic by-products accumulate, and cells in nearby muscle and subcutaneous tissues begin to die. Muscle and fat are less tolerant of interruptions in blood flow than skin. Consequently, by the time signs of impending necrosis appear on the skin, underlying tissue has probably suffered substantial damage. Keep this 'tip of the iceberg' effect in mind when assessing the size of a pressure ulcer. (See *Pressure points*, page 292.)

The pressure mounts

When external pressure exceeds venous capillary refill pressure (about 12 mmHg), capillaries begin to leak. The resulting ooedema increases the amount of pressure on blood vessels, further impeding circulation. When interstitial pressure surpasses arterial intravascular pressure, blood is forced into nearby tissues (non-blanchable erythema). Continued capillary occlusion, lack of oxygen and nutrients and buildup of toxic waste leads to necrosis of muscle, subcutaneous tissue and, ultimately, the dermis and epidermis.

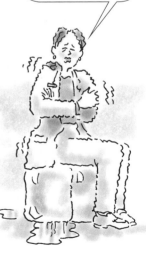

When assessing the size of a pressure ulcer, don't forget that it may just be the tip of the iceberg!

Pressure points

Pressure points are likely areas for ulcer formation. These illustrations show the areas at highest risk for ulcers when the patient is in different positions.

Sitting

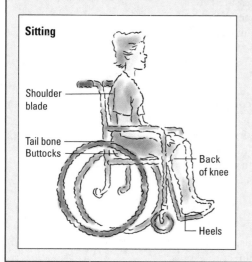

Shoulder blade

Tail bone
Buttocks

Back of knee

Heels

Lying

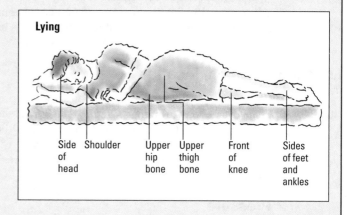

Side of head

Shoulder

Upper hip bone

Upper thigh bone

Front of knee

Sides of feet and ankles

Spreading the load

The force associated with any given pressure increases as the amount of body surface exposed to the pressure decreases. For example the force exerted on the buttocks of a person lying in bed is about 70 mmHg. However, when the same person sits on a hard surface, the force exerted on the ischial tuberosities can be as much as 300 mmHg. Consequently, bony prominences are particularly susceptible to pressure ulcers. However, they aren't the only areas at risk. Ulcers can develop on any soft tissue subjected to prolonged pressure. Therefore, spreading the pressure over a larger area may help prevent pressure ulcer development.

Between a bone and a hard place

When blood vessels, muscle, subcutaneous fat and skin are compressed between a bone and an external surface, for instance a bed or a chair, pressure is exerted on the tissues from the external surface and the bone. In effect, the external surface produces pressure and the bone produces counter-pressure. These opposing forces create a cone-shaped pressure gradient. (See *Understanding the pressure gradient*.) Although the pressure affects all tissues between these two points, tissues closest to the bony prominence suffer the greatest damage.

Understanding the pressure gradient

In this illustration, the V-shaped pressure gradient results from the upward force exerted by the supporting surface and the downward force of the bony prominence. Pressure is greatest on tissues at the apex of the gradient and lessens to the right and left of this point.

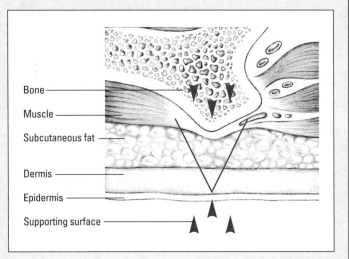

Bone

Muscle

Subcutaneous fat

Dermis

Epidermis

Supporting surface

Time and pressure

Over time, pressure causes a growing discomfort that prompts a person to change position before tissue ischaemia occurs. In ulcer formation, an inverse relationship exists between time and pressure. Typically, low pressure for long periods is far more damaging than high pressure for short periods. For example a pressure of 70 mmHg sustained for 2 hours or longer almost always causes irreversible tissue damage, whereas a pressure of 240 mmHg can be endured for a short time with little or no tissue damage. Furthermore, after the time-pressure threshold for damage passes, damage continues even after the pressure stops. Although pressure ulcers can result from one period of sustained pressure, they're more likely to result from repeated ischaemic events without adequate intervening time for recovery.

Shear

Shearing force intensifies the pressure's destructive effects. Shear is a mechanical force that runs parallel, rather than perpendicular, to an area of skin; deep tissues feel the brunt of the force.

The shear truth of it

Shearing force is most likely to develop during repositioning or when a patient slides down after being placed in the sitting position. However, simply elevating the head of the bed increases shear and pressure in the sacral and coccygeal areas; gravity pulls the body down but the skin on the back resists the motion because of friction between the skin and the sheets. The result

Shearing force

Shear is a mechanical force parallel, rather than perpendicular, to an area of tissue. In this illustration, gravity pulls the body down the incline of the bed. The skeleton and attached tissues move, but the skin remains stationary, held in place by friction between the skin and the bed linen. The skeleton and attached tissues actually slide within the skin, causing skin to pucker in the gluteal area.

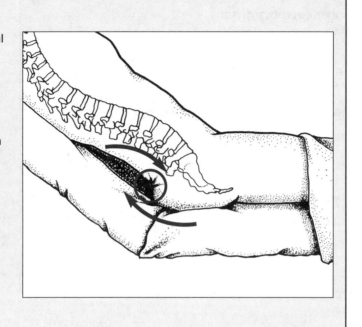

is that the skeleton (and attached tissues) actually slides somewhat beneath the skin (evidenced by the puckering of skin in the gluteal area), generating shearing force between outer layers of tissue and deeper layers. The force generated is enough to obstruct, tear, or stretch blood vessels. (See *Shearing force*.)

Shearing force reduces the length of time that tissue can endure a given pressure before ischaemia or necrosis occurs. A sufficiently high level of shearing force can halve the amount of pressure needed to produce vascular occlusion. Research indicates that shearing force is responsible for the high incidence of triangular-shaped sacral ulcers and the large areas of tunnelling or deep sinus tracts beneath these ulcers.

Friction

Friction is another potentially damaging mechanical force. Friction develops as one surface moves across another surface, for example the patient's skin sliding across the bedsheet. Abrasions are wounds created by friction.

Those at particularly high risk for tissue damage due to friction include patients who have uncontrollable movements or spastic conditions, patients who wear braces or appliances that rub against the skin and older patients. Friction is also a problem for patients who have trouble lifting themselves during repositioning. Rubbing against the sheet can result in an abrasion, which increases the potential for deeper tissue damage. Elevating the head of the bed, as discussed earlier, generates friction between the patient's skin and the bed linen as gravity tugs the patient's body downwards. As the skeleton moves inside the skin, friction and shearing force combine to increase the risk of tissue damage in the sacral area. The use of skin protectants and adherent dressings with slippery backings can help reduce the impact of friction. The most important aspect of reducing friction is the proper use of moving and handling equipment.

Excessive moisture

Prolonged exposure to moisture can waterlog, or macerate, skin. Maceration contributes to pressure ulcer formation by softening the connective tissue. Macerated epidermis erodes more easily, degenerates and eventually sloughs off. In addition, damp skin adheres to bed linen more readily, making friction's effects more profound. Consequently, moist skin is five times more likely to develop ulcers than dry skin. Excessive moisture can result from perspiration, wound drainage, bathing or faecal or urinary incontinence.

Risk factors

Factors that increase the risk of developing pressure ulcers include advancing age, immobility, incontinence, infection, poor nutrition and low blood pressure. High-risk patients, whether in an institution or at home, should be assessed regularly for pressure ulcers.

Age

With advancing age, the skin becomes more fragile as epidermal turnover slows, vascularisation decreases and skin layers adhere less securely to one another. Older adults have less lean body mass and less subcutaneous tissue cushioning bony areas. Consequently, they're more likely to suffer tissue damage due to friction, shear and pressure. (See *Aging and skin function*, page 296.)

Other common problems include poor nutrition, poor hydration and impaired respiratory or immune systems.

Immobility

Immobility may be the greatest risk factor for pressure ulcer development. The patient's ability to move in response to pressure sensations as well as the frequency with which their position is changed should always be considered in risk assessment.

Incontinence

Incontinence increases a patient's exposure to moisture and, over time, increases the risk of skin breakdown. Urinary and faecal incontinence create problems as a result of excessive moisture and chemical irritation. Due to pathogens in stools, faecal incontinence can cause more skin damage than urinary incontinence. The risk increases even higher if the patient is doubly incontinent, there is a chemical reaction between the faeces and urine causing more damage to the skin.

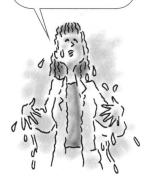

Prolonged exposure to moisture can waterlog, or *macerate*, skin, contributing to pressure ulcer formation.

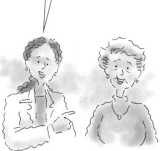

Older adults are more likely to suffer tissue damage due to friction, shear, and pressure.

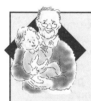

Ages and stages

Aging and skin function

Over time, skin loses its ability to function as efficiently or as effectively as it once did. As a result, the golden years of life place a person at greater risk for such injuries as pressure ulcers and tumours as well as various other skin conditions. This chart outlines the major changes that take place in the skin during the aging process and the implications of those changes for older people.

Change	Implications
50% reduction in the cell turnover rate in the stratum corneum (outermost layer) and a 20% reduction in dermal thickness	• Higher risk of infection because thinner skin is a less effective barrier to germs and allergens
Generalised reduction in dermal vascularisation and an associated drop in blood flow to the skin	• Bruising more easily and increasing tendency of oedema around wounds
Redistribution of subcutaneous tissue, which contains fewer fat cells in older people, to the stomach and thighs	• Risk of hyperthermia or hypothermia • Higher incidence of ischaemia (cell damage resulting from too little oxygen reaching cells) in compressed tissue of bony areas
Flattening of papillae in the dermoepidermal junction (meeting of the epidermis and dermis), which reduces adhesion between layers	• Much higher incidence of shear and tear injuries
Drop in the number of Langerhans' cells (immune macrophages that attack invading germs) present in the skin	• Higher risk of infection • Slower sensitisation response (redness, heat, discomfort), resulting in overuse of topical medications and more severe allergic reactions (because signs aren't evident early on)
50% decline in the number of fibroblasts and mast cells (cells that play a key role in the inflammatory response)	• Higher risk of infection
Marked reduction in the ability to sense pressure, heat, and cold, even though the same number of nerve endings in the skin are retained	• Higher incidence of pressure and thermal (hot and cold) damage to the skin • Higher incidence of ischaemia (cell damage resulting from too little oxygen reaching cells) in compressed tissue • Higher incidence of skin tears
Significant decline in the number of sweat glands	• Difficulty with thermoregulation and increased risk of hyperthermia due to decreased production of sweat
Poorer absorption through the skin	• Risk of overdose of transdermal medications due to too frequent application
Reduction in the skin's ability to synthesise vitamin D	• Skin loses elasticity and wrinkles develop

Nutrition

Proper nutrition is vitally important to tissue integrity. A strong correlation exists between poor nutrition and pressure ulceration, yet nutrition is all too commonly overlooked during treatment. NICE guidelines on the management of pressure ulcers (NICE, 2003) recommend the use of a recognised nutritional assessment tool.

Albumin acumen

Increased protein is required for the body to heal itself. Albumin is one of the key proteins in the body. A patient's serum albumin level is an important indicator of their protein levels. A sub-normal serum albumin level is a late manifestation of protein deficiency. Normal serum albumin levels range from 3.5 to 5 g/dl. Serum albumin deficits are ranked as:

- mild—3 to 3.5 g/dl
- moderate—2.5 to 3 g/dl
- severe—less than 2.5 g/dl.

> Extra protein can help a patient's body heal itself. I think I need some extra healing so I'll help myself to another piece.

Blood pressure

Low arterial blood pressure is clearly linked to tissue ischaemia, particularly in vascular patients. When blood pressure is low, the body shunts blood away from the peripheral vascular system that serves the skin and towards vital organs to ensure their health. As perfusion drops, the skin is less tolerant of sustained external pressure, and the risk of damage due to ischaemia rises.

Assessing risk factors

NICE (2005) recommend that all patients' pressure ulcer risk is assessed within 6 hours of being admitted to a care institution and whenever their condition changes.

There are assessment tools available to help determine a patient's risk of developing pressure ulcers and, when used with clinical judgement, can help to identify a patient's risk of developing a pressure ulcer. Those available include the Norton score, the Braden scale and, most widely used, the Waterlow score, revised in 2005 to the Waterlow pressure ulcer prevention treatment policy. It is a detailed policy which helps detect the risk of a pressure ulcer developing and indicates the prevention options.

Common denominators

Most scales use the following factors to determine a patient's risk of developing pressure ulcers:
- immobility
- inactivity
- incontinence
- malnutrition
- impaired mental status or sensation.

Each category receives a value based on the patient's condition. The sum of these values determines the patient's score and level of risk. Scores for each category as well as the assessment as a whole help the care team develop appropriate interventions.

The Norton scale
The Norton score assesses five aspects which include the patient's physical condition, mental state, their mobility, whether they are active and whether they are incontinent. The scoring from each aspect is 4 to 1, 1 being the highest risk. This scale does not include nutrition or age as Norton did not intend for this scale to be used in isolation.

The Braden scale
This tool scores aetiologic factors that contribute to prolonged pressure as well as factors that contribute to diminished tissue tolerance for pressure. Factors scored in this assessment include sensory perception, moisture, activity, mobility, nutrition and friction and shear. The lower the score, the higher the patient's risk of pressure ulceration. A score of 18 or lower denotes a risk of pressure ulcers.

Early does it
In nursing home populations, most pressure ulcers develop during the 2 weeks immediately following admission, so early identification of at-risk patients is crucial. No definitive guidelines exist for how often to reassess a patient; however, a common-sense approach would be to reassess the patient when their condition changes or in the event that they become chair-bound or confined to bed.

Memory jogger

To remember the five factors commonly used to determine a patient's risk of developing pressure ulcers, think of the five is:

immobility
inactivity
incontinence
improper nutrition (malnutrition)
impaired mental status or sensation

Pressure ulcer prevention

Pressure ulcer prevention focuses on compensating for prevailing risk factors and addressing the underlying pathophysiology. When planning interventions, be sure to adopt a holistic approach and consider all of the patient's needs.

Managing pressure

Managing the intensity and duration of pressure is a fundamental goal in prevention, especially for the patient with mobility limitations. Frequent, careful repositioning helps the patient avoid the damaging repetitive pressure that can cause tissue ischaemia and subsequent necrosis. When repositioning the patient, it's important to reduce the duration and the intensity of pressure.

Positioning
Any time that you reposition the patient, check for any signs of reddened skin especially over boney prominences. Avoid the use

Overall assessment and scores for each category of pressure ulcer risk help the team develop appropriate interventions.

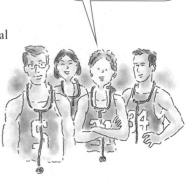

of donut-shaped supports or ring cushions that encircle the ischaemic area because these can reduce blood flow to an even wider expanse of tissue. If the affected area is on an extremity, use pillows to support the limb and reduce pressure. As noted earlier, avoid raising the head of the bed more than 30 degrees to prevent tissue damage due to friction and shearing force.

Little steps

Inactivity increases a patient's risk of ulcer development. To the degree that the patient is physically able, encourage activity. Start with a short step—help them out of bed and into a chair. As their tolerance improves, help them walk around the bedspace and then longer distances.

Positioning a patient in bed

When the patient is on their side, never allow weight to rest directly on the greater trochanter of the femur. Instead, have the patient rest their weight on their buttocks and use a pillow or foam wedge to maintain the position (a 30 degree tilt). This position ensures that no pressure is placed on the trochanter or sacrum. Also, a pillow placed between the knees or ankles minimises the pressure exerted when one limb lies on top of the other. Make sure the patient is comfortable in this position. (See *Repositioning a reclining patient*.)

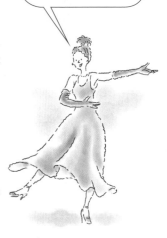

Ballroom dancing is great, but not the right activity to start your patient on! Try something a little more basic.

Repositioning a reclining patient

When repositioning a reclining patient, use the Rule of 30—that is, raise the head of the bed 30 degrees (as shown top right). Avoid raising the head of the bed more than 30 degrees to prevent the buildup of shearing pressure. When you must raise it more—at mealtimes, for instance—keep the periods brief.

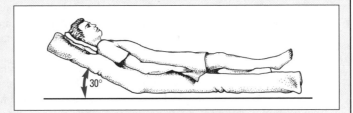

As you reposition the patient from one side to the other, make sure the weight rests on their buttock, not hip bone. Resting weight on the buttock reduces pressure on the trochanter and sacrum. The angle between the bed and an imaginary lateral line through their hips should be about 30 degrees. If needed, use pillows or a foam wedge to help the patient maintain the proper position (see illustration bottom right). Cushion pressure points, such as the knees and shoulders, with pillows as well.

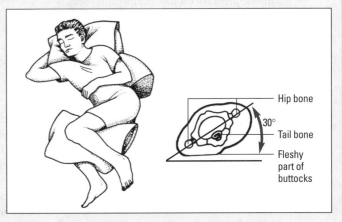

Hip bone
30°
Tail bone
Fleshy part of buttocks

Heel appeal

Heels present a particularly difficult challenge. Even with the aid of specially designed mattresses, reducing the pressure on heels to below capillary refill pressure is almost impossible. Instead, suspend the patient's foot so the bony prominence on the heel is under no pressure. Gel pads can be used to relieve pressure on the heels. Placing a pillow or foam cushion under the length of the patient's leg can permit a comfortable position while suspending the foot. Take care to avoid knee contraction, however.

Positioning a seated patient

Unlikely as it seems, a patient is more likely to develop pressure ulcers from sitting than from reclining. Sitting tends to focus all of the patient's weight on the relatively small surface areas of the buttocks, thighs and soles. Much of this weight is focused on the small area of tissue covering the ischial tuberosities. Proper posture and alignment help ensure that the weight of the patient's body is distributed as evenly as possible. NICE (2003) recommend that sitting time for individuals who are at risk should be less than 2 hours until their condition changes.

Posture perfect

Proper posture alone can significantly reduce the patient's risk of ulcers at the ankles, elbows, forearms, wrists and knees. Explain proper posture to your patient, if necessary, as described here:
• Sit with back erect and against the back of the chair, thighs parallel to the floor, knees comfortably parted and arms horizontal and supported by the arms of the chair. This posture distributes weight evenly over the available body surface area.
• Keep feet flat on the floor to protect the heels from focused pressure and distribute the weight of the legs over the largest available surface area—the soles.
• Avoid slouching, which causes shearing force and friction and places undue pressure on the sacrum and coccyx.
• Keep the thighs and arms parallel to ensure that weight is evenly distributed all along the thighs and forearms, instead of being focused on the ischial tuberosities and elbows, respectively.
• Part the knees to keep knees and ankles from rubbing together.

Feet up

If the patient likes to use a footstool, check to see if their knees are above the level of their hips. If so, it means that the weight has shifted from the back of their thighs to the ischial tuberosities—and that they need a different footstool. The same problem—knees above hips—can occur if the chair itself is too short for the patient.

Patients should be encouraged to reposition themselves every 15 minutes while sitting, if they can. Patients with spinal cord injuries can perform wheelchair push-ups to intermittently relieve pressure on the buttocks and

---

Pressure reduction devices

Here are some special pads, mattresses and beds that help relieve pressure when a patient is confined to one position for long periods:

- *Gel pads* disperse pressure over a wide surface area.
- *Alternating-pressure air mattress* involves alternating deflation and inflation of mattress tubes that changes areas of pressure.
- *High-specification foam* mattress, cushion skin, minimising pressure.
- *Low-air-loss bed* has a surface that consists of inflated air cushions. Each section is adjusted for optimal pressure relief for the patient's body size.
- *Air-fluidised bed* contains beads that move under an airflow to support the patient, thus reducing shearing force and friction.
- *Moving and handling devices*, including glide sheets and other devices, prevents shearing by lifting the patient rather than dragging them across the bed.
- *Padding*, including pillows and soft blankets, can reduce pressure in body hollows.
- *Foot cradle* lifts the bed linen to relieve pressure over the feet.

---

sacrum. This requires a fair amount of upper body strength, however, and some patients might not have the strength. Others may have injuries that preclude using this technique.

Support aids and cushions

Pillows may be used as support tools, but they're no longer the only options available. Today, people can choose from a vast array of support surfaces and cushioning aids. Special beds, mattresses and seating options that employ foams, gels, water and air as cushioning agents make it possible to tailor a comprehensive and personal system of supports for your patient.

Effective care depends on knowledge of the classes and types of products. In the course of your work, take time to learn as much as you can about these products. (See *Pressure reduction devices*.)

False security

Be informed, but be cautious as well. Using these devices can instill a false sense of security. It's important to remember that as helpful as these devices may be, they aren't substitutes for attentive care. Patients require individual turning schedules, regardless of the equipment used, and this schedule depends on your assessment of the patient's tolerance for pressure.

Beds and mattresses

When we discuss horizontal support surfaces we are, for the most part, talking about beds, mattresses and mattress overlays. These products employ foams, gels, water and air to minimise the pressure a patient experiences while lying in bed.

Beds

Specialty beds, such as oscillating and rotating beds, relieve pressure by turning the patient or help lift the patient to reduce the risk of friction and shear. However, they're expensive and are rarely an option for a patient returning home. The use of electronic beds has grown and are available in both the hospital and home settings. These enable the patient or care to alter the position of the patient at the press of a button.

Mattresses

Most mattresses and overlays use some form or manipulation of foam, gel, air or water to cushion the patient. Low-tech mattresses and overlays spread the pressure over a larger area, they include the high-specification foam mattresses, gel, fluid or fibre filled mattresses or overlays. High-tech devices include low-air-loss mattresses which support the patient on air filled sacs, they remain at a constant pressure and air is able to pass air over the patient's skin. These mattresses promote evaporation and are especially useful when skin maceration is a problem. Alternating-pressure uses air evenly distributes pressure under the patient, by alternately inflating and deflating tubes within the mattress to distribute pressure (NICE, 2003).

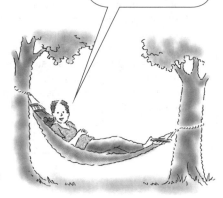

This is probably not the best for your patient in terms of support surfaces. Works fine for a quick nap for me though!

Support aids for sitting

Products designed to help prevent pressure ulcers while sitting fall into two broad categories: products that relieve pressure and products that ease re-positioning.

Ambulatory and wheelchair-dependent patients should use seat cushions to distribute weight over the largest possible surface area. Wheelchair-dependent patients require an especially rugged seat cushion that can stand up to the rigors of daily use. In most instances, a good foam cushion 7.5 to 10 cm thick

---

Saftey first!

- Make sure that mattresses and overlays don't make the bed too high for your patient.
- Check the mattress used is suitable for the weight of your patient.
- Assess the patient's risk of developing a pressure ulcer and select the right mattress.

Extra care with children

- Suitable mattresses must be selected for small children, ensuring that the mattress has the correct cell size.
- The pressure sensors on some mattresses may not detect the child's position on it, causing inappropriate pressure. Also, the head area on an AP mattress tends to remain inflated which can cause too much pressure on the back of their head.

(Adapted from NICE, 2005.)

suffices. However, many wheelchair-seating clinics now use computers to create custom seating systems tailored to fit the physiology and needs of each patient. For patients with spinal cord injuries, the selection of wheelchair seating is based on pressure evaluation, lifestyle, postural stability, continence and cost. Custom seats and cushions are more expensive; however, in this case, the added expense is justifiable. Encourage wheelchair patients to replace seat cushions as soon as their current one begins to deteriorate.

A position on repositioning

Repositioning is just as important when the patient is sitting as when they are lying in bed. For a patient requiring assistance, various devices are available. Such devices include overhead frames, trapezes, walkers and canes; these can help the patients reposition themself as necessary. Health-care personnel can help manoeuvre I.V. poles and other support equipment.

Managing skin integrity

An effective skin integrity management plan includes regular inspections for tissue breakdown, routine cleaning and moisturising and steps to protect the skin from incontinence, if this is an issue.

Inspecting the skin

The patient's skin should be routinely inspected for damage by pressure, depending on the patient's assessed risk and their ability to tolerate pressure. Check for pallor and areas of redness—both signs of ischaemia. Be aware that redness that occurs after the pressure is removed (called reactive hyperaemia) is commonly the first external sign of ischaemia due to pressure. Remember to remove anti-emboli stockings daily to check for any skin damage on the legs and heels.

With patients who have darker skin, dectecting pressure damage is more difficult and it important to assess any localised pain or temperature difference of the skin together with any colour change.

Cleaning the skin

Usually, cleaning with a gentle soap and warm water suffices for daily skin hygiene. Use a soft cloth to pat, rather than rub, the skin dry. Avoid scrubbing or the use of harsh cleaning agents.

Moisturising the skin

Skin becomes dry, flaky and less pliable when it loses moisture. Dry skin is more susceptible to damage. There are a considerable number of skin moisturising products available, it is difficult to know which to choose. The simpler the better, choose ones without perfumes as they may cause skin irritation.

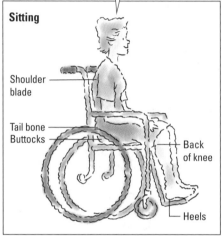

Important! Wheel chair users should be assessed by a physiotherapist or occupational therapist.

Sitting

Shoulder blade

Tail bone
Buttocks

Back of knee

Heels

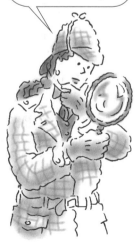

Effective management of skin integrity requires regular inspections as well as routine cleaning and moisturising and protecting the skin from incontinence. It's elementary!

Lotions

Lotions are dissolved powder crystals held in suspension by surfactants. Lotions have the highest water content and evaporate faster than any other type of moisturiser. Consequently, lotions must be applied more often. The high water content is why lotions feel cool when they're applied.

Creams

Creams are preparations of oil and water; they're more occlusive than lotions. Creams don't have to be applied as often as lotions; three or four applications per day should do the trick. Creams are better for preventing moisture loss due to evaporation than for replenishing skin moisture.

Ointments

Ointments are preparations of water in oil (typically lanolin or petrolatum). They're the most occlusive and longest-lasting form of moisturiser. They can be quite greasy and take time for the skin to absorb them.

Protecting the skin

Although some moisture is good, too much is a problem. Waterlogged skin is easily eroded by friction and is more susceptible to irritants and bacteria colonisation than dry skin. Close monitoring helps head off problems before they escalate.

Skin protection is particularly important if the patient is incontinent. Urine and faeces introduce chemical irritants and bacteria as well as moisture, which can speed skin breakdown. To effectively manage incontinence, first determine the cause and then plan interventions that protect skin integrity while addressing the underlying problem.

In older adults, don't assume that incontinence is a normal part of aging. It isn't. Instead, consider factors that can precipitate incontinence, such as:
- faecal impaction and tube feeding (can cause diarrhoea)
- reaction to a medication (can cause urinary incontinence)
- urinary tract infection
- mobility problems (can keep the patient from reaching the bathroom in time)
- confusion or embarrassment (can keep the patient from asking for a bedpan or help getting to the bathroom).

Lend a helping hand

Whether the underlying cause is reversible or not, encourage the patient to ask for help when they need a bedpan or needs to go to the bathroom. Make sure the patient does not have to walk too far. Use incontinence pads and skin barriers, as appropriate, to minimise skin damage. Step up the frequency of inspections, cleaning and moisturising for these patients.

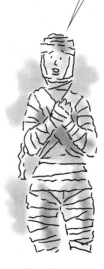

I wouldn't advise this method for protecting the skin. For your patient, determine the cause and plan interventions that protect skin integrity.

Assessing pressure ulcers

Pressure ulcers can occur even with the best preventive measures. Effective treatment depends on a thorough assessment of the developing wound. Meaningful ulcer assessment requires a systematic, objective approach. The European Pressure Ulcer Advisory Panel (EPUAP) advise that an assessment of the ulcer should include:

- location
- grade
- size (length, width and depth in centimeters)
- wound bed (necrotic tissue, granulation or epithelialisation tissue present)
- amount of exudate
- apperance of surrounding skin
- pain.

On the border

Ulcer borders can provide clues to healing potential. Assess skin around the ulcer for:

- redness
- warmth
- induration or hardness
- swelling
- signs of infection.

Before you examine the ulcer, assess the patient's pain. In most cases, pressure ulcers cause some degree of pain; in some cases, pain is severe. Have the patient rate their pain on a visual analogue scale of 0 to 10, with 0 representing no pain and 10 representing severe pain. Similarly, ask the patient whether the pain interferes with their ability to function normally and, if so, to what degree.

Location

Common locations for pressure ulcers include:

- sacrum
- coccyx
- ischial tuberosities
- greater trochanters
- elbows
- heels
- scapulae
- occipital bone
- sternum
- ribs
- iliac crests

- patellae
- lateral malleoli
- medial malleoli.

Characteristics

Tissue involvement ranges from blanchable erythema to the deep destruction of tissue associated with a full-thickness wound. Pressure against tissue interrupts blood flow and causes pallor due to tissue ischaemia. If prolonged, ischaemia causes irreversible and extensive tissue damage.

Reactive hyperemia

Usually, reactive hyperemia is the first visible sign of ischaemia. When the pressure causing ischaemia is released, skin flushes red as blood rushes back into the tissue. This reddening is called reactive hyperemia, and it's due to a protective mechanism in the body that dilates vessels in the affected area to increase the blood flow and speed oxygen to starved tissues. Reactive hyperemia first appears as a bright flush that lasts about one-half or three-quarters as long as the ischaemic period. If the applied pressure is too high for too long, reactive hyperemia fails to meet the demand for blood and tissue damage occurs.

Blanchable erythema

Blanchable erythema (redness) can signal imminent tissue damage. Erythema results from capillary dilation near the skin's surface. In the patient with pressure ulcers, the redness results from the release of ischaemia-causing pressure. Blanchable erythema is redness that blanches—turns white—when pressed with a fingertip and then immediately turns red again when pressure is removed. Tissue exhibiting blanchable erythema usually resumes its normal colour within 24 hours and suffers no long-term damage. However, the longer it takes for tissue to recover from finger pressure, the higher the patient's risk of developing pressure ulcers.

In dark-skinned patients, erythema is hard to discern. Use bright light and look for taut, shiny patches of skin with a purplish tinge. Also, assess carefully for localised heat, induration, or oedema, which can be better indicators of ischaemia than erythema.

Non-blanchable erythema

Non-blanchable erythema can be the first sign of tissue destruction. In high-risk patients, non-blanchable tissue can develop in as little as 2 hours. The redness associated with non-blanchable erythema is more intense and doesn't change when compressed with a finger. If recognised and treated early, non-blanchable erythema is reversible. It may be difficult to see on darker skin, compare the surrounding skin for warmth, pain and hardness as it may indicate tissue damage and appropriate action can be taken.

What you can't see

In many cases, the full extent of ulceration can't be determined by visual inspection because there may be extensive undermining along fascial planes. For example, tunneling can connect ulcers over the sacrum to ulcers over the trochanter of the femur or the ischial tuberosities. These cavities can contain extensive necrotic tissue.

Size

Using a disposable measuring tape, measure wound length (in centimeters) as the longest dimension of the wound and width as the longest distance perpendicular to the length. Alternatively, carefully trace the wound margins on a piece of paper. In addition, a growing number of areas now use wound photography. Measure the ulcer's depth at its deepest point by inserting a gloved finger or a cotton-tipped swab. If you're using a probe other than your finger, be very careful; it's easy to cause further damage. Note any visible tunnels or undermining. If possible, use a gloved finger to gauge the extent.

Colour

Wound colour is a good indication of wound status. Record wound colour using the red–yellow–black classification system. If more than one colour is evident, classify the wound using the least healthy colour.

Base

The type of tissue in the ulcer base determines the potential for healing and the type of treatment. Know how to identify necrotic tissue, granulation tissue and epithelial tissue.

Necrotic tissue

Necrotic tissue may appear as a moist yellow or gray area of tissue that's separating from viable tissue. When dry, necrotic tissue appears as thick, hard and leathery black eschar. Areas of necrotic or devitalised tissue may mask underlying abscesses and collections of fluid. Before the ulcer can begin to heal, necrotic tissue, drainage and metabolic wastes must be removed from the wound.

Granulation tissue

Granulation tissue appears as beefy red, bumpy, shiny tissue in the base of the ulcer. As it heals, a full-thickness ulcer develops more and more granulation tissue. Such factors as tissue oxygenation, tissue hydration and nutrition can alter the colour and quality of granulation tissue.

Epithelial tissue

Epithelialisation is the regeneration of epidermis across the ulcer surface. It appears as pale or dark pink skin, first becoming evident at ulcer borders in full-thickness wounds and as islands around hair follicles in partial-thickness wounds. Wound healing can be assessed and quantified by the percentage of surface covered by new epithelium.

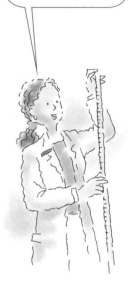

Measure wound length in centimetres as the longest dimension of the wound and width as the longest distance perpendicular to the length.

Exudate

Ulcers with exudate (drainage) take longer to heal. Exudate characteristics include amount, colour, consistency and odour. Record the amount as scant, moderate, large or copious. Describe the colour and consistency together with clear, descriptive terms, such as:

- serous—clear, watery
- sanguineous—bloody
- serosanguineous—clear red or reddish brown
- purulent—thick, yellow, cloudy.

The nose knows

Odour is a subjective observation—one that can suggest infection. It's important to clean the wound thoroughly before assessing the colour and odour of drainage. Otherwise, perceived drainage may be, in actuality, a combination of dressing residue and dead cells—a combination that always produces a noxious odour. However, putrid odour that remains after wound cleaning may indicate anaerobic infection.

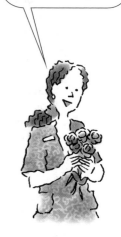

Your nose knows. Although these roses smell lovely, your patient's wound may have a putrid odour if it's infected. Keep your nose on the job!

Margins

Pressure ulcer edges have distinct characteristics, including colour, thickness and degree of attachment to the wound base. Assess the epithelial rim as an integral part of the wound base. Ideally, there should be a free border of epithelial cells. These are the cells that proliferate and migrate across the wound bed during healing. When epidermis at the ulcer edges thickens and rolls under, it impairs migration of epithelial cells.

Tunnel troubles

In undermining, which occurs when necrosis of subcutaneous fat or muscle occurs, a pocket extends beneath the skin at the ulcer's edge. Tunneling differs from undermining in that both ends of a tunnel emerge through the skin's surface. In many cases, a tunnel connects two otherwise distinct pressure ulcers, and it may be necessary to open the tunnel before the ulcer can heal.

Sometimes full-thickness pressure ulcers form tracts along fascial planes. When extensive, external palpation is the only way to determine the direction and length of the tracts. It may be helpful to outline the tract on the outer skin using a felt tipped pen which will be useful in determing whether the ulcer is responding to treatment in future assessments.

Surrounding skin

Assess intact skin surrounding the ulcer for redness, warmth, induration (hardness), swelling and signs of infection. Feel for heat, pain and oedema. The ulcer bed should be moist, but the surrounding skin should be dry. The skin should be adequately moisturised, but neither macerated nor eroded. Macerated skin appears waterlogged and may turn white at the wound's edges.

Inappropriate dressings can cause maceration of surrounding skin, since the dressing may not absorb all of the exudate. Other causes of maceration include urine or faeces contamination and poor technique during dressing changes may result in irritation or stripping of the surrounding skin.

Grading pressure ulcers

The most widely used system for grading pressure ulcers is the classification system developed by the European Pressure Ulcer Advisory Panel (EPUAP). These guidelines identify a grading system, which defines four stages, which aides the health-care worker to assess and describe the pressure ulcer according to accepted criteria.

Grading

Grading reflects the depth and extent of tissue involvement. Regrading isn't needed unless deeper layers of tissue are exposed by treatments such as debridement. Keep in mind that although grading is useful for classifying pressure ulcers, it's only one part of a comprehensive assessment. Ulcer characteristics and the condition of the surrounding skin provide equally important clues to the ulcer's prognosis. (See *Grading pressure ulcers*, page 310.)

Closed pressure ulcers

Closed pressure ulcers are unique and potentially life-threatening pressure ulcers. They begin when shearing force causes ischaemic necrosis in subcutaneous tissue. No surface defect marks this event. In time, pressure from inflammation in the cavity of necrotic debris causes a small, unremarkable ulcer to form on the skin. This ulcer drains a large contaminated base. There are no signs of systemic infection either.

A class of their own

Closed pressure ulcers can't be classified by grade because the extent of damage can't be determined until the defect is surgically opened. In addition, surgery is the only viable treatment.

Patients confined to wheelchairs because of spinal cord injury are at highest risk for this type of pressure ulcer, and the ulcers occur most commonly in the pelvic region. Prompt recognition is crucial. The only viable treatment is wide surgical excision and closure with a muscle rotation flap.

Stay on the ball

Grading pressure ulcers

You can use pressure ulcer characteristics gained from your assessment to stage the pressure ulcer, as described here. Staging reflects the anatomic depth of exposed tissue. Keep in mind that if the wound contains necrotic tissue, you won't be able to determine the grade until you can see the wound base.

Grade 1

A grade 1 pressure ulcer is an area of skin with observable pressure-related changes when compared with an adjacent area or the same region on the other side of the body. This ulcer presents clinically as a defined area of persistent redness in patients with light skin or persistent red, blue or purple in patients with darker skin. Indicators include a change in one or more of the following characteristics:

- skin temperature (warmth or coolness)
- tissue consistency (boggy or firm)
- sensation (pain or itching).

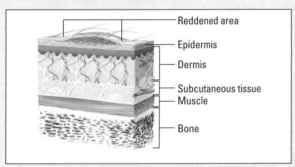

Reddened area
Epidermis
Dermis
Subcutaneous tissue
Muscle
Bone

Grade 2

A grade 2 pressure ulcer is a superficial partial-thickness wound that appears as an abrasion, a blister or a shallow crater involving the epidermis and dermis.

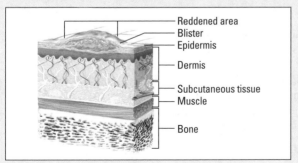

Reddened area
Blister
Epidermis
Dermis
Subcutaneous tissue
Muscle
Bone

Grade 3

A grade 3 pressure ulcer is a full-thickness wound with tissue damage or necrosis of subcutaneous tissue that can extend down to, but not through, underlying fasciae. The ulcer appears as a deep crater with or without undermining of adjacent tissue.

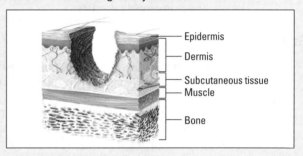

Epidermis
Dermis
Subcutaneous tissue
Muscle
Bone

Grade 4

A grade 4 pressure ulcer involves full-thickness skin loss with extensive damage, destruction or necrosis to muscle, bone and supporting structures (such as tendons and joint capsule). Undermining and sinus tracts may be present as well.

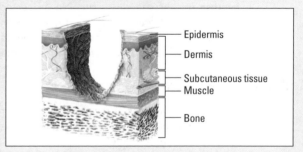

Epidermis
Dermis
Subcutaneous tissue
Muscle
Bone

Treating pressure ulcers

Treatment of pressure ulcers follows the four basic steps common to all wound care:

- Debride necrotic tissue and clean the wound to remove debris.
- Provide a moist wound-healing environment through the use of proper dressings.
- Protect the wound from further injury.
- Provide nutrition that's essential to wound healing.

A key element in all pressure ulcer treatment plans is identifying and treating, when possible, the underlying pathophysiology. If the cause of the ulcer remains, existing ulcers don't heal and new ulcers develop.

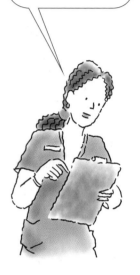

Topical agents can be used to treat some issues of wounds. Usually, cleaning, debriding and dressings are part of treatment as well.

That's so typical

Typically, wound care involves cleaning the wound, debriding necrotic tissue and applying a dressing that keeps the wound bed moist. Topical agents are used to resolve various issues.

Wound cleaning

Wound cleaning removes wound debris, old dressing materials and necrotic tissue from the wound surface. Pressurised wound irrigation is adequate for almost all wound cleaning.

Debridement

Debridement removes non-viable tissue and is the most important factor in wound management. Healing can't take place until necrotic tissue is removed.

Dressings

Dressings serve to:

- protect the wound from contamination
- prevent trauma
- provide compression (if bleeding or swelling occurs)
- apply medications
- absorb drainage or debride necrotic tissue.

The cardinal rule

When choosing a dressing for a pressure ulcer, the cardinal rule remains the same: keep moist tissue moist and dry tissue dry. Wound characteristics dictate the type of dressing used. The dressing selected should protect wound integrity and keep the wound surface moist but prevent an excessive build-up of moisture, which can cause maceration and bacterial colonisation. The frequency of dressing changes depends on the amount and type of wound drainage, as well as the characteristics of the dressing.

Keep it light

Wound cavities may require light packing or fill to prevent areas from walling off and developing into abscesses. Be careful with packing though; too much packing can generate more pressure and cause additional tissue damage.

Patient education

Remember that the goal of patient education is to improve the outcome. For any care plan to succeed after the patient leaves the hospital, the patient or caregiver must understand the care plan and be physically capable of carrying it out at home. Therefore, education and goal establishment should take into consideration the preferences and lifestyles of the patient and their family whenever possible.

Teach the patient and their family how to prevent pressure ulcers and what to do when they occur. (See *Pressure ulcer dos and don'ts*.) Explain repositioning, and show them what a 30 degree laterally inclined position looks like. If the patient needs assistance with repositioning, make sure they know the types of devices available and where to obtain them.

Pressure ulcer dos and don'ts

With proper skin care and frequent position changes, patients and their caregivers can keep the patient's skin healthy—a crucial element in pressure ulcer prevention. Here are some important dos and don'ts to pass along to patients:

Dos
- Change position at least once every 2 hours while reclining. Follow a schedule. Lie on your right side, then your left side, then your back and then your stomach (if possible). Use pillows and pads for support. Make small turns between the 2-hour changes.
- Check your skin for signs of pressure ulcers twice daily. Use a mirror to check areas you can't inspect directly, such as the shoulders, tail bone, hips, elbows, heels and the back of the head. Report any breaks in the skin or changes in skin temperature to your nurse.
- Use oil-free lotions.
- Follow the prescribed exercise program, including range-of-motion exercises every 8 hours, or as recommended.
- Eat a well-balanced diet, drink lots of fluids, and strive to maintain the recommended weight.

Don'ts
- Don't use commercial soaps or skin products that dry or irritate your skin.
- Don't sleep on wrinkled bedsheets or tuck your covers tightly into the foot of your bed.

Mirror, mirror . . .

Show the patient how they can inspect their back and other areas using a mirror. If the patient can't do this, a family member can help. Make sure they understand the importance of inspecting skin over bony prominences for pressure related damage every day.

If the patient needs to apply dressings at home, make sure they know the proper ways to apply and remove them. Tell them where they can get further supplies if they run low. Provide them with written information where possible and how to contact a health-care professional if they need more help or advice.

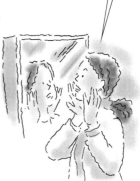

Teach the patient how to inspect their back and other areas using a mirror.

Proper nutrition

Ensuring proper nutrition can be difficult, but the patient and their family need to know how important proper nutrition is to the healing process. Provide materials on nutrition and maintaining an ideal weight, as appropriate. Refer the patient or carer to a dietician for more advice, if necessary.

Pressure ulcers should be reassessed at least weekly or when the patient's condition changes. Measure progress by the reduction in necrotic tissue and drainage and the increase in granulation tissue and epithelial growth. Clean, vascularised pressure ulcers should show evidence of healing within 2 weeks. If they don't, and the patient has followed the guidelines for nutrition, repositioning, use of support surfaces and wound care, it's time to re-evaluate the care plan.

Quick quiz

1. The main functions of the skin include:
    A. support, nourishment and sensation.
    B. protection, sensory perception and temperature regulation.
    C. fluid transport, sensory perception and aging regulation.
    D. support, protection and communication.

Answer: B. The skin's main functions involve protection from injury, noxious chemicals and bacterial invasion; sensory perception of touch, temperature and pain; and regulation of body heat.

2. Which type of wound closes by primary intention?
    A. Second-degree burn
    B. Pressure ulcer
    C. Traumatic injury
    D. Surgical incision

Answer: D. A surgical incision is an example of a wound that closes by primary intention, in which there's no deep tissue loss and the wound edges are well approximated.

3. Which wound bed colour indicates normal, healthy granulation tissue?
    A. Red
    B. Yellow
    C. Tan
    D. Black

Answer: A. Red tissue indicates healthy granulation tissue.

4. Which intervention is most appropriate for preventing excessive heel pressure?
    A. Flexing the knees
    B. Placing a donut-shaped cushion under the feet
    C. Suspending the heels by placing a pillow under the lenghth of the leg
    D. Putting a pressure-reducing foam mattress under the heels

Answer: C. Suspending the heels using a pillow under the lenghth of leg is the best way to protect heels from pressure ulceration.

Scoring

✩✩✩   If you answered all four questions correctly, superb! You have a lot of integrity when it comes to knowledge of skin and wounds.

✩✩   If you answered three questions correctly, great! You're holding up well under the pressure.

✩   If you answered fewer than three questions correctly, relax! Just take a load off, review the chapter, and try again.

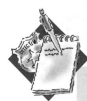

14 Mobility, activity and exercise

Just the facts

In this chapter, you'll learn:

♦ factors that affect musculoskeletal functioning

♦ proper patient positioning

♦ use of alignment

♦ legal and professional responsibilities

♦ principles of moving and handling

♦ methods of transferring a patient

♦ walking-frame use

♦ ways to perform range of movement (ROM) exercises.

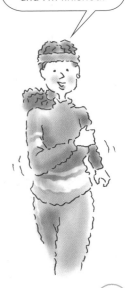

It's all about mobility. Another 30 minutes of mobility and I'm finished!

A look at mobility, activity and exercise

Mobility is defined as an individual's ability to move within, and interact with, the environment and the ability to move from one location to another. A patient's mobility or ability to move and be active affects not only their physical but also their emotional well-being. Mobility is essential to an individual's independence. Many older adults experience loss of mobility, along with functional loss and a lowered activity level. However, younger patients can also be affected by immobility from prolonged bed rest due to the physical restraints secondary to fractures or traction, or from loss of strength due to illness.

Actively active

Activity keeps the mind and body active. Musculoskeletal inactivity or immobility adversely affects all body systems. Exercise, even passive ROM exercises, helps prevent muscle atrophy, prevent muscle contractures and maintain circulation. Exercise increases muscle strength, tone and mass. It also enhances the condition of other body systems.

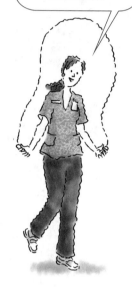

Exercise helps maintain circulation.

A look at the musculoskeletal system

Muscles, bones, joints, tendons and ligaments give the human body its shape and ability to be mobile, perform such activities as those of daily living, and exercise. The three main components of the musculoskeletal system are:

 bones

 joints

 muscles.

Bones

The 206 bones of the skeleton form the body's framework, supporting and protecting organs and tissues. The bones also serve as storage sites for minerals and contain bone marrow, the primary site for blood production. (See *A close look at the skeletal system*.)

Joints

The junction of two or more bones is called a *joint*. Joints stabilise the bones and allow a specific type of movement. The two types of joints are:

 non-synovial

 synovial.

Non-synovial

In non-synovial joints, the bones are connected by fibrous tissue, also called *cartilage*. The bones may be immovable, such as the sutures in the skull, or slightly movable, such as the vertebrae.

Synovial

Synovial joints move freely; the bones are separate from each other and meet in a cavity filled with synovial fluid, a lubricant. In synovial joints, a layer of resilient cartilage covers the surfaces of opposing bones. This cartilage cushions the bones and allows full joint movement by making the surfaces of the bones smooth. These joints are surrounded by a fibrous capsule that stabilises the joint structures. The capsule also surrounds the joint's ligaments, the tough, fibrous bands that join one bone to another.

A close look at the skeletal system

Of the 206 bones in the human skeletal system, 80 form the axial skeleton (skull, facial bones, vertebrae, ribs, sternum and hyoid bone) and 126 form the appendicular skeleton (arms, legs, shoulders and pelvis). Shown here are the body's major bones.

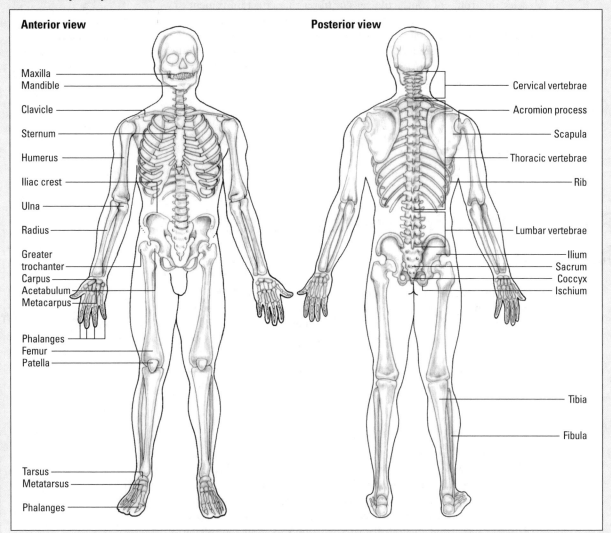

Anterior view

Maxilla
Mandible
Clavicle
Sternum
Humerus
Iliac crest
Ulna
Radius
Greater trochanter
Carpus
Acetabulum
Metacarpus
Phalanges
Femur
Patella
Tarsus
Metatarsus
Phalanges

Posterior view

Cervical vertebrae
Acromion process
Scapula
Thoracic vertebrae
Rib
Lumbar vertebrae
Ilium
Sacrum
Coccyx
Ischium
Tibia
Fibula

Popular joints

Synovial joints come in several types, including ball-and-socket joints and hinge joints. Ball-and-socket joints, the shoulders and hips being the only examples of this type, enable flexion, extension, adduction and abduction. These joints also rotate in their sockets and are assessed by their degree of internal and external rotation. Hinge joints, such as the knee and elbow, typically move in flexion and extension only. (See *Synovial joint*.)

Muscles

Muscles are groups of contractile cells or fibres that effect movement of an organ or a part of the body. Skeletal muscles, the focus of this chapter, contract and produce skeletal movement when they receive a stimulus from the central nervous system (CNS). The CNS is responsible for involuntary and voluntary muscle function. Tendons, the tough fibrous portions of muscle, attach the muscles to bone.

Where would we be without bursae?

Bursae are sacs filled with friction-reducing synovial fluid; they're located in areas of high friction such as the knee. Bursae enable adjacent muscles or muscles and tendons to glide smoothly over each other during movement.

Factors affecting musculoskeletal function

When an individual has limited mobility and movement, one's health can deteriorate and multiple complications can occur. The signs and symptoms of inactivity can include decreased muscle strength and tone, lack of co-ordination, altered gait, falls, decreased joint flexibility, pain on movement and decreased activity tolerance.

Lifestyle and habits can affect a person's mobility. Regular exercise helps maintain musculoskeletal functioning and mobility. Inactivity due to age, disease or trauma can alter that mobility.

Major or minor trauma

Anything that interferes with bone resiliency and strength or muscle strength may impair the musculoskeletal system's capacity to assist mobility. Trauma can result in injury to tendons, ligaments, joints, bones or muscles. This damage can be minor or major and can affect mobility for a short time, or for a longer time if it involves a dislocated joint, broken bone, torn tendons or joint replacement.

Diseases such as rheumatoid arthritis, osteoporosis, gout and osteoarthritis can also limit mobility. Bone tumours can cause pain and may require amputation of the affected limbs.

The nerves have it

Any disorder that impairs the nervous system's ability to control movement of the muscles and co-ordination hinders mobility. Such diseases as muscular

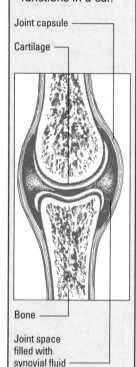

Synovial joint

Normally, bones fit together. Cartilage, a smooth, fibrous tissue, cushions the end of each bone, and synovial fluid fills the joint space. This fluid lubricates the joint and eases movement, much as the brake fluid functions in a car.

Joint capsule

Cartilage

Bone

Joint space filled with synovial fluid

dystrophy, Parkinson's disease, and multiple sclerosis slowly erode and destroy the patient's capacity for co-ordinated movement.

Two or four

Brain or spinal cord injuries can result in a severed or severely damaged spinal cord, causing paralysis below the injury. Decreased motor and sensory function to the legs is referred to as *paraplegia* and paralysis of the arms and the legs is called *quadriplegia*.

O₂ needed

Oxygen is needed for the muscles to function properly. Any disease that limits the oxygen supply affects muscle contraction and movement. Lung conditions reduce the amount of oxygen delivered to the cells, including skeletal muscles.

Ouch! That hurts!

Activity intolerance may be associated with pain or oedema. Alternatively, the patient's activity may be severely restricted by such conditions as fractures requiring skeletal traction, rheumatoid arthritis, vertebral fractures, neurogenic arthropathy, Paget's disease, muscular dystrophy and other disorders.

Treating immobility

Impaired physical mobility is related to many musculoskeletal disorders that involve joint inflammation as well as fractures, bone disorders and other disorders that cause decreased mobility.

Proper positioning

Proper positioning (*see Positioning patients*, page 320) and alignment and pressure-reducing devices help maintain correct body positioning and prevent complications that can occur with prolonged bed rest. When a patient is weak, in pain, frail, paralyzed, immobilised or unconscious, they can't readily position and reposition themselves. Thus, they need your assistance to help or provide position changes. Assessing the skin and providing skin care before and after re-positioning is also important.

Change is good

Frequent position changes help prevent muscle discomfort, damage to superficial nerves and blood vessels, prolonged pressure resulting in pressure ulcers and muscle contractures.

Positioning patients

Supine position

In the supine position, the patient is placed on their back with the knees slightly flexed. Place a pillow beneath their head for comfort. This position immobilises the spine. It's commonly used for a spinal cord injury, urinary catheter insertion or, in women, a vaginal examination.

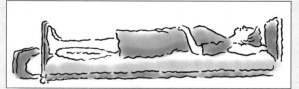

Semi-recumbent position

For a semi-recumbent position, elevate the head of the bed to 30 degrees and raise the bed section under the patient's knees, flexing the knees slightly. This position promotes drainage, cardiac output and ventilation. It also prevents aspiration of food and secretions. It's commonly used for a patient who has a head injury, increased intracranial pressure or dyspnoea; has undergone abdominal surgery, cranial surgery, thyroidectomy or eye surgery; or is vomiting.

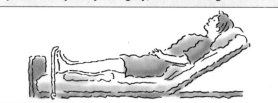

Prone position

The prone position is used to promote gas exchange and enable examination of the back. It's accomplished by placing the patient on their stomach with the head turned to one side and positioning the arms at the side or above their head. Make sure that the legs are extended. This position is commonly used for immobilisation, acute respiratory distress syndrome and after lumbar puncture or a myelogram.

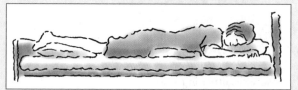

Lateral position

The lateral position promotes safety and prevents atelectasis, pressure ulcers and aspiration of food and secretions. Place the patient on their side, with their weight supported mostly by the lateral aspect of the lower scapula and the lower ilium. Support this position by placing pillows as needed. This position is commonly used for administering an enema or a suppository and for a patient who has undergone abdominal surgery, is in a coma or has pressure ulcers.

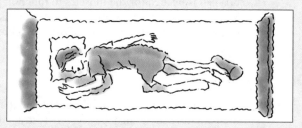

Semi-prone position

The semi-prone position enables examination of the back and rectum and can help prevent atelectasis and pressure ulcers. Position the patient on their side with a small pillow placed beneath the head. Flex one knee towards their abdomen, with the other knee only slightly flexed. Place one arm behind their body and the other in a comfortable position. Support the patient in this position with pillows as needed. This position is commonly used for a patient who has sustained rectal injuries or is in a coma.

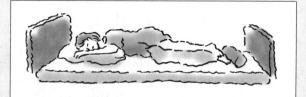

Using alignment devices

Alignment devices include abduction pillows (triangular shaped wedge placed between the legs) or wedges to help prevent internal hip rotation after femoral fracture, hip fracture or surgery; trochanter rolls or T-rolls to help prevent external hip rotation; and hand rolls to help prevent hand contractures. Several of these devices—trochanter rolls, hand rolls etc.—are especially useful when caring for patients who have a loss of sensation, mobility or consciousness or following a neuromuscular incident such as stroke.

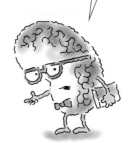

A disorder affecting the nervous system can impair a person's ability to co-ordinate movement.

What you need

Abduction pillow ✳ trochanter rolls ✳ hand rolls (see *Common preventive devices*, page 322)

Getting ready

If you're using a device that's available in different sizes, select the appropriate size for the patient.

How you do it

• Explain the purpose and steps of the procedure to the patient.

Applying an abduction pillow

• Place the patient in a supine position and put the pillow between their legs. Slide the pillow towards the groin so that it touches their legs all along their length.
• Place the upper part of both legs in the pillow's lateral indentations, and secure the straps *to prevent the pillow from slipping*.

Applying a trochanter roll

• Position one roll along the outside of the thigh, from the iliac crest to midthigh. Then place another roll along the other thigh. Make sure neither roll extends up to the knee *to avoid peroneal nerve compression and palsy, which can lead to footdrop*.

Applying a hand roll

• Place one roll in the patient's hand *to maintain the neutral position*. Then secure the strap, if present, or apply roller gauze and secure with hypoallergenic or adhesive tape.
• Place another roll in the other hand.
• Remember that the use of assistive devices doesn't preclude regularly scheduled patient positioning, ROM exercises and skin care.
• Contractures and pressure ulcers may occur with the use of a hand roll and, possibly, with other assistive devices. *To avoid these problems*, remove a soft hand roll every 4 hours (every 2 hours if the patient has hand spasticity); remove a hard hand roll every 2 hours.

Common preventive devices

These illustrations show different devices used to help maintain positioning, depending upon the patient's needs.

Trochanter roll

The trochanter roll prevents external hip rotation and is made of sponge rubber.

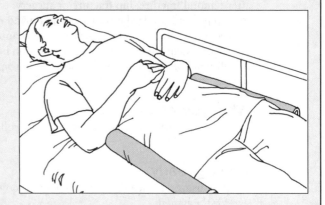

Abduction pillow

The abduction pillow prevents internal hip rotation. It's a wedge-shaped piece of sponge rubber with lateral indentations for the patient's thighs. Its straps wrap around the thighs to maintain correct positioning. Although a properly shaped bed pillow may temporarily substitute for the commercial abduction pillow, it's difficult to apply and fails to maintain the correct lateral alignment.

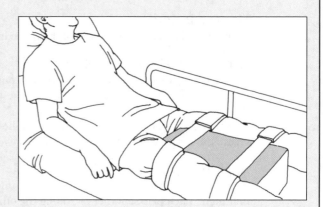

Hand roll

The hand roll prevents hand contractures. It's available in hard and soft materials and is held in place by fixed or adjustable straps

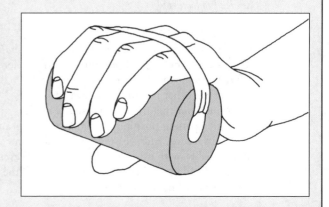

Legal and professional responsibilities

If you are moving and handling people or equipment, it is essential that you have a practical understanding of legal and professional responsibilities. When moving and handling people, the law has two objectives: injury prevention and compensation for the injured handler. This law also operates in the context of meeting a person's health and social care needs and observing their human rights. Health-care staff and student nurses need to be aware of: the main legal and professional responsibilities. These are explained under the following headings:

- Legal responsibilities
- Professional responsibilities
- The people in your care—their safety.

Legal responsibilities

The Manual Handling Operations Regulations (1992) referred to as MHOR 92, govern the moving and handling of people in the workplace. These regulations are part of the framework of health and safety legislation and have been significant when moving and handling policies and practices are reviewed.

The MHOR 92 states that employers should avoid, so far as reasonably practicable, the need for employees to undertake moving and handling which involves a risk of injury. Failing this, your duty (and your employer's) is to take appropriate steps to reduce the risk of injury to the lowest level reasonably practicable, and to provide information about the *task* and *load*.

It is important that
- you avoid manual handling operations involving a risk of injury, so far as reasonably practicable.
- where hazardous manual handling operations cannot with reasonable practicability be avoided, you assess them, taking into account the task, the load, the working environment and the individual capabilities of the handlers.
- on the basis of the information supplied by the assessment, the employer must reduce the risk of injury to the lowest level that is reasonably practicable.

Where the task is unavoidable you should undertake a risk assessment. The risk assessment recommended by *The Guide to the Handling of People*, known as HOP 5 (Smith, 2005) is easily remembered by the acronym TILE.

TILE stands for:
T = **T**ask (what you need to do)
I = **I**ndividual capability (of the staff)
L = **L**oad (the patient or object)
E = **E**nvironment

Once the assessment is completed, it must be kept up to date, recorded and readily available. By adhering to the MHOR 92, and taking reasonable care, this should protect employees from injury and protect the people in your care from moving and handling incidents.

The Management of Health and Safety at Work Regulations (1999) also refers to risk assessments being reviewed, taking into account individual capabilities information, training, co-operation and co-ordination.

The *Health and Safety at Work Act (1974)* (known as HSWA 74) refers to a safe system of work, information, training, instruction and supervision. The safe use, handling, storage and transport of equipment are also included in this Act. Section 3 of this Act does contain an explicit duty in respect of the health and safety of non-employees (patients, clients and staff of other organisations). These legal provisions are sometimes used by the health and safety executive to take action where there is an 'unsafe system of work', for example a piece of equipment has not been checked properly, or been properly maintained.

Lifting Operations and Lifting Equipment Regulations (1998), often referred to as LOLER (1998) relate to lifting equipment used at work, such as hoists—their strength, stability, positioning/installation and inspection.

Provision and Use of Work Equipment Regulations (1998) or PUWER (1998) relates to the state of the equipment being used (profiling beds, hoists, sliding sheets, transfer boards etc.), their purpose, maintenance, information, instruction and training.

Professional responsibilities

As a professional, you are personally accountable for actions and omissions in your practice and must always be able to justify your decisions. You need to ensure that you follow local moving and handling policies and *The Code: Standards of Conduct, Performance and Ethics for Nurses and Midwives* (NMC, 2008).

The people in your care cannot use health and safety at work legislation to bring compensation claims in court. They must use the common law of negligence. It is easier to bring a negligence case to court after harm has occurred, if they can demonstrate that it was caused by a carelessly taken or implemented moving and handling decision or action.

Professional competence is examined closely in negligence cases; sometimes this is easy to examine, such as a patient being dropped by two ill-trained care staff, or not using the correct sling for the patient size, ability and/or weight.

The people in your care—their safety

The Human Rights Act (1998) may have an impact upon moving and handling and the health and safety needs of yourself and for the people in your care. In respect of manual handling issues, the courts have to date referred to three in particular. These concern the right to life, the right not to be subjected to inhuman or degrading treatment, and the right to respect for home, private and family life. Therefore, we must consider the issues mentioned in the Humans Rights Act, 1998, balancing the safety and human rights of paid staff with the assessed needs and human rights of service users.

The Mental Capacity Act (2005), which came into force in April 2007, states that we can assume people have capacity. The people we care for can state through advanced directives how they would like to be cared for when they are unwell—this can include how they would like to be moved.

This Act also gave guidance for all those working with or caring for people who lack capacity to make their own decisions. In other words, the person you are caring for cannot do one or more of the following things:
* Understand information given to them.
* Retain that information long enough to make a decision.
* Weigh up the information to make a decision.
* Communicate that decision.

So you must:
* keep your skills and knowledge up to date.
* recognise and work within the limits of your competence.
* keep your knowledge and skills up to date throughout your working life.
* take part in appropriate learning and practice activities that maintain and develop your competence and performance.

Principles of moving and handling

Safe patient handling is a skilled activity, which necessitates sound underpinning theoretical knowledge combined with practical experience. Applying safe moving and handling principles will help to prevent you from developing any musculoskeletal injury (See *Twenty one principles of moving and handling*, page 326.).

Within the health-care profession, there are high rates of lower back, neck and shoulder pain that have been attributed to patient moving and handling activities. It was hoped that that the Manual Handling Operations Regulations (HSE, 2004) and related mandatory training in Moving & Handling would reduce the frequency of these accidents.

However, moving and handling activities continue to be a key cause of sickness absence across all sectors of the NHS. Dangerous patient handling practices also continue to be used by some clinically-based health-care staff, which increases their risk of injury. Poor work technique is also likely to affect the patient's safety and their experience of comfort.

It is important to be aware of the principles of moving and handling. By learning these principles you will then be able to apply them to any moving and handling situation. They are important in making moving and handling practices safer for you, your colleagues and your patient.

The principles are not in any order of importance as they are all thought to be important! However, the following are applied more frequently in moving and handling situations:
* Adopt a stable base (feet shoulder-width apart).
* Bend your knees, instead of your back.

- Never twist during the moving and handling procedure.
- Only carry out a moving and handling task if it is necessary.
- Assess every person and object task before you begin.
- Know your own individual capabilities.
- Instructions should be clear and straightforward.
- Make sure the correct equipment is chosen for the task and patient.
- Ensure equipment is in good working order and that you are trained to use it.

Twenty-one principles of moving and handling

1. If a patient can stand without assistance, let them.
2. Make sure you are aware of the risks involved in the task and that you know how to safely manage them.
3. Do not lift heavy or awkwardly-shaped objects which you feel may cause you injury. Do not move patients who may require more assistance than you are capable of delivering. Also if you have any concerns about your health or fitness (e.g. you are pregnant or have hurt yourself playing a sport, gardening etc.), you must mention this to a senior person on shift.
4. This person should be the most experienced person. They should lead and co-ordinate the move to avoid confusion. This should ensure that a safe moving and handling transfer takes place.
5. Check that everyone knows what is to happen and how the moving and handling task is to take place before commencing. Do *not* give instructions such as "1, 2, 3" but *instead say*, 'Ready, . . . steady, . . . move/sit/stand/slide'.
6. Make sure the brakes on a bed (or trolley) are applied before rolling or sliding a patient.
7. Before using a hoist, check that it is the correct type for the patient/task and that any sling to be used is suitable for the patient and transfer that is to be undertaken. The sling must be the one recommended to be used with the hoist.
8. A hoist should be serviced every six months (LOLER 1998) and recorded in an appropriate place. Do not use equipment that you are not trained to use.
9. Use handles and handling belts to help improve your grasp. Test your grip to ensure you can maintain it safely. Do *not* grab the patient's clothing.
10. Hold boxes/equipment at your waist height (in front of your lower torso).
11. Use small rocking movements with the patient (if they are playing an active part such as with a 'sit-to-stand' transfer) and anyone else involved in the task. These should follow the direction of movement. This helps prepare muscles and the body for movement and ensures that you are all in time with each other.
12. Do not use bending, reaching, stooping or twisting movements during a moving and handling task.
13. Keep knees flexed, not locked, so that you are able to lower yourself without bending your back and maintaining your centre of gravity.
14. If you wish to stand up and walk towards something, you will automatically and naturally lead with your head. It should be no different when doing a moving and handling task.
15. Standing with your feet together means you can easily loose your balance. Stand with your feet shoulder-width apart and you reduce your chance of rotating your spine or loosing your balance.
16. Wear clothing that does not restrict natural body movement or get in the way. Shoes should be closed toe, non-slip, supportive and low-heeled.
17. Clear away clutter. Make sure there is enough room to carry put the moving and handling task without risk of injury.
18. Make sure you position your feet and move your body (and sometimes feet) when performing a moving and handling task to avoid twisting your lower back.
19. Do not perform a standing technique if a lateral transfer is more suitable for the patient.
20. Do not move loads or patients if your field of vision is restricted.
21. If you are in any doubt, seek advice.

Ambulating patients

Many patient care activities require you to push, pull, lift and carry. By using proper body mechanics, you can avoid your own musculoskeletal injury and fatigue and reduce the risk of injuring patients. *Please remember that a risk assessment and relevant principles for moving and handling must be carried out before you undertake any moving and handling. For the rest of this chapter, we assume this has taken place.*

Using proper body mechanics

Correct body mechanics can be summed up in three principles:

Keep a low centre of gravity by flexing the hips and knees instead of bending at the waist to distribute weight evenly between the upper and lower body and maintain balance.

Create a wide base of support by spreading your feet apart to provide lateral stability and lower your body's centre of gravity.

Maintain proper body alignment and keep your body's centre of gravity directly over the base of support by moving your feet rather than twisting and bending at the waist.

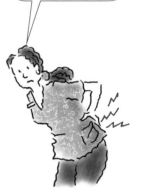

Spare your back. Know the proper way to push, pull and carry!

Do it right

In addition to the three basic principles, follow the directions below to push, pull, stoop, lift and carry correctly.

Pushing and pulling correctly

• Stand close to the object, and place one foot slightly ahead of the other, as in a walking position. Tighten your leg muscles and set your pelvis by simultaneously contracting your abdominal and gluteal muscles. This is known as a 'stable base'.
• To push, place your hands on the object and flex your elbows. Lean into the object by shifting weight from your back leg to your front leg, and apply smooth, continuous pressure.
• To pull, grasp the object and flex your elbows. Lean away from the object by shifting weight from your front leg to your back leg. Pull smoothly, avoiding sudden, jerky movements.
• For pushing and pulling, it's advisable to start slowly; when you work fast your body has to cope with enormous forces at once.
• After you've started to move the object, keep it in motion; *stopping and starting uses more energy.*

• Use your body weight, lean forward when you push and backwards when you pull. Pushing is preferable to pulling.
• Never push/pull and twist at the same time (only one movement at a time).

Maintaining a stable base
• Stand with your feet apart and one foot slightly ahead of the other *to widen the base of support.*
• Lower yourself by flexing your knees, and place more weight on the front foot than on the back foot. Keep your upper body straight by not bending at the waist.
• To stand up again, straighten your knees and keep your back straight.
• Always look in the direction of where you are moving.

Moving and handling objects correctly
• Assume a stable base directly in front of the object *to minimise back flexion and avoid spinal rotation when lifting.*
• Lower yourself by flexing your knees, and place more weight on the front foot than on the back foot. Keep your upper body straight by not bending at the waist. Don't lose your balance at this stage.
• Get a secure hold of the object and test it to see if you can pick it up.
• Grasp the object, and tighten your abdominal muscles.
• Don't twist, especially while your back is bent.
• Stand up by straightening your knees, using your leg and hip muscles. Remember to look up when you stand up.
• Carry the object close to your body at waist height, near the body's centre of gravity, *to avoid straining your back muscles.*

Transfer from bed to stretcher/trolley

Transfer from bed to stretcher, one of the most common transfers, can require the help of one or more colleagues, depending on the patient's size and condition. Techniques for achieving this transfer include the combination of both pushing and pulling, which is effective in laterally moving your patient from one surface to another.

What you need
Stretcher ✳ slide sheet ✳ pat slide

Getting ready
Adjust the bed to the same height as the stretcher/trolley.

Pat slide and slide sheet transfer *(this transfer should be carried out with a minimum of three nurses)*
• Tell the patient that you're going to move him from the bed to the stretcher/trolley, and place him in the supine position.

- Ask team members to remove watches and rings *to avoid scratching the patient during transfer.*
- With one nurse on either side of the bed, one nurse rolls the patient on the bed and the other inserts the pat slide and the single full-length slide sheet on top of the pat slide.
- Return the patient onto their back, so they're laying half on the pat slide and half on the bed.
- Place the stretcher parallel to the bed (so that they're touching), and lock the wheels of both *to ensure patient safety.*
- Turn the patient's head to the direction they'll be moving. If their head is on a pillow ensure the slide sheet goes underneath.

Making the transfer

- The nurses (ideally two) on the pulling side are to grasp the extension handles of the slide sheet and tension the sheet evenly.
- On the other side of the bed, the nurse will be pushing when the command is given.
- The nurse standing nearest the patient's head will be giving the verbal commands for this transfer. Check that everyone knows what is to happen and how the moving and handling task is to take place before commencing. Do *not* give instructions such as '1, 2, 3' but *instead say* 'Ready, steady, slide'.
- At this point, the nurses should follow the guidelines for pushing and pulling, depending on what their role is.

Getting him settled

- Remove the pat slide and slide sheet using the rolling technique, identified earlier.
- Position the patient comfortably on the stretcher/trolley and secure the side rails.

Special circumstances

If the patient is obese

- Depending on the patient's size, this transfer can require two to seven people.
- If available, consider using a mechanical lift to transfer the patient.

Transfer from bed to wheelchair

For a patient with diminished or absent lower-body sensation or one-sided weakness, immobility or injury, transfer from bed to wheelchair may require partial support to full assistance, initially by at least two persons. After transfer, proper positioning helps prevent excessive pressure on bony prominences, which predisposes the patient to skin breakdown.

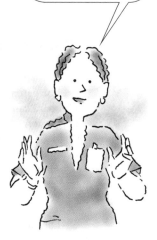

Make sure you secure the side rails after any patient transfer.

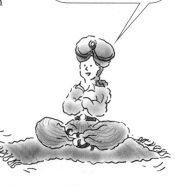

Sure, this looks easy. A slide sheet transfer is nothing like this. It takes at least two people and can take up to seven, depending on the size of the patient.

What you need

Wheelchair with brakes ✳ shoes or slippers with non-slip soles ✳ slide board

Getting ready

- Explain the procedure to the patients and demonstrate their role.
- Set the bed low, but not lower than the wheelchair.

How you do it

- Raise the head of the bed, and allow the patient to rest briefly *to adjust to posture changes, in a sitting position*.
- The patient should be encouraged to rock their body to one side so that the board can be placed under one buttock (the side closest to the surface to be transferred on to).
- Place the wheelchair parallel to the bed, facing the foot of the bed, and lock its wheels (remove one armrest and both leg rests *to avoid interfering with the transfer*). Make sure the bed wheels are also locked.

Out of the bed . . .

- The patients push themselves bit by bit over the sliding board.
- The patients pull their feet along after each movement (or the nurse can do this for them). Using a slide sheet under the patient's feet will make this process much easier.
- The patients support themselves and slowly slide across onto the wheelchair.
- Remove the slide board and replace arm and foot supports.

. . . and into the chair

- Position, position, position.
- If the patients can't position himself correctly, help them move their buttocks against the back of the chair *so that the ischial tuberosities, not the sacrum, provide the base of support*.
- Place the patients' feet flat on the footrests, pointed straight ahead.
- Position the knees and hips with the correct amount of flexion and in appropriate alignment.
- If appropriate, use elevating leg rests to flex the patient's hips at more than 90 degrees; *this position relieves pressure on the popliteal space (the back of the knee) and places more weight on the ischial tuberosities*.
- If the patient starts to fall during transfer, ease them to the closest surface. Never stretch to finish the transfer. *Doing so can cause loss of balance, falls, muscle strain and other injuries to you and the patient*.

Compensating for weakness

- If the patient has one-sided weakness, follow the preceding steps, but place the wheelchair on their unaffected side. Instruct them to pivot and bear as much weight as possible on the unaffected side. Support the affected side *because they'll tend to lean to this side*. If the patient is hemi-plegic, use pillows to support their affected side *to prevent slumping in the wheelchair*.

Types of walking frame

Various types of walking frames are available. The standard walking frame is used by the patient with unilateral or bilateral weakness or an inability to bear weight on one leg. It requires arm strength and balance. Platform attachments may be added to a standard walking frame for the patient with arthritic arms or a casted arm, who can't bear weight directly on their hand, wrist or forearm.

Got wheels

Wheels may be placed on the front legs of the standard walking frame to allow the extremely weak or poorly co-ordinated patient to roll the device forward, instead of lifting it. The rolling walking frame, used by the patient with very weak legs, has four wheels and may also have a seat.

- If from your risk assessment the patient requires more help consider using a hoist.

Using a walking frame (zimmer frame)

A walking frame consists of a metal frame with handgrips and four legs that buttresses the patient on three sides; one side remains open. *Because this device provides greater stability and security than other ambulatory aids*, it's recommended for the patient with insufficient strength and balance or with weakness requiring frequent rest periods to use crutches or a cane.

Attachments for standard walking frame and modified walking frames help meet special needs. For example, a walking frame may have a platform added to support an injured arm.

What you need

Walking frame ✳ platform or wheel attachments, as necessary (see *Types of walking frame*)

Getting ready

- Obtain the appropriate walking frame with the advice of a physical therapist, and adjust it to the patient's height; their elbows should be flexed at a 15-degree angle when standing comfortably within the walking frame with their hands on the grips.
- To adjust the walking frame, turn it upside down, and change the leg length by pushing in the button on each shaft and releasing it when the leg is in the correct position.
- Make sure the walking frame is level before the patient attempts to use it.

How you do it

- Help the patient stand within the walking frame, and instruct them to hold the handgrips firmly and equally. Stand behind them, closer to the involved leg.

Teacher's lounge

Teaching safe use of a walking frame

To teach a patient how to sit down and get up safely using a walking frame, follow the steps outlined here.

Sitting down

- First, tell the patient to stand with the back of their stronger leg against the front of the chair, their weaker leg slightly off the floor, and the walking frame directly in front.
- Tell them to grasp the armrests on the chair, one arm at a time, while supporting most of their weight on the stronger leg. (In the illustrations below, the patient has left leg weakness.)
- Tell the patients to lower themselves into the chair and slide backwards. After they're seated, they should place the walking frame beside the chair.

Getting up

- After bringing the walking frame to the front of their chairs, tell the patients to slide forward in the chair. Placing the back of their stronger leg against the seat, they should then advance the weaker leg.
- Next, with both hands on the armrests, the patient can push themselves to a standing position. Supporting themselves with the stronger leg and the opposite hand, the patient should grasp the walking frame's handgrip with their free hand.
- Then the patient should grasp the free handgrip with their other hand.

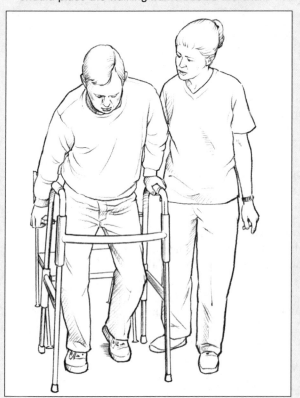

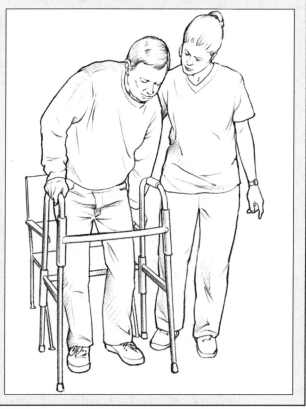

• If the patients have one-sided leg weakness, tell them to advance the walking frame 15 to 20 cm, step forward with the involved leg, and follow with the uninvolved leg, supporting themselves on their arms. Encourage them to take equal strides. If they have equal strength in both legs, instruct them to advance the walking frame 15 to 20 cm and step forward with either leg. If they can't use one leg, tell them to advance the walking frame 15 to 20 cm and swing onto it, supporting their weight on their arms.

For more information, *The Handbook of Transfers'* (Knibbe et al., 2008) was adapted from the Dutch transfers manual and has been written with direct reference to relevant UK legislation and the HOP 5.

Helping patients exercise

Exercise maintains or increases muscle strength and endurance and helps maintain cardiopulmonary function. *Because an immobilised patient may not be able to perform these exercises by himself*, learning how to assist a patient in exercise is an essential part of proper care and health promotion. You may think that this is solely the role of the physiotherapist but actually helping your patient regain their mobility or preventing deterioration is an important nursing role and allows you to assess your patient's abilities. Ideally, if your patient has limited movement, you should be performing these passive exercises prior to any moving and handling situations.

Passive then active

Passive ROM exercises help prevent deterioration of the muscles and tissues of a patient who can't independently exercise. Later, as this type of patient gains strength and no longer needs passive exercise, they can perform isometric (static contraction of a muscle, with no visible movement of the joint) or active ROM exercises.

> Passive ROM exercises help prevent deterioration of muscles and tissues. Later, the patient may be able to perform isometric or active ROM exercises.

Passive ROM exercises

Passive ROM exercises improve or maintain joint mobility and help prevent contractures. Performed by a nurse, a physiotherapist, or a caregiver of the patient's choosing, these exercises are indicated for the patient with temporary or permanent loss of mobility, sensation or consciousness. Passive ROM exercises require recognition of the patient's limits of motion and support of all joints during movement.

Just say no

Passive ROM exercises are contraindicated in patients with septic joints, acute thrombophlebitis, severe arthritic joint inflammation, or recent trauma with possible hidden fractures or internal injuries.

Equal opportunity exercises

The exercises discussed here treat all joints, but they don't have to be performed in the order given or all at once. You can schedule them over the course of a day, whenever the patient is in the most convenient position. Remember to perform all exercises slowly, gently and to the end of the normal ROM or to the point of pain, but no further. (See *Types of joint motion*.)

Getting ready
• Determine the joints that need ROM exercises, and consult the doctor or physiotherapist about limitations or precautions for specific exercises.
• Before you begin, raise the bed to a comfortable working height.

How you do it
Use the following steps to perform ROM on the patient's neck, shoulder, elbow, forearm, wrist, fingers and thumb, hip and knee, ankle, and toes.

Exercising the neck
• Support the patient's head with your hands and extend their neck, flex their chin to their chest, and tilt their head laterally towards each shoulder.
• Rotate their head from right to left.

Exercising the shoulder
• Support the patient's arm in an extended, neutral position; then extend their forearm and flex it back. Abduct their arm outwards from the side of their bodies, and adduct it back to their sides.
• Rotate their shoulder so that their arm crosses their midline, and bend their elbow so that the hand touches their opposite shoulder and then the mattress of the bed for complete internal rotation.
• Return their shoulder to a neutral position and, with the elbow bent, push their arm backwards so that the back of the hand touches the mattress for complete external rotation.

Exercising the elbow
• Place the patient's arm at their side with the palm facing up.
• Flex and extend their arm at the elbow.

Exercising the forearm
• Stabilise the patient's elbow, and then twist their hand to bring the palm up (supination).
• Twist it back again to bring the palm down (pronation).

Exercising the wrist
• Stabilise the patient's forearm, and flex and extend their wrist. Then rock the hand sideways for lateral flexion, and rotate the hand in a circular motion.

Types of joint motion

These illustrations show various areas of the body and the types of movements their joints allow.

Circumduction

Moving in a circular manner

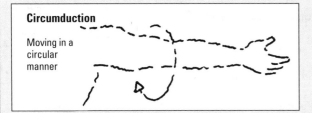

Flexion
Bending, decreasing the joint angle

Extension
Straightening, increasing the joint angle

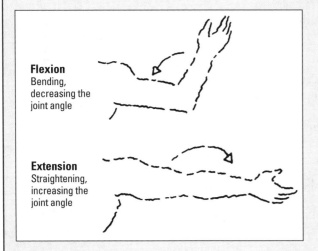

Abduction
Moving away from midline

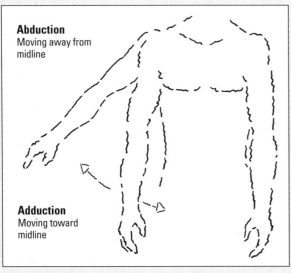

Adduction
Moving toward midline

Retraction and protraction
Moving backward and forward

Pronation
Turning downward

Supination
Turning upward

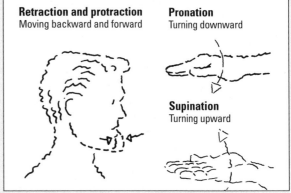

Internal rotation
Turning toward midline

External rotation
Turning away from midline

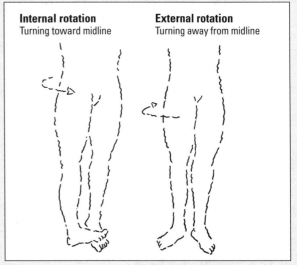

Eversion
Turning outward

Inversion
Turning inward

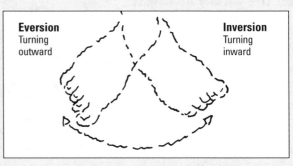

Exercising the fingers and thumb

• Extend the patient's fingers, and then flex the hand into a fist; repeat extension and flexion of each joint of each finger and thumb separately.
• Spread two adjoining fingers apart (abduction), and then bring them together (adduction).
• Oppose each fingertip to the thumb, and rotate the thumb and each finger in a circle.

Exercising the hip and knee

• Fully extend the patient's leg, and then bend their hip and knee towards the chest, allowing full joint flexion.
• Next, move their straight leg sideways, out and away from the other leg (abduction), and then back, over and across it (adduction).
• Rotate their straight leg internally towards their midline, then externally away from their midline.

Exercising the ankle

• Bend the patient's foot so that the toes push upwards (dorsiflexion), and then bend the foot so that the toes push downwards (plantar flexion).
• Rotate their ankle in a circular motion.
• Invert their ankle so that the sole of the foot faces their midline, and then evert their ankle so that the sole faces away from their midline.

Exercising the toes

• Flex the patient's toes towards the sole, and then extend them back towards the top of their foot.
• Spread two adjoining toes apart (abduction), and then bring them together (adduction).

Time is of the essence

• *Because joints begin to stiffen within 24 hours of disuse*, start passive ROM exercises as soon as possible, and perform them at least once per shift, particularly while bathing or turning the patient. Use proper body mechanics, and repeat each exercise at least three times.

Get the family involved

• If the disabled patient requires long-term rehabilitation after discharge, consult a physiotherapist, and teach a family member or caregiver to perform passive ROM exercises. (See *Documenting passive ROM exercises*.)

Isometric and active ROM exercises

Patients on prolonged bed rest or with limited activity without profound weakness can also be taught to perform ROM exercises on their own (called *active ROM*) or they may benefit from isometric exercises. (See *Learning about isometric exercises*.)

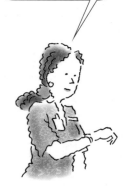

Start passive ROM exercises as soon as possible, and perform them at least once per shift.

Take note!

Document-ing passive ROM exercises

To document passive range of movement (ROM) exercises, include in your notes:

• which joints were exercised
• patient's tolerance of the exercises
• oedema or pressure areas
• pain from the exercises
• ROM limitation.

Learning about isometric exercises

A patient can strengthen and increase muscle tone by contracting muscles against resistance (from other muscles or from a stationary object, such as a bed or wall) without joint movement. These exercises require only a comfortable position, standing, sitting or lying down and proper body alignment. For each exercise, instruct the patient to hold each contraction for 2 to 5 seconds and to repeat it three to four times daily, below peak contraction level for the first week and at peak level thereafter.

Neck rotators

The patient places the heel of their hand above one ear. Then they push their head towards the hand as forcefully as possible, without moving the head, neck or arm. They repeat the exercise on the other side.

Neck flexors

The patient places both palms on their forehead. Without moving their neck, they push their head forwards while resisting with their palms.

Neck extensors

The patient clasps their fingers behind their head, and then pushes their head against the clasped hands without moving the neck.

Shoulder elevators

Holding their right arm straight down at their side, the patient grasps their right wrist with their left hand. They then try to shrug their right shoulder, but prevent it from moving by holding their arm in place. They repeat this exercise, alternating arms.

Shoulder, chest and scapular musculature

The patient places their right fist in their left palm and raises both arms to shoulder height. They push their fist into their palm as forcefully as possible without moving either arm. Then, with their arms in the same position, they clasp their fingers and try to pull their hands apart. They repeat the pattern, beginning with the left fist in the right palm.

Elbow flexors and extensors

With their right elbow bent 90 degrees and the right palm facing upward, the patient places their left fist against their right palm. They try to bend their right elbow further while resisting with their left fist. They repeat the pattern, bending their left elbow.

Abdomen

The patient assumes a sitting position and bends slightly forward, with their hands in front of the middle of their thighs. They try to bend forward further, resisting by pressing their palms against their thighs.

Alternatively, in the supine position, they clasp their hands behind their head. Then they raise their shoulders about 2.5 cm, holding this position for a few seconds.

Back extensors

In a sitting position, the patient bends forward and places their hands under the buttocks. They try to stand up, resisting with both hands.

Hip abductors

While standing, the patient squeezes their inner thighs together as tightly as possible. Placing a pillow between the knees supplies resistance and increases the effectiveness of this exercise.

Hip extensors

The patient squeezes their buttocks together as tightly as possible.

Knee extensors

The patient straightens their knee fully. Then they vigorously tighten the muscle above the knee so that it moves the kneecap upward. They repeat this exercise, alternating legs.

Ankle flexors and extensors

The patient pulls their toes upward, holding briefly. Then they push them down as far as possible, again holding briefly.

Quick quiz

1. Exercises performed without any effort by the patient are called:
  A. strengthening exercises.
  B. easy exercises.
  C. active ROM exercises.
  D. passive ROM exercises.

Answer: D. Passive ROM exercises are performed to test muscle tone and if the patient can't do active ROM exercises.

2. Your patient can't move their right arm toward the midline, so you document this as impaired:
  A. supination.
  B. abduction.
  C. adduction.
  D. eversion.

Answer: C. Adduction is the ability to move a limb toward the midline.

3. Which patient position requires that the head of the bed be elevated to 30 degrees?
  A. Supine
  B. Semi-recumbent
  C. Prone
  D. Lateral

Answer: B. In the semi-recumbent position the head of the bed is elevated to 30 degrees and the bed section under the patient's knees is also raised to flex the knees slightly.

Scoring

☆☆☆ If you answered all three questions correctly, wonderful! Your knowledge of mobility, activity and exercise is going strong.

☆☆ If you answered two questions correctly, great! Your brain exercises are really paying off.

☆ If you answered fewer than two questions correctly, don't fret! Do some extra ROM (reading on mobility) and try again!

15 Self-care and hygiene

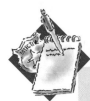

Just the facts

In this chapter, you'll learn:

♦ various methods for determining a patient's ability to perform activities of living

♦ factors that affect self-care

♦ ways that hygiene affects health

♦ common hygiene practices.

Learning about self-care and hygiene

Hygiene means performing practices that promote health through personal cleanliness. Those practices include bathing, cleaning and maintaining fingernails and toenails, shampooing and grooming hair, oral care, feeding and toileting. Hygiene also refers to caring for assistive devices, including hearing aids, eyeglasses, contacts, and such dental appliances as dentures and removable dental bridges.

Many factors influence a person's hygiene practices and ability to perform them. A person's age, gender, personal preferences, socioeconomic status, and religious or cultural practices commonly affect their approach to self-care. Physical limitations, body image or changes in health status can also affect a person's ability to attend to personal care needs. Nurses need to be mindful of how these factors affect self-care yet encourage patients to perform hygiene and self-care whenever possible. It is important not to impose your own standards of hygiene onto patients; for example, some older people may only bathe once a week and we must respect that. Where infection control is an issue careful explanation of the need for more frequent bathing must be undertaken in a private area so as not to embarrass the patient.

> Hygiene practices can vary because of a person's age, gender, religion, culture, physical limitations and changes in health.

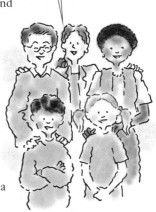

I want to do it myself!

The inability to perform self-care and attend to hygiene needs can be very embarrassing as well as frustrating for patients, especially when they are adults. A young child is accustomed to having an adult help with brushing teeth, combing hair, toileting or bathing, but an older adult may feel a loss of dignity and independence when needing assistance.

The ability to independently perform self-care and hygiene procedures enhances a person's emotional well-being and health status. In fact, one of the goals of nursing is to help patients to learn or relearn self-care activities to achieve as much independence as possible with activities of daily living.

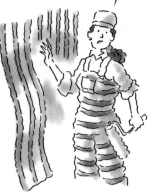

Look, I did this all by myself! I feel great!

Normal self-care patterns

Daily self-care and hygiene routines are largely based on personal and cultural preferences. Many patients are accustomed to a morning routine of rising from sleep, then brushing their teeth, bathing and dressing. Men may shave or trim facial hair and women may put on makeup as part of this routine.

Throwing a monkey wrench into the works

Illness and hospitalisation can affect how and when these daily practices are carried out. Paying attention to a patient's usual routine schedule or what they consider normal self-care activity can help you determine which areas are problematic and when the patient needs your assistance. By doing so, you'll help the patient establish a routine that's as close to normal as possible.

Factors affecting self-care

Many factors can affect a patient's ability to perform self-care and hygiene, including:
- vision impairment
- activity intolerance or weakness from a past medical condition or a current illness
- mental impairment due to age or a psychiatric condition that alters cognitive ability
- pain or discomfort from surgery or disease
- neuromuscular impairment such as a stroke
- skeletal impairment, such as a fracture or joint replacement
- medically prescribed activity restriction such as a patient on bed rest
- therapeutic procedure that restrains physical activity, such as a cast application or an I.V. infusion that restricts their movement
- environmental barriers, such as financial restraints that may prevent them from affording shampoo, shaving supplies, or clean clothes or the resources to wash them
- psychological barriers such as a reluctance to ask for help.

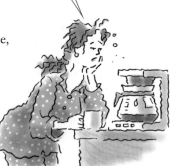

I don't do mornings well... especially on weekends and holidays!

Hygiene and the body

Most hygiene practices help to maintain or restore healthy skin, mucous membranes, hair and nails.

The skin

The skin covers the internal structures of the body and protects them from the external world. Intact, healthy skin is important for preventing infection. Regular bathing removes excess oil, perspiration and bacteria from the skin surface.

> I've always had the feeling I was missing out on something, but I could never put a finger on it.

The skinny on skin

The skin is the body's largest organ and carries out several important functions, including:
- protecting the tissues from trauma and bacteria
- preventing the loss of water and electrolytes from the body
- sensing temperature, pain, touch and pressure
- regulating body temperature through sweat production and evaporation
- synthesising vitamin D
- promoting wound repair by allowing cell replacement of surface wounds.

Layers of the skin

The skin consists of two distinct layers: the epidermis and the dermis. Subcutaneous tissue lies beneath these layers. The epidermis—the outer layer—is made of squamous epithelial tissue. It's thin and contains no blood vessels. The two major layers of the epidermis are the stratum corneum— the most superficial layer—and the deeper basal cell layer, or stratum germinativum. (See *What's in your skin*, page 342.)

Migration

The stratum corneum is made up of cells that form in the basal cell layer, then migrate to the skin's outer surface and die as they reach the surface. However, because epidermal regeneration is continuous, new cells are constantly being produced.

Melon colour's all the rage this season!

The basal cell layer contains melanocytes, which produce melanin and are responsible for skin colour. Hormones, environment and heredity influence melanocyte production. Because melanocyte production is greater in some people than in others, skin colour varies considerably.

What's in your skin

This cross-section of the skin illustrates major skin structures.

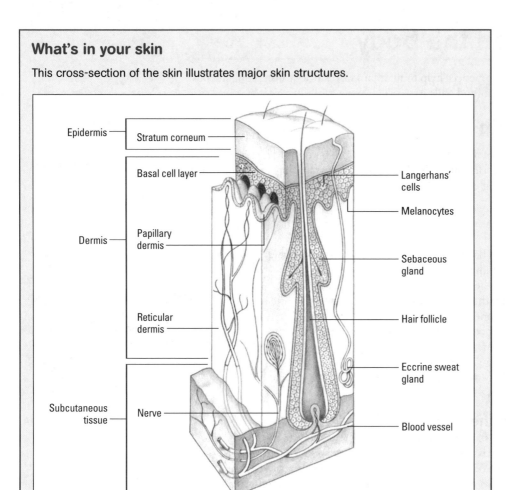

- Epidermis
  - Stratum corneum
  - Basal cell layer
- Dermis
  - Papillary dermis
  - Reticular dermis
- Subcutaneous tissue
  - Nerve
- Langerhans' cells
- Melanocytes
- Sebaceous gland
- Hair follicle
- Eccrine sweat gland
- Blood vessel

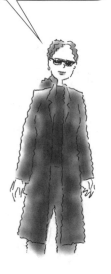

You don't need an oracle to understand how integral the matrix and connective tissue are to a person's dermis.

Laying it on thick

The dermis—the thick, deeper layer of the skin—consists of connective tissue and an extracellular material called matrix, which contributes to the skin's strength and pliability. Blood vessels, lymphatic vessels, nerves and hair follicles are located in the dermis, as are sweat and sebaceous glands. Because it's well supplied with blood, the dermis delivers nutrition to the epidermis. In addition, wound healing and infection control take place in the dermis.

Give the glands a hand!

Sebaceous glands, found primarily in the skin of the scalp, face, upper body and genital region, are part of the same structure that contains the hair follicles. Their main function is to produce sebum, which is secreted onto the skin or into the hair follicle to make the hair shiny and pliant.

There are two types of sweat glands:

- *Eccrine glands* are located over most of the body. In response to thermal stress, eccrine glands produce a watery fluid that helps regulate body temperature. Eccrine glands in the palms and soles secrete fluid in response to emotional stress.
- *Apocrine glands* secrete a milky substance and open into the hair follicle. They're located mainly in the axillae and the genital areas. Inadequate hygiene allows bacteria to break down the fluid causing body odour.

Hair

Hair is formed from keratin and produced by matrix cells in the dermal layer. Each hair lies in a hair follicle and receives nourishment from a papilla, a loop of capillaries at the base of the follicle. At the lower end of the hair shaft is the hair bulb. The hair bulb contains melanocytes, which determine hair colour.

Each hair is attached at the base to a smooth muscle called the arrector pili. This muscle contracts during emotional stress or exposure to cold and elevates the hair, causing goose bumps.

Hair today, gone tomorrow

As a person ages, melanocyte function declines, producing light or grey hair, and the hair follicle itself becomes drier as sebaceous gland function decreases. Hair growth declines, so the amount of body hair decreases. Balding, which is genetically determined in younger individuals, occurs in many people as a normal result of aging.

Nails

Nails are formed when epidermal cells are converted into hard plates of keratin. The nails are made up of the nail root (or nail matrix), nail plate, nail bed, lunula, nail folds and cuticle.

What's on your plate?

The nail plate is the visible, hardened layer that covers the fingertip. The plate is clear with fine longitudinal ridges. The pink colour results from blood vessels underlying vascular epithelial cells.

What is the matrix?

The nail matrix is the site of nail growth. It's protected by the cuticle. At the end of the matrix is the white, crescent-shaped area, the lunula, which extends beyond the cuticle.

Not hard as nails anymore

With age, nail growth slows and the nails become brittle and thin. Longitudinal ridges in the nail plate become more pronounced, making the nails prone to splitting. Also, the nails lose their lustre and become yellowed.

Oral cavity

The mouth (also called the buccal cavity or oral cavity) contains glands that secrete saliva to moisten food for mechanical breakdown. Proper hygiene practices in the care of mucous membranes and teeth also contribute to optimal health.

Teeth

Teeth are considered accessory digestive organs. Upper teeth are anchored in the alveoli or sockets of the left and right maxillae; lower teeth, in the alveoli of the mandible. The tooth consists of enamel, dentin and pulp.

Those pearly whites

All exposed surfaces of the teeth are covered with enamel, the hardest tissue of the body. Enamel protects the underlying layers from food acids, heat and cold. It's a shiny, hard, non-living tissue that can't repair itself after being damaged.

Second hardest

Dentin is the second-hardest tissue in the body. It's the yellow substance under tooth enamel. Millions of tiny canals contain nerve fibres and cells that form the dentin. Dentin has a slight flexibility that protects teeth from breaking during chewing.

Deep inside

Pulp is the innermost part of the tooth. It holds tiny nerves and blood vessels. The root canal is a conduit for nerve vessels between the tooth socket and the pulp area. A thin protective layer of cementum covers each tooth root. Cementum is similar to bone; it's alive and can repair itself.

Performing hygiene practices

Hygiene practices help maintain personal cleanliness and healthy skin. Most patients routinely perform bathing, shaving, brushing the teeth, shampooing and caring for nails. Always ask the patient their personal hygiene practices before planning their care.

Consent

Consent must be gained before undertaking any aspects of hygiene. If the patient refuses, gentle questioning may highlight issues you are unaware of; if the patient continues to refuse, make sure you document this in their notes, and also tell their relatives at the earliest opportunity so that a solution may be found.

Giving a bed bath

A complete bed bath cleans the skin, stimulates circulation, provides mild exercise and promotes comfort. Bathing also allows you to assess your patient's skin condition, joint mobility and muscle strength. Depending on their overall condition and duration of hospitalisation, your patient may have a complete or partial bath daily. A partial bath—including hands, face, axillae, back, genitalia and anal region—may be more suitable than a complete bath for someone with dry, fragile skin or extreme weakness. It also can be given to supplement a complete bath when a patient has diaphoresis or incontinence.

> Most people routinely perform bathing and other hygiene practices. I know I bathe as often as I can—purely for the health effects, of course!

What you need
Bowl ✳ towels ✳ soap or skin lotions ✳ flannel ✳ disposable washcloth ✳ gloves ✳ apron ✳ yellow waste bag ✳ fresh linen

Getting ready
• Explain the procedure and gain consent.
• Offer the patient a bedpan or urinal.
• Close any doors or windows to prevent drafts.
• Draw curtains to ensure privacy.
• Determine the patient's preference for soap or other hygiene aids because some patients are allergic to soap or prefer bath oil or lotions.
• Assemble the equipment by the patient's bedside.
• Put on apron, and wear gloves only if the patient has been incontinent or has a known infection.

> Try to get your patient to help with their bath. It's one way to provide exercise and promote independence.

How you do it
• If the patient's condition permits, encourage them to assist with bathing to provide exercise and promote independence.
• Fill the bath basin two-thirds full of warm water and bring it to the patient's bedside, ensuring there are no spillages. Test the water temperature to avoid scalding or chilling the patient; the water should feel comfortably warm.
• Raise the patient's bed to a comfortable working height to avoid back strain. Keep the side rail away from you raised.
• Position the patient on their back, if possible.
• Remove the patient's gown and other articles, such as antiemboli stockings. Cover the patient with a towel and blanket to provide warmth and maintain dignity.

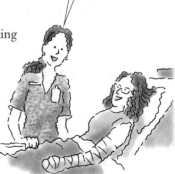

Wash, rinse and dry

- Place a towel under the patient's chin.
- If the patient uses soap, apply it to the flannel or disposable washcloth, and wash the face, ears and neck, using firm, gentle strokes. Rinse thoroughly because residual soap can cause itching and dryness. Then dry the area thoroughly, taking special care in skin folds and creases. Observe the skin checking for any abnormalities.

No tickling

- Turn down the blanket, and cover the patient's chest with a towel; uncover one side of the chest at a time, beginning with the far side. While washing, rinsing and drying the chest and axillae observe the patient's respirations. Use firm strokes to avoid tickling the patient. Apply deodorant if the patient wishes.
- Place a towel beneath the patient's arm farthest from you. Then wash the arm, using long, smooth strokes and moving from wrist to shoulder to stimulate venous circulation.
- If possible, soak the patient's hand in the basin to remove any dirt and soften nails. Clean the patient's fingernails with an orangewood stick, if necessary. Follow the same procedure for the other arm and hand.
- Turn down the blanket to expose the patient's abdomen and groin, keeping a towel across their chest to prevent chilling and maintain dignity. Bathe, rinse and dry the abdomen and groin while checking for abdominal distension or tenderness. Cover the patient's chest and abdomen.
- Uncover the leg farthest from you, and place a bath towel under it. Use the blanket to cover the perineum. Rinse and dry the leg. Repeat with the other leg.
- Wash and dry the feet, paying particular attention to between the toes. Note any redness or oedema.
- Check the toenails and cut if necessary. (See *Performing foot care*, page 354.)

> Remember! Change the water at any point it is getting too cool or excessively dirty. Also, using disposable washcloths will help prevent transferring bacteria to any breaks in the skin.

Remember front to back

- Apply gloves, wash the genitals and perineal area from front to back, with a new disposable washcloth, to avoid contaminating the perineum. Rinse and dry the area well.

> Many patients may be able to wash the genitalia with minimal assistance so should be encouraged to do so, as this will help maintain dignity and lessen embarrassment.

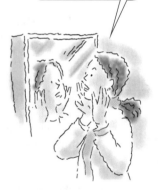

Observe the skin for irritation, scaling or other abnormalities. Unfortunately, ladies, for most of us, wrinkles aren't abnormal—so they don't count!

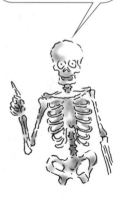

While you're at it, you might want to check those bony prominences. Just a suggestion!

- If the patient has an indwelling urinary catheter, perform catheter care at this point using clean water and disposable washcloth, wash away from the meatus, being careful not to pull the catheter but firm enough to remove any secretions or encrustations.
- Remove gloves.

Nearly finished
- Roll the patient away from you, using the correct moving and handling technique, place a towel beneath the patient, and cover to prevent chilling and maintain dignity. Wash, rinse and dry their back and buttocks using disposable washcloth.
- Check for redness, abrasions and pressure ulcers, paying special attention to bony prominences.

Tight bottom sheet!
- At this stage, while the patient is lying on their side, change the bottom sheet by pushing the soiled sheet towards the patient, roll the clean sheet lengthways and place it alongside, secure it to the mattress using hospital corners, assist the patient to roll over the sheets using the correct moving and handling technique, pull through the sheets taking care not to contaminate the clean one, secure the corners of the clean sheet to the mattress. This will help prevent pressure ulcers, by reducing the risk of friction, and will be more comfortable for the patient who has to remain in bed.
- Dispose soiled linen into the linen skip.
- Dress the patient in a clean gown, and reapply antiemboli stockings if necessary.
- Remake the top of the bed, ensure the linen is not too tight by putting a pleat in the foot of them or are pulled up from the toes to reduce pressure on the toes and feet.
- Brush or comb hair.
- Return the bed to its original position, and make the patient comfortable.
- Ensure call bell is within reach.

Practice pointers
- Change the water as often as necessary to keep it warm and clean.
- Remove and dispose of gloves appropriately. Wash your hands.

Watch the powder puff

- Carefully dry creased skin-fold areas—for example, under breasts, in the groin area, and between fingers, toes and buttocks. If the patient uses talcum powder, use sparingly to avoid caking and irritation and provoking coughing in patients with respiratory disorders.
- If the patient has very dry skin, use bath oil instead of soap. No rinsing is necessary.
- To improve circulation, maintain joint mobility and preserve muscle tone, move the body joints through their full range of motion during the bath.

Remember, a little powder goes a long way. Use with care if the patient requests it.

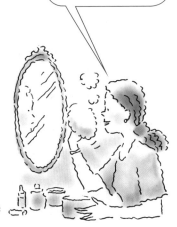

Performing perineal care

Perineal care, which includes care of the external genitalia and the anal area, should be performed during the daily bath and, if necessary, at bedtime and after urination and bowel movements. The procedure promotes cleanliness and prevents infection. It also removes irritating and odorous secretions, such as smegma, a cheese-like substance that collects under the foreskin of the penis and on the inner surface of the labia.

Standard precautions must be followed when providing perineal care, with due consideration given to the patient's privacy.

What you need

Gloves * washcloths * bowl * mild soap * towel * blanket * toilet tissue * absorbent pad * yellow waste bag

Following genital or rectal surgery, you may need to use sterile supplies, including sterile gloves and gauze.

Getting ready

- Explain the procedure to the patient and gain consent.
- Fill the basin two-thirds full with warm water.
- Assemble equipment at the patient's bedside, and provide privacy.
- Wash your hands thoroughly, and put on apron and gloves.

How you do it

- Adjust the bed to a comfortable working height to prevent back strain.
- Provide privacy and help the patient to lie on their back. Place an absorbent pad under the patient's buttocks to protect the bed from stains and moisture.

Perineal care for the female patient

- To minimise the patient's exposure and embarrassment, keep them covered with a blanket or sheet only exposing the perineum.
- Ask the patient to bend their knees slightly and to spread their legs. Separate the labia with one hand and wash with the other, using gentle downward strokes from the front to the back of the perineum to prevent intestinal organisms from contaminating the urethra or vagina. Avoid the area around the anus, and use a clean section of washcloth for each stroke by folding each used section inwards. This prevents the spread of contaminated secretions or discharge.

Rinse and pat dry

- Using a clean washcloth, rinse thoroughly from front to back because soap residue can cause skin irritation. Pat the area dry with a towel because moisture can also cause skin irritation and discomfort.
- Turn the patient on their side to expose the anal area.
- Clean, rinse and dry the anal area, wiping from front to back.

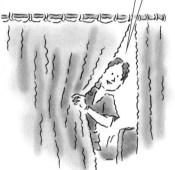

It's important to maintain your patient's privacy and dignity during bath time. So, if you'll excuse us for a few minutes…

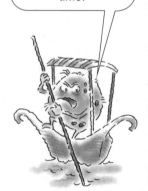

'Downward strokes… front to back… fold each section inwards….' Nurses—always coming up with some new scheme to ruin my good time!

Perineal care for the male patient
- Keep the patient covered and only expose the genital area.
- Hold the shaft of the penis with one hand and wash with the other. Use a clean section of washcloth for each stroke to prevent the spread of contaminated secretions or discharge.
- Rinse thoroughly.

Retract and replace

- For the uncircumcised patient, gently retract the foreskin and clean beneath it. Rinse well but don't dry because moisture provides lubrication and prevents friction when replacing the foreskin. Replace the foreskin to avoid constriction of the penis, which causes oedema and tissue damage.
- Wash the rest of the penis, using downward strokes towards the scrotum. Rinse well and pat dry with a towel.
- Wash the scrotum; rinse thoroughly and pat dry.
- Turn the patient on their side. Wash the bottom of the scrotum and the anal area. Rinse well and pat dry.

After providing perineal care
- Reposition the patient and make them comfortable. Remove the blanket and absorbent pad, and replace the bed linen.
- Clean the bowl and dispose of soiled articles, including gloves and apron, into the clinical waste bin. Wash your hands.

Practice pointers
- Give perineal care in a matter-of-fact way to minimise embarrassment.
- Only apply ointment or creams if prescribed.

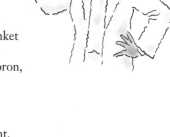

To minimise embarrassing a male patient when providing perineal care, cover his legs to ensure privacy and begin cleaning in a matter-of-fact way.

Eye Care

Unconscious patients will need to have their eye care performed for them to help prevent infection and promote comfort. Some areas may have their own eye care policies so remember to follow these.

What you need
Sterile low-lint gauze pads ✳ sterile gallipot ✳ sterile 0.9% saline solution ✳ sterile dressing towel ✳ small alcohol wipe ✳ clinical waste bag

How you do it
- Wash hands and put on apron.
- Open sterile dressing towel onto a clean surface and use this as the sterile field.
- Tip out all sterile equipment, wipe along the tearline of the sachet of saline and pour saline into the gallipot.

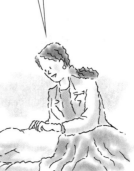

Application of warmed lotion prevents chilling or startling the patient.

• Soak gauze swab in the saline, squeeze out excess fluid and gently wipe from the inner canthus (corner) to the outer canthus. This will remove any debris.
• Use a separate piece of gauze for each wipe to prevent cross-contamination. Clean each eye separately.
• Dispose of equipment in the clinical waste bag, remove apron and wash hands.

Hair care

Hair care includes combing, brushing and shampooing. Combing and brushing stimulate scalp circulation, remove dead cells and debris and distribute hair oils to produce a healthy sheen. Shampooing removes dirt and old oils and helps prevent skin irritation. Hair care also enhances self-esteem and body image.

> For some people, it's wash and set once a week. For me, it's daily shampoos and a trip to the hair dresser every 5 weeks.

1 week for most

Frequency of hair care depends on the length and texture of the patient's hair, the duration of hospitalisation and the patient's condition. Usually, hair should be combed and brushed daily and shampooed according to the patient's normal routine. Typically, no more than 1 week should elapse between washings. Patient's hair can be washed when they are having a shower, a bath or when they are in bed. Showering is much easier and most patients will be able to wash their hair themselves.

Patients who need to remain in bed will need assistance to wash their hair. If the patient can sit upright the hair can be washed over a bowl placed on a bedtable; for those patients who cannot, the hair can washed from the supine position.

What you need
Shampoo ✳ towels ✳ comb or brush ✳ bowl ✳ large jug of warm water ✳ plastic sheet if available, or absorbent pads ✳ flannel or disposable washcloth ✳ chair

> Make sure the comb and brush are clean and, perhaps, a little less pointy than a pitch fork.

How you do it
• Remove the head of the bed and store it safely to prevent injury to others.
• Adjust the bed height to ensure safe moving and handling technique for your back.
• Place the empty bowl on the chair at the head of the bed.
• Protect the bed with the plastic sheet or absorbent pads. If long enough, lay the end of these into the bowl to help prevent spillage.
• Assist the patient to lie flat with their head at the end of the bed.
• Check the temperature of the water, then pour over the hair, taking care not to pour over the face; a flannel can be placed on the forehead to protect the eyes.

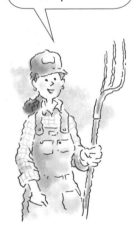

- Apply sufficient shampoo, as required for the length of hair, and massage the scalp.
- Ensure all the shampoo is rinsed off
- Apply conditioner if requested by patient, comb through.
- Rinse well.
- Cover the hair with a towel until you have removed the equipment and repositioned the patient.

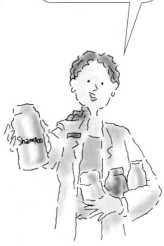

You need to gather more than just shampoo when you're shampooing a patient's hair!

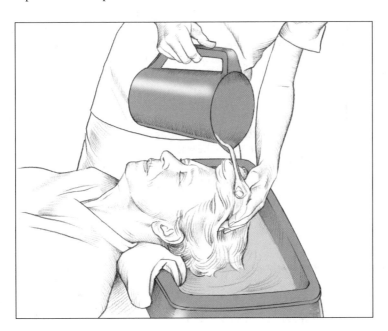

It's a wrap!

- Dry the patient's hair by gently rubbing it with a towel; a hair dryer can be used if available.
- Style the hair as the patient wishes.
- Remake the bed or change the linen, if needed, and remove the bath blanket.
- Reposition the patient comfortably.
- Wash and dry the bowl and jug.
- Remove your apron. Wash your hands.
- Document care given.

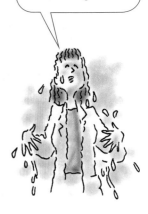

Shampooing a bedridden patient's hair is usually a fairly simple procedure—a little wet, but easy enough.

Practice pointers

- When giving hair care, check the patient's scalp carefully for signs of scalp disorders, head lice or skin breakdown, particularly if the patient is confined to bed. Make sure each patient has their own comb and brush to avoid cross-contamination.
- Empty the bowl frequently to prevent overflow.

Remember that this position can be uncomfortable for the patients, so don't take too long!

Shaving a patient

Performed with a straight, safety, or electric razor, shaving is part of the male patient's usual daily care. In addition to reducing bacterial growth on the face, shaving promotes patient comfort by removing whiskers that can itch and irritate the skin and produce an unkempt appearance. Shaving may also promote positive self-esteem.

Do the electric slide

Because nicks and cuts are most common with use of a straight or safety razor, shaving with an electric razor is indicated for the patient with a clotting disorder or the patient undergoing anticoagulant therapy. Shaving may be contraindicated in the patient with a facial skin disorder or wound.

Wet shave

What you need

Razor ✳ soap or shaving cream ✳ towel ✳ washcloth ✳ bowl

Getting ready

• Make sure the blade is sharp, clean, even and rust-free. If necessary, insert a new blade securely into the razor. A razor may be used more than once, but only by the same patient. Assemble the equipment at the bedside; if he's ambulatory, assemble it at the sink. When the patient is ready to shave, fill the basin or sink with warm water.

A little privacy, please

• Ask the patient if he wants a shave, gain consent and provide privacy. Ask them to assist you as much as possible to promote their independence.
• Unless contraindicated, sit the patient upright. If the patient is unconscious, elevate their head to prevent soap and water from running behind it.

How you do it

Using a straight or safety razor
• Place a towel under the patient's chin to protect the bed from moisture and to catch falling whiskers.

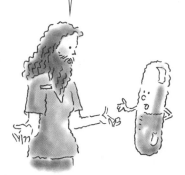

An unfortunate temporary adverse effect, I know! But, hey, look at the bright side... at least you'll get some first hand experience with a straight razor and aftershave lotion.

Stay sharp as a razor's edge

• Fill the basin with warm water. Using the washcloth, wet the patient's entire beard with warm water. Let the warm cloth soak the beard for at least 1 minute to soften whiskers.
• Apply shaving cream to the beard. Or, if you're using soap, rub to form lather.
• Gently stretch the patient's skin taut with one hand and shave with the other, holding the razor firmly. Ask the patient to puff their cheeks or turn their head, as necessary, to shave hard-to-reach areas.
• Begin at the sideburns and work towards the chin using short, firm, downward strokes in the direction of hair growth to reduce skin irritation and help prevent nicks and cuts.
• Rinse the razor often to remove whiskers. Apply more warm water or shaving cream to the face, as needed, to maintain adequate lather.

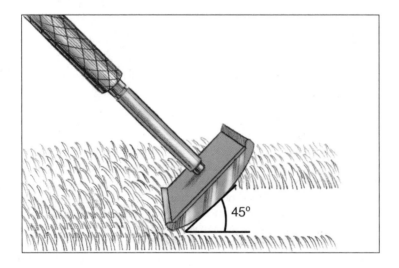

45°

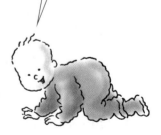

Done correctly, shaving should leave your patient's face smooth as a baby's bottom.

Smooth as a baby's bottom

• Shave across the chin and up the neck and throat. Use short, gentle strokes for the neck and the area around the nose and mouth to avoid skin irritation.
• Change the water, and rinse any remaining lather and whiskers from the patient's face. Then dry their face with a towel and, if the patient desires, apply aftershave lotion.
• Rinse the razor and return it to its storage area.
• Wash and dry the bowl.

Using an electric or battery razor

• Plug in the razor and apply preshave lotion, if available, to remove skin oils. If the razor head is adjustable, select the appropriate setting.

- Using a circular motion and pressing the razor firmly against the skin, shave each area of the patient's face until smooth.
- If the patient desires, apply aftershave lotion.
- Clean the razor head, and return the razor to its storage area.

Practice pointers
- If the patient is conscious, find out their usual shaving routine. Although shaving in the direction of hair growth is most common, the patient may prefer the opposite direction.

No borrowing allowed

- Don't interchange patients' shaving equipment to prevent cross-contamination.
- Care must be taken if patient is on anticoagulant therapy. Check your local policy.

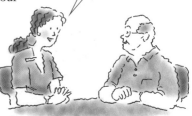

Do you prefer a straight, safety or electric razor? And do you usually go with or against the grain?

Performing foot care

Daily bathing of feet and regular trimming of toenails promotes cleanliness, prevents infection, stimulates peripheral circulation and controls odour by removing debris from between toes and under toenails.

Put your foot down . . . it's important!

Foot care is particularly important for all patients, especially those susceptible to foot infection, such as patients with peripheral vascular disease, diabetes mellitus, poor nutritional status, arthritis or a condition that impairs peripheral circulation. In such patients, proper foot care should include meticulous cleanliness and regular observation for signs of skin breakdown. (See *Foot care for diabetic patients.*)

What you need
Bowl ✻ soap ✻ warm water ✻ disposable wash cloths ✻ absorbent pad ✻ towel ✻ nail clippers ✻ disposable nail file ✻ apron

Getting ready
- Assemble equipment at the patient's bedside. Wash your hands and put on apron.

Guaranteed to make them smile

- Tell the patient that you'll be washing their feet and providing foot and toenail care.
- If possible, sit the patient in a chair at the side of the bed.
- Place an absorbent pad and a towel under the patient's feet.

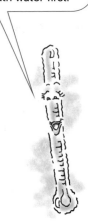

Remember that a patient with diminished peripheral sensation can burn his feet in hot water without feeling any warning pain. Always test bath water first.

Foot care for diabetic patients

Redness, drying, cracking, blisters, discoloration or any evidence of traumatic injury to the feet could be a sign of infection or gangrene.

- Refer the patient to see a doctor or podiatrist if any problems are found.

Because diabetes mellitus can reduce blood supply to the feet, normally minor foot injuries can lead to dangerous infection. When caring for a diabetic patient, keep these foot-care guidelines in mind:

- Exercising the feet daily can help improve circulation. While the patient is sitting on the edge of the bed, ask them to point their toes upwards, then downwards, 10 times. Then have them make a circle with each foot 10 times.
- A diabetic patient's shoes must fit properly. Instruct the patient to break in new shoes gradually by increasing wearing time by 30 minutes each day. Also tell them to check old shoes frequently in case they develop rough spots in the lining.

- Tell them to change their socks daily, and to avoid socks with holes, darned spots or rough, irritating seams.
- Advise the patient to wear warm socks or slippers and to use extra blankets to avoid cold feet. The patient shouldn't use heating pads and hot water bottles because these can cause burns.
- Teach the patient to regularly inspect the skin on their feet for cuts, cracks, blisters and red, swollen areas. Even slight cuts on the feet should receive a doctor's attention. As a first-aid measure, tell them to wash the cut thoroughly and apply a mild antiseptic. Urge the patient to avoid harsh antiseptics, such as iodine, because they can damage tissue.
- Advise the patient to avoid tight-fitting garments or activities that can decrease circulation. They should avoid sitting with their knees crossed, picking at sores or rough spots on their feet, walking barefoot or applying adhesive tape to the skin on their feet.

How you do it
- Place the feet into the bowl of warm soapy water and allow them to soak for about 5 minutes. Soaking softens the skin and toenails, loosens debris under toenails and comforts and refreshes the patient.
- After soaking, rinse the feet with a washcloth, remove them from the bowl and place it on the towel.

Soft-cloth touch

- Dry the feet thoroughly, especially between the toes, to prevent skin breakdown. Blot gently to dry because harsh rubbing may damage the skin.
- Do one foot at a time if the bowl is too small.

Trimming nails

- If the nails are long, trim them to prevent them from causing injury by cutting into other toes or scratching.
- Nails should not be cut immediatley following soaking as this can lead to them being cut too short.
- Do not cut into the sulci (the side of the nail) but follow the curve of the nail and file the edges.
- Consult a podiatrist if nails are thickened or disformed.
- Remove and clean all equipment. Dispose of apron and wash your hands.

If your patient's skin is dry, moisten it with lotion.

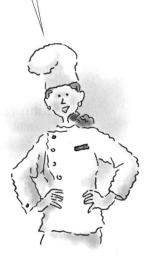

Practice pointers

• While providing foot care, observe the colour, shape and texture of the toenails. If you see redness, drying, cracking, blisters, discolouration or other signs of traumatic injury, especially in patients with impaired peripheral circulation, notify the doctor. Because such patients are vulnerable to infection and gangrene, they need prompt treatment.

• Refer ingrown toenails to a podiatrist.

Tailoring care to those patients confined to bed

• If patients are unable to sit out of bed, the feet can be washed using a washcloth; pay particular attention to washing and drying between the toes.

• When giving the patient foot care, perform range-of-motion exercises unless contraindicated to stimulate circulation and prevent foot contractures and muscle atrophy. Tuck folded 2″ × 2″ gauze pads between overlapping toes to protect the skin from the toenails. Check heels at least daily.

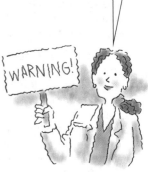

Redness, drying, cracking, blisters, discolouration or any evidence of traumatic injury to the feet could be a sign of infection or gangrene.

Performing mouth care

Given in the morning, at bedtime or after meals, mouth care entails brushing and flossing the teeth and inspecting the mouth. Mouth care removes soft plaque deposits and calculus from the teeth, cleans and massages the gums, reduces mouth odour and helps prevent infection. Patient comfort and self-esteem are increased by freshening the patient's mouth. Appreciation of food is enhanced, thereby aiding appetite and nutrition.

A mouthful of attention

Although most patients can usually perform mouth care alone, some may require partial or full assistance. An unconscious patient requires use of suction equipment to prevent aspiration during oral care.

What you need

Towel or facial tissues ✳ vomit bowl ✳ clinical waste bag ✳ toothbrush and toothpaste ✳ disposable cup ✳ water ✳ pen torch ✳ disposable tongue depressor ✳ small mirror, if necessary

Getting ready

• Assemble equipment at the patient's bedside.

• If using oral suction equipment, connect the tubing to the suction bottle and suction catheter, insert the plug into an outlet and check for correct operation.

• Explain the procedure to the patient, gain consent and provide privacy.

• Wash your hands and put on apron.

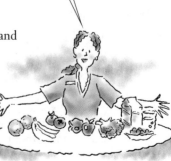

A clean mouth is a healthy mouth, and that means being able to enjoy eating all types of food.

How you do it
- If the patient is confined to bed but capable of self-care, encourage them to perform their own mouth care.
- If allowed, sit patient upright. Place the bedtable in front of them and arrange the equipment on it.
- Place a towel over the patient's chest to protect their gown.

Performing mouth care
- If the patient is unconscious or conscious, but incapable of self-care, perform mouth care on them. If they wear dentures, clean them thoroughly. (See *Dealing with dentures*.)

Prepping the patient

- Raise the bed to a comfortable working height to prevent back strain. Position the patient on their side, with their face extended over the edge of the pillow to facilitate drainage and prevent fluid aspiration. If the patient is conscious, sit them upright.
- Arrange the equipment on the bedtable or trolley.
- Place the towel under the patient's chin to absorb or catch drainage.

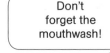

Don't forget the mouthwash!

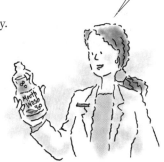

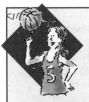

Stay on the ball

Dealing with dentures

Dentures require proper care to remove soft plaque deposits and calculus and to reduce mouth odour. Such care involves removing and rinsing dentures after meals, daily brushing and removal of tenacious deposits, and soaking in a commercial denture cleaner. Dentures must be removed from the unconscious or pre-surgical patient to prevent possible airway obstruction.

Equipment and preparation

Start by assembling the following equipment at the patient's bedside: vomit bowl ✳ labelled denture pot ✳ toothbrush or denture brush ✳ gloves ✳ toothpaste ✳ commercial denture cleaner ✳ paper towel ✳ mouthwash ✳ gauze ✳ optional: adhesive denture liner

Removing dentures

- Wash your hands and put on gloves.
- To remove a full upper denture, grasp the front and palatal surfaces of the denture with your thumb and forefinger. Position the index finger of your opposite hand over the upper border of the denture, and press to break the seal between denture and palate. Grasp the denture with gauze because saliva can make it slippery.
- To remove a full lower denture, grasp the front and lingual surfaces of the denture with your thumb and index finger and gently lift up.
- To remove partial dentures, first ask the patient or caregiver how the prosthesis is retained and how to remove it. If the partial denture is held in place with clips or snaps, then exert equal pressure on the

(continued)

Dealing with dentures (continued)

border of each side of the denture. Avoid lifting the clasps, which can easily bend or break.

Oral and denture care

- After removing dentures, place them in a properly labelled denture pot. Add warm water and a commercial denture cleaner to remove stains and hardened deposits. Follow package directions. Avoid soaking dentures in mouthwash containing alcohol because it may damage a soft liner.
- Instruct the patient to rinse with mouthwash to remove food particles and reduce mouth odour. Then gently brush the palate, buccal surfaces, gums and tongue with a soft toothbrush to clean the mucosa and stimulate circulation. Check for irritated areas or sores because they may indicate a poorly fitting denture.
- Carry the denture pot, vomit bowl, toothbrush and toothpaste to the sink. After lining the basin with a paper towel, fill it with water to cushion the dentures in case you drop them. Hold the dentures over the basin, wet them with warm water and apply toothpaste to a denture brush or long-bristled toothbrush. Clean the dentures using only moderate pressure to prevent scratches and using warm water to prevent distortion.
- Clean the denture pot, and place the dentures in it. Rinse the brush, and clean and dry the vomit bowl. Return all equipment to the patient's bedside locker.

Wearing dentures

- If the patient desires, apply adhesive liner to the dentures. Moisten them with water, if necessary, to reduce friction and ease insertion.
- Encourage the patient to wear their dentures to enhance their appearance, facilitate eating and speaking, and prevent changes in the gum line that may affect denture fit.

Brushing them clean

- Wet the toothbrush with water. If necessary, use hot water to soften the bristles. Apply toothpaste.
- Brush the patient's lower teeth from the gum line up; the upper teeth, from the gum line down.

Covering all the angles

- Place the brush at a 45-degree angle to the gum line, and press the bristles gently into the gingival sulcus. Using short, gentle strokes to prevent gum damage, brush the buccal surfaces (towards the cheek) and the lingual surfaces (towards the tongue) of the bottom teeth; use just the tip of the brush for the lingual surfaces of the front teeth. Using the same technique, brush the buccal and lingual surfaces of the top teeth. Brush the biting surfaces of the bottom and top teeth, using a back-and-forth motion.
- Hold the vomit bowl under the patient's cheek, and wipe their mouth and cheeks with facial tissues as needed.

After mouth care

- Use the pen torch and tongue depressor to assess the patient's mouth for cleanliness and tooth and tissue condition.
- Rinse the toothbrush.

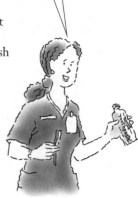

Follow the proper brushing technique, and use gentle strokes to prevent damaging tooth and gum surfaces.

- Discard disposable equipment in the clinical waste bag. Remove apron and gloves.
- Wash hands.

Making an unoccupied bed

Although considered routine, daily changing and periodic straightening of bed linen promotes patient comfort and prevents skin breakdown. When preceded by hand washing, performed using clean technique, and followed by proper handling and disposal of soiled linen, this procedure helps control nosocomial (hospital-acquired) infections.

What you need

Two sheets ✳ pillowcase ✳ blanket and or bedspread ✳ apron ✳ gloves (only if bed linen is soiled with bodily fluids) ✳ linen skip

Getting ready

- Obtain clean linen. The bottom sheet should be folded so that the rough side of the hem is face down when placed on the bed to help prevent skin irritation caused by the rough hem edge rubbing against the patient's heels. The top sheet should be folded similarly so that the smooth side of the hem is face up when folded over the spread, giving the bed a neat appearance and protecting the patient's skin.

Vacating the premises

- Wash your hands and put on apron. Bring clean linen to the patient's bedside. If the patient is present, tell them that you're going to change the bed. Help them to a chair, if necessary.
- Move any furniture away from the bed to provide ample working space.
- Lower the head of the bed to make the mattress level and to ensure tight-fitting, wrinkle-free linen. Then raise the bed to a comfortable working height to prevent back strain. Make sure the wheels of the bed are locked.

How you do it

- When stripping the bed, watch for any belongings that may have fallen among the linen.
- Remove the pillowcase and place it in the linen skip.
- Set the pillow aside.

It's in the bag

- Lift the mattress edge slightly and work around the bed, untucking the linen. If you plan to reuse the top linen, fold them down to the blanket rest, at the bottom of the bed. Otherwise, carefully remove them and put them in the linen skip.
- Remove the soiled bottom sheet and place it in the linen skip. To avoid spreading microorganisms, don't fan the linen or place them on the floor.

Oops, it's sliding!

- If the mattress has slid downward, push it to the head of the bed.
- Place the bottom sheet with its centre fold in the middle of the mattress. Align the end of the sheet with the foot of the mattress, and use hospital corners to keep the sheet firmly tucked under the mattress.

Hospital corners

- Firstly tuck the top end of the sheet evenly under the mattress at the head of the bed. Then lift the side edge of the sheet about 30 cm from the mattress corner and hold it at a right angle to the mattress. Tuck in the bottom edge of the sheet hanging below the mattress. Lastly, drop the top edge and tuck it under the mattress, as shown below (mitred corners).

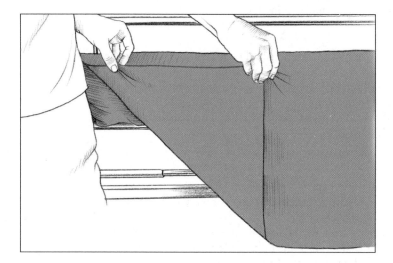

Neatly does it!

- Place the top sheet with its centre fold in the middle of the bed and its wide hem even with the top of the bed. Position the rough side of the hem face up so that the smooth side shows after folding. Allow enough sheet at the top of the bed to form a cuff over the blanket.
- Place the blanket over the top sheet, with its centre fold in the middle of the bed.

Heel and 'toe'

- Make a toe pleat, or vertical tuck, in the top linen to allow room for the patient's feet and to prevent pressure that can cause discomfort, skin breakdown and footdrop.
- Tuck the top sheet and spread under the foot of the mattress. Then mitre the bottom corners.

Who 'taut' you how to do that?

• After fitting all corners of the bottom sheet or tucking them under the mattress, pull the sheet at an angle from the head towards the foot of the bed. Pulling the sheet tightens the linen, making the bottom sheet taut and wrinkle-free and promoting patient comfort.
• Fold the top sheet over the spread at the head of the bed to form a cuff and give the bed a neat appearance.

You don't have to go to finishing school to give a bed a finished look!

'Seams' like a good plan

• Slip the pillow into a clean case, tucking in the corners.
• Lower the bed making sure the wheels remained locked to ensure the patient's safety.

Getting carried away
• Place soiled linen in the linen skip.
• After disposing of the linen, remove apron and gloves, if used.
• Wash hands.

Practice pointers
• Because a hospital mattress is covered with plastic to protect it and to facilitate cleaning, the bottom sheet tends to loosen and become untucked. Use a fitted sheet, if available, to prevent this.
• Many pressure-relieving mattresses used now rely on air movement within the mattress and therefore require that sheets are not tucked under them.

Making an occupied bed

For the patient confined to bed, daily linen changes promote comfort and help prevent skin breakdown and nosocomial infection.

It takes two

To maintain the safety of the patient making an occupied bed requires two people. It also entails loosening the bottom sheet on one side and fanfolding it to the centre of the mattress instead of loosening the bottom sheet on both sides and removing it, as in an unoccupied bed. Also, the foundation of the bed must be made before the top sheet is applied.

A simple demonstration of what *not* to do with soiled bed linens... and what I'll be wearing to this year's Halloween party.

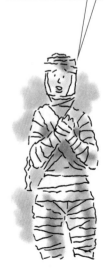

What you need
Two sheets (one fitted, if available) ✳ pillowcase ✳ blanket and/or bedspread ✳ apron ✳ linen skip ✳ gloves (only if the linen is soiled)

Keep it clean

• Explain the procedure and gain consent.
• Wash your hands and put on apron, bring clean linen to the patient's bedside.
• Draw the curtains around the bedspace to provide privacy and maintain dignity.

- Move any furniture away from the bed to ensure ample working space.
- Adjust the bed to a comfortable working height to prevent back strain. Make sure the wheels are locked.
- If allowed, lower the head of the bed to ensure tight-fitting, wrinkle-free linen.

How you do it
- When stripping the bed, check for belongings among the linen.
- Pull out the blanket rest at the foot of the bed.
- Cover the patient with a blanket to avoid exposure and provide warmth and privacy.

Gather ye linen

- Loosen the top linen at the foot of the bed, and remove them separately. If reusing the top linen, fold each piece and hang it on the blanket rest, at the bottom of the bed making sure none of the linen is touching the floor. Otherwise, place it in the linen skip.

Roll 'em, roll 'em, roll 'em

- Roll the patient to the far side of the bed using the correct moving and handling techniques. Move the pillow under the patient's head to support the neck.
- Loosen the soiled bottom linen on the side of the bed nearest you. Then roll the linen towards the patient's back in the middle of the bed, as shown below.

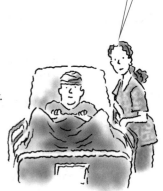

Tell the patient that you'll be changing his bed linens, and explain how he can help if he's able.

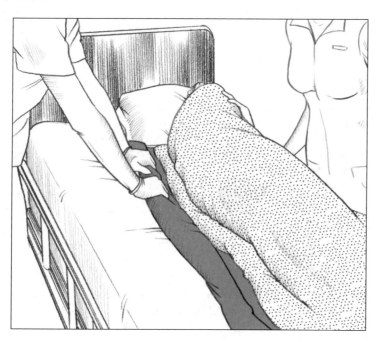

- Place a clean bottom sheet on the bed, with its centre fold in the middle of the mattress. Use hospital corners (mitre) as you would for an unoccupied bed, to keep linen firmly tucked under the mattress, preventing wrinkling.
- Roll the patient to the clean side of the bed.

Loosen and remove

- Loosen and remove the soiled bottom sheet and place in the linen skip.
- Pull the clean bottom sheet taut and secure in place using hospital corners.
- Assist the patient to sit up, if their condition permits.
- Remove the soiled pillowcase, and place it in the laundry bag. Then slip the pillow into a clean pillowcase. Place the pillow beneath the patient's head.

No "cuff" links

- Unfold the clean top sheet over the patient with the rough side of the hem facing away from the bed to avoid irritating the patient's skin. Allow enough sheet to form a cuff over the spread.
- Remove the blanket from beneath the sheet, and centre the spread over the top sheet.

Be kind to your patient's feet

- Make a toe pleat, or vertical tuck, in the top linen to allow room for the patient's feet and prevent pressure that can cause discomfort, skin breakdown and footdrop.
- Tuck the top sheet and spread under the foot of the bed, and mitre the bottom corners. Fold the top sheet over the spread to give the bed a neat appearance.

Lock and load

- Raise the head of the bed to a comfortable position, raise side rails if required, and then lower the bed and lock its wheels to ensure the patient's safety.
- Place the call button within the patient's easy reach.
- Remove and discard apron, and gloves if used, wash your hands to prevent the spread of nosocomial infections.

Practice pointers

To every sheet, turn, turn

- If the patient can't help you move or turn them, use an appropriate moving and handling device.

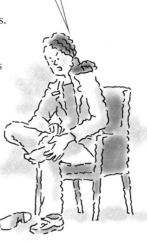

Remember the golden rule… Do unto your patient's feet as you would have them do unto yours (or something along those lines)!

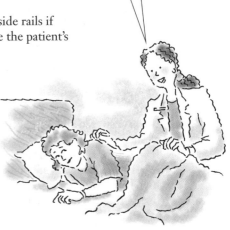

Remember! A glide sheet can help in bed making and repositioning. Now, if only I could use one to get teenagers off the sofa!

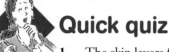

Quick quiz

1. The skin layers from outside in are:
   A. dermis, epidermis, subcutaneous tissue.
   B. epidermis, subcutaneous tissue, dermis.
   C. epidermis, dermis, subcutaneous tissue.

Answer: C. The subcutaneous tissue lies beneath the dermis and epidermis.

2. When performing personal hygiene on a female patient, it's important to wash the genital area in what direction?
   A. Back to front
   B. Side to side
   C. In a circular motion
   D. Front to back

Answer: D. It's best to wash the female genital area from the front to back to avoid contaminating the urethral orifice with faecal material from the anal area.

3. Which of the following is the correct position to perform mouth care on a unconscious patient?
   A. Semi-recumbent
   B. Side-lying
   C. Prone
   D. Supine

Answer: B. The side-lying position with the head of the bed lowered will help water and debris drain from the patient's mouth and prevent aspiration.

4. When providing morning care to a patient, which of the following is the correct direction for washing the patient's eye?
   A. Outer canthus to inner canthus
   B. Lower canthus to upper canthus
   C. Inner canthus to outer canthus
   D. Upper canthus to lower canthus

Answer: C. The eye should be cleaned from the inner canthus to the outer canthus.

Scoring

☆☆☆ If you answered all four questions correctly, congratulations! You really cleaned up!

☆☆ If you answered three questions correctly, great! You're fundamentally prepared to take care of yourself.

☆ If you answered fewer than three questions correctly, don't despair! Just review the chapter and you'll be a whiz at patient care in no time.

16 Comfort, rest and sleep

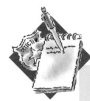

Just the facts

In this chapter, you'll learn:

♦ sleep stages and circadian rhythms

♦ types of sleep disorders and their causes.

A look at comfort, rest and sleep

Comfort is described as the absence of stress, which promotes rest, relaxation and sleep. *Sleep* is a natural state of rest during which muscle movements and awareness of surroundings diminish. Sleep restores energy and well-being, enabling us to function optimally.

Unlike other states resembling sleep (such as coma), sleep is easily interrupted or prevented by external stimuli, such as noise and light, or by internal factors, such as stress and anxiety. According to the BBC Science and Nature article 'A Hard Night's Sleep', 25% of the UK population suffer some form of sleep disorder, and snoring affects around 3.5 million people in the UK. Sleep disturbances can also have a direct impact on other family members' sleep patterns. For example, someone snoring may awaken their spouse or prevent the spouse from falling asleep in the first place.

Primary or secondary

Sleep disorders may be primary or may arise secondary to a medical or psychiatric disorder, substance use or environmental factors.

Medical conditions that can cause sleep disorders include Parkinson's disease, Huntington's disease, viral encephalitis, brain disease, thyroid disease and hormonal imbalances.

A psychiatric disorder, such as depression or an anxiety disorder, is the most common cause of chronic insomnia. High levels of stress may also contribute to sleep disorders.

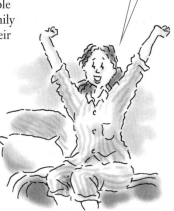

Sleep restores energy and well-being—two pretty important elements in my job!

Substances that can disrupt sleep include alcohol, caffeine and prescription medications, most notably anti-histamines, corticosteroids and central nervous system drugs.

Fuel for family feuds

Someone who doesn't sleep well is likely to feel tense, unhappy and even depressed. These feelings can compromise healthy family relationships.

Sleep stages

Sleep occurs in five stages. With each stage, sleep becomes deeper and brain waves grow progressively larger and slower.

Stage 1

The lightest stage of sleep, stage 1, occurs as a person falls asleep. The muscles relax and brain waves are fast and irregular. Called *theta waves*, these spike like waves have low–medium amplitude and occur three to seven times per second. Stage 1 accounts for approximately 5% of an adult's total sleep time.

Stage 2

During stage 2, a relatively light stage of sleep, theta waves continue but become interspersed with sleep spindles (sudden increases in wave frequency) and K complexes (sudden increases in wave amplitude). Stage 2 makes up about 50% of total sleep time.

Stages 3 and 4

Stages 3 and 4 are the deepest stages of sleep. Delta waves, large, slow waves of high amplitude and low frequency, appear on the EEG. Stages 3 and 4 differ only in the percentage of delta waves seen; during stage 3, delta waves account for less than 50% of brain waves, whereas during stage 4, they account for more than 50%.

Conserve as you sleep

Arousing a sleeping person from stage 3 or 4 is harder than during any other stage. Because these stages are marked by decreased body temperature and metabolism, researchers believe they function to conserve energy. They account for 10% to 20% of total sleep time.

As night fades into morning, stages 3 and 4 get progressively shorter. During the last few cycles of the sleep period, no delta-wave sleep occurs at all.

Stage 5

Stage 5 is a deep sleep called *rapid-eye movement (REM) sleep*. During this stage, the sleeping person shows darting eye movements, muscle twitching and short, rapid brain waves resembling those seen during the waking state. (See *Sleep stages and brain waves*.)

Sleep stages and brain waves

Each sleep stage generates distinctive brain waves, as measured by EEG:

- During stage 1, which occurs as a person falls asleep, fast, irregular brain waves called *theta waves* appear on the EEG.
- During stage 2, theta waves are interspersed with wave phenomena called *sleep spindles* and *K complexes*.
- During stages 3 and 4, the EEG shows large, slow waves of high amplitude and low frequency waves, called *delta waves*.
- During stage 5, called *rapid-eye movement (REM) sleep*, short, rapid brain waves appear.

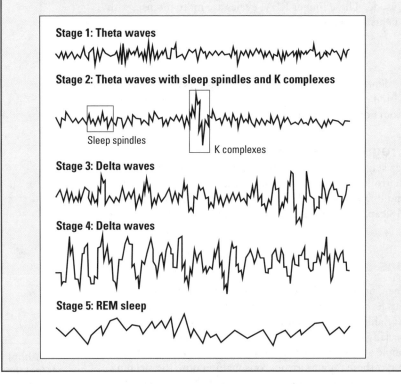

REM sleep usually begins about 90 minutes after sleep onset. Over the course of the night, REM periods lengthen. Overall, REM sleep accounts for 20% to 25% of total sleep time.

To sleep, perchance to dream

Most story-like dreams take place during REM sleep. People awakened from REM sleep commonly report vivid dreams. In contrast, people awakened during stages 1 through 4 rarely report vivid dreams.

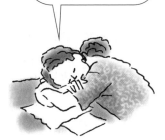

Sshhh! People awakened from REM sleep commonly report vivid dreams, and I'm in the middle of a good one!

Alternating sleep cycles

Throughout the night, REM (stage 5) and non-REM (NREM) (stages 1 through 4) sleep alternate in cycles of about 90 minutes each. Stages 3 and 4 occur during the first one-third to first one-half of the night. REM sleep increases towards the morning.

Functions of REM and NREM sleep

Scientists believe REM and NREM sleep serve different biological functions, although they don't know exactly what these functions are. REM sleep may stimulate brain growth or consolidate memory.

A person deprived of REM sleep tends to have longer REM cycles during the next sleep episode. These longer REM cycles are more intense, with more eye movements per minute.

Make-up sleep

Similarly, people deprived of NREM sleep have longer NREM sleep during the next sleep period and the 'make-up' NREM sleep produces different EEG patterns from normal NREM sleep.

Neurologic regulation of sleep stages

The various sleep stages are influenced by different parts of the brain. REM sleep is controlled by the pons (a part of the brain stem) and adjacent portions of the midbrain. Chemical stimulation of the pons may induce long periods of REM sleep, whereas damage to the pons may reduce or prevent REM sleep.

Paralysis and the pons

During REM sleep, neurons in the pons and midbrain that control muscle tone show various levels of activity: some are active whereas others aren't. Reflecting this variable activity, certain body muscles remain inactive during REM sleep, especially those of the back, neck, arms and legs. As a result, during sleep, people are effectively paralysed so they can't act out their dreams. However, if these regulatory neurons malfunction, the sleeping person may be more active during dreams, thrashing about or becoming violent.

Baths and the basal forebrain

The basal forebrain, located in front of the hypothalamus, controls NREM sleep. Damage to this region of the brain may cause difficulty falling asleep or staying asleep. Some neurons in the basal forebrain are activated by heat, which may explain the sleep-promoting benefits of taking a warm bath in the evening.

Ahhh! I can just feel the neurons in my basal forebrain getting happy!

Factors that affect sleep

Factors affecting sleep quality and quantity include the patient's age, lifestyle, sleep environment and medication use.

Age

Amounts and patterns of sleep differ at each major stage of the life cycle. Both REM and NREM sleep periods decrease with age.

Neonates and toddlers

Neonates sleep the most; averaging 17 to 18 hours a day, with REM accounting for roughly one-half of total sleep time.

Go to sleep-y, little baby

At first, a neonate sleeps in episodes of 3 to 4 hours. Gradually, by about age 3 or 4 months, they get more sleep at night. A 6-month old typically sleeps 12 hours at night and naps 1 to 2 hours each day.

Toddlers sleep about 11 or 12 hours a night, with a 1- to 2-hour nap after lunch. Nap requirements vary, with some children taking naps up to age 5. By age 5, children typically sleep 10 to 12 hours a day, with REM sleep accounting for about 20% of the total.

Tweens and teens

Pre-adolescents need about 10 hours of sleep. Adolescent requirements aren't well defined. Many teenagers get too little sleep because of their busy schedules and academic pressures.

Young adults

A typical young adult needs about 8 hours of sleep, though the requirement varies widely. Some young adults need as little as 6 or 7 hours, whereas others may need 9 or 10 hours to function optimally. Lifestyle choices make this group vulnerable to sleep disturbances.

Middle-aged adults

In middle-aged adults, sleep requirements may remain unchanged from those of the young adult years. Typical sleep disturbances during middle age may stem from hormonal changes in women, breathing-related disorders and insomnia.

Elderly adults

Sleep problems are common among elderly adults. Besides taking longer to fall asleep, they spend less time in deep NREM sleep, so their sleep is more easily interrupted or fragmented. (See *Sleep requirements of elderly adults*, page 370.)

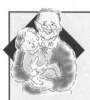

Ages and stages

Sleep requirements of elderly adults

It's a common misconception that elderly adults need much less sleep than younger adults. On the contrary, sleep requirements increase in elderly people because they tend to get decreased amounts of deep sleep and suffer frequent sleep interruptions.

Bathroom breaks

Early awakening is also common in elderly adults and may result from an earlier rise in body temperature. Lastly, many seniors have trouble falling back to sleep after awakening to urinate.

Lifestyle

Travel, shift work, stress and anxiety can greatly influence sleep. A person who travels through different time zones may suffer jet lag, which is worse when travelling west to east. They will typically try to sleep when they aren't tired (travelling west to east) and try to stay awake when it's daylight (travelling east to west).

Night-shift blues

In addition, it is suggested that some night-shift workers experience sleep problems resulting from disruption of the body's natural rhythms.

Environment

Sleep environment can greatly affect sleep quality. Environmental influences on sleep include noise, bright lights or sunlight, excessive activity and an uncomfortable room temperature. When these influences are prominent, sleep can be difficult even for someone who's sleepy. Removing such stimuli produces an environment that's more conducive to sleeping.

Hospital blues

Hospitalised patients commonly have trouble sleeping. First of all, they aren't in their own bed and the noises of everyday hospital routine can be disruptive. If they're in a special care unit, such as intensive and cardiac care, the bells and whistles of equipment can disturb sleep or prevent a patient from getting to sleep. In addition, the stress of hospitalisation and the fear of a bad prognosis or new procedures can also disrupt routine sleeping patterns. Lastly, the routines of regular vital signs measurement, doctor visits and medication regimens can also disrupt sleep.

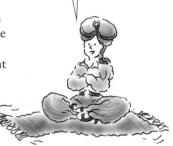

Travel, shift work, stress and anxiety can greatly influence sleep. A person who travels through different time zones may suffer jet lag.

Medications and substances

Medications of any kind may alter sleep patterns. Prescription drugs may cause somnolence (drowsiness) at inappropriate times; some may cause insomnia. Illicit drugs and other substances may also disturb established sleep patterns.

Alcohol

Alcohol's effect on sleep varies with the amount and time of consumption. In non-alcoholics, alcohol may have a sedative effect, increasing the amount of slow-wave sleep for the first 4 hours after sleep onset. After alcohol's effects wear off, sleep may be disrupted, with an increased amount of REM sleep and anxiety-causing dreams. Alcoholics may have trouble falling asleep and staying asleep. Many have REM sleep disturbances.

Withdrawal woes

During alcohol withdrawal, sleep deprivation is common. When sleep occurs, it's usually fragmented and accompanied by nightmares and anxiety-causing dreams.

No nite-nite

The most important symptoms of sleep disturbances are insomnia at night (the most common symptom) and sleepiness during waking hours. A thorough medical and psychological history should be obtained from a patient who complains of sleep problems. You may also need to question the family because the patient may be unaware of their sleep behaviour.

Sometimes, a physical examination is also warranted. Because sleep disorders are commonly linked to mood disorders, psychological tests may be administered as well.

Common sleep disorders

Some of the most common sleep disorders include circadian rhythm disorders, breathing-related sleep disorders, narcolepsy, primary hypersomnia and primary insomnia.

Circadian rhythm disorders

Circadian refers to biological rhythms with a cycle of about 24 hours. (*Circadian* comes from the Latin phrase 'circa diem', meaning 'about a day'.) The circadian rhythm functions as the body's internal 'clock', regulating the 24-hour sleep-awake cycle and other body functions, such as body temperature, hormones and heart rate. (See *Tick tock, it's the body clock*, page 372.)

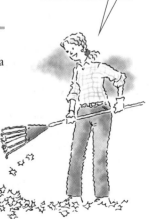

My circadian rhythms can help me adjust to disturbances like seasonal changes. Now if they could only help me enjoy raking these leaves!

Tick tock, it's the body clock

The human body has an internal 'clock' that follows a 24-hour cycle of wakefulness and sleepiness. This clock runs on circadian rhythms, which are linked to nature's cycle of light and darkness.

Critical organs, such as the heart, liver and kidneys, have their own 'clocks' that work in a coordinated fashion with the body's master clock. Researchers know, for example, that certain cardiac events, such as heart attacks and sudden cardiac death, occur more commonly during specific times of the circadian cycle.

Lark vs. owl

The body's clock keeps us alert during daylight hours and makes us sleepy when night falls. All of our physiologic functions are geared towards being active during the day and resting at night. The desire to sleep is strongest between 12 and 6 a.m.

Nonetheless, individual patterns of alertness vary, explaining why some people are relatively more alert during the day ('larks') while others are more alert at night ('night owls').

Mighty melatonin

The body's internal clock is regulated by melatonin, a hormone that causes sleepiness. Melatonin is secreted by the pineal gland, a structure located in the roof of the brain's third ventricle. Influenced by light, the pineal gland slows melatonin production during daylight hours to promote alertness and increases production when darkness falls, causing sleepiness.

With age, the body produces less melatonin. Not surprisingly, many elderly adults suffer from sleep disorders.

The body's internal clock can reset itself to help a person adjust to such disturbances as seasonal changes, transitions to or from daylight savings time or the start of a new workingweek. However, it can't always overcome longer lasting disruptions resulting from shift work or jet lag.

Weirded-out rhythms

Disruption of circadian rhythms may cause sleep difficulties, fatigue, a short attention span, impaired cognitive abilities (such as poor judgment and decision making) and even GI disorders.

There are three main types of circadian rhythm sleep disorders:

- delayed sleep phase
- jet lag
- shift-work disorders.

Delayed sleep phase sleep disorder

In *delayed sleep phase sleep disorder*, the patient sleeps according to a delayed clock time, relative to the light–dark cycle and social, economic and family demands. Typically, they have trouble falling asleep until the early hours of morning and end up sleeping through much of the day. This disorder commonly begins in childhood and is relatively common among adolescents.

Jet lag sleep disorder

The *jet lag sleep disorder* results from rapid travel across more than one time zone. Until the body's clock fully adjusts to the new time zone, the patient feels sleepy or alert at an inappropriate time of day relative to local time. Jet lag commonly requires a recovery period of 1 day for every time zone passed over.

Shift-work sleep disorder

In *shift-work sleep disorder*, night-shift work or frequently changing shift work causes insomnia during the major sleep period or excessive sleepiness during the major awake period. The patient typically suffers chronic sleep disruption.

Breathing-related sleep disorders

Breathing-related sleep disorders are marked by abnormal breathing during sleep. Obstructive sleep apnoea syndrome (OSAS) is the most common breathing-related sleep disorder. Other disorders in this category include central sleep apnoea syndrome and central alveolar hypoventilation syndrome.

Breathing blockade

In OSAS, the upper airway becomes blocked during sleep, impeding airflow. Reduced airway muscle tone and the pull of gravity in the supine position further limit airway size during sleep. As tissue collapse worsens, the airway may become completely obstructed.

With partial or complete airway obstruction, the patient struggles to breathe. Blockage of airflow lasts 10 seconds to 1 minute and arouses the patient from sleep as the brain responds to decreased blood oxygen levels. (However, arousal is commonly partial and goes unrecognised by the patient.)

Snoring, then silence

This pattern causes disturbed and fragmented sleep, with periods of loud snoring or gasping when the airway is partly open, alternating with silence when the airway is blocked. (However, not everyone who snores has OSAS.)

People with severe, untreated sleep apnoea have two to three times the risk of motor vehicle accidents. That is, unless the car falls asleep first!

With arousal, the muscle tone of the tongue and airway tissues increases, causing the patient to awaken just enough to tighten the upper airway muscles and open the trachea. However, when they fall back to sleep, the tongue and soft tissue relax again—and the cycle begins anew. This cycle may be repeated hundreds of times each night.

Repetitive cycles of snoring, airway collapse and arousal may lead to cardiovascular problems—high blood pressure, arrhythmias and even myocardial infarction or stroke. In some high-risk patients, sleep apnoea may lead to sudden death from respiratory arrest during sleep.

Drowsy, irritable and indifferent

Frequent awakenings leave the patient sleepy during the day and can cause irritability or depression. The patient may suffer morning headaches, decreased mental functioning and a reduced sex drive.

Narcolepsy

Narcolepsy is characterised by sudden, uncontrollable attacks of deep sleep lasting up to 20 minutes. These 'sleep attacks' come on without warning and may be accompanied by paralysis and hallucinations. Although the brief sleep is refreshing, the urge to sleep soon returns.

Sleep paralysis and hallucinations typically occur during sleep onset (hypnagogic hallucinations) or during the transition from sleep to wakefulness (hypnopompic hallucinations). Mostly visual, these hallucinations are intense, dreamlike images commonly involving the immediate environment.

Confounding cataplexy

A large proportion of patients with narcolepsy experience attacks of cataplexy, sudden loss of muscle tone and strength. (In more subtle forms of cataplexy, the patient's head may drop or his jaw may slacken.)

Cataplexy is commonly triggered by emotions, for example, the knees may buckle after the patient laughs, gets angry or feels elated or surprised. Cataplexy typically lasts just a few seconds and the patient remains alert during the episode. However, in severe cases, the patient falls down and becomes completely paralysed for up to several minutes.

Narcoleptic sleep attacks may occur at any time of day. All too commonly, they occur during activities that call for undivided attention, such as driving.

Image problems

Besides causing accidents, narcolepsy can be disabling, impairing work performance and disrupting leisure activities and interpersonal relationships. Co-workers may perceive the patient as lazy; an employer may suspect them of illegal drug use. It has been known for narcoleptic patients to give up working because of the disease.

Jeers from their peers

In children, narcolepsy impairs school performance and social relationships and invites ridicule from peers. Teenagers with the disorder are at increased risk for car accidents.

Primary hypersomnia

Primary hypersomnia is a condition of excessive sleepiness characterised by prolonged sleep periods at night or daytime sleep episodes occurring nearly every day. During long periods of drowsiness, the patient may exhibit automatic behaviour, acting in a semi-controlled fashion. They may have trouble meeting morning obligations, commonly arriving late.

Symptomatic categories

Primary hypersomnia can be monosymptomatic or polysymptomatic:
• In the *monosymptomatic* form, the patient has isolated excessive daytime sleepiness unrelated to abnormal nocturnal awakenings.
• The *polysymptomatic* form involves abnormally long night-time sleep and signs of sleep 'drunkenness' (difficulty awakening completely, confusion, disorientation, poor motor coordination and slowness) on awakening. Usually, the patient falls asleep easily at night and can stay asleep but seems out of sorts or even combative on awakening in the morning.

Primary insomnia

The most common sleep disorder, *primary insomnia*, encompasses many types of problems: difficulty falling asleep, sleeping too lightly, frequent awakenings during the night, inability to fall back to sleep once awakened and waking up in the early morning and being unable to fall back to sleep. These problems aren't attributable to another sleep disorder or psychiatric disorder, a general medical condition or substance use. (See *Key questions to ask about insomnia*, page 376.)

Obsessing over insomnia

Insomnia can be acute or chronic. With chronic insomnia, the person may become pre-occupied with getting enough sleep. The more they try to sleep, the greater their sense of frustration and distress and the more elusive sleep becomes.

Insomnia commonly leads to daytime drowsiness that causes poor concentration, memory impairments, difficulty coping with minor problems and reduced ability to enjoy family and social relationships.

You don't snooze, you lose

Insomniacs are more than twice as likely as the general population to have a fatigue-related motor vehicle accident. Those who sleep fewer than 5 hours per night may have a higher death rate, too.

Key questions to ask about insomnia

When a patient complains of insomnia, ask the following questions:

- When did the problem begin?
- Do you have a medical or psychiatric illness that might affect your ability to sleep?
- What's your sleep environment like? Is it dark? Quiet? Bright? Noisy? Does it have a comfortable room temperature?
- What time do you usually go to bed?
- What time do you usually get up in the morning on weekdays? On weekends?
- Do you drink alcohol or smoke? Are you taking prescribed medications? Non-prescription preparations? Illegal drugs?
- What's your typical work schedule?
- How do you feel the day after a poor night's sleep?

Family inquiries

If possible, ask the patient's spouse or other family members if the patient snores or has unusual limb movements when asleep.

Treatments for sleep disturbances

Various therapies can be used to treat sleep disorders, depending on the source of the disorder.

Circadian rhythm disorders

Treatments for circadian rhythm disorders include chronotherapy, luminotherapy, chronopharmacotherapy and melatonin.

Chronotherapy

Chronotherapy is most commonly used to treat delayed sleep phase sleep disorder. *Chronotherapy* involves manipulating the patient's sleep schedule by progressively delaying bedtime by one or more hours each night, until the patient can go to sleep and wake up at appropriate times.

Luminotherapy

Luminotherapy is the use of bright light to manipulate the circadian system. Typically administered with light boxes, it's safe and effective when used according to recommendations.

Here comes the sun

For patients with delayed sleep phase sleep disorder, some doctors recommend exposure to bright light on awakening. Sunlight exposure for

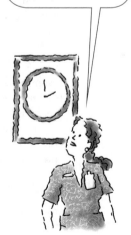

In chronotherapy, manipulation of the patient's sleep schedule helps the patient go to sleep and wake up at appropriate times.

night-shift workers or jet travellers at their destination may help reset the circadian clock to environmental time.

Chronopharmacotherapy

Chronopharmacotherapy involves the use of drugs to induce sleep or promote wakefulness when desired. Short-acting sedative-hypnotic drugs may be used to promote sleep, especially in jet lag sleep disorder.

Many night-shift workers use caffeine to keep themselves awake on the job. However, some become unresponsive to caffeine's effects over time.

Melatonin

Melatonin is a hormone released by the pineal gland to help the body regulate sleep–wake cycles. Supplemental melatonin therapy has been studied recently as a treatment for circadian rhythm sleep disorders. However, it hasn't been proven safe or effective in long-term use. Also, because melatonin is a hormone, it may have unpredictable effects.

Breathing-related disorders

Treatments for breathing-related disorders, such as OSAS, include lifestyle changes, continuous positive airway pressure (CPAP) and dental devices.

Lifestyle changes

Lifestyle changes, especially weight loss, are used to treat OSAS. Weight loss reduces the amount of excess tissue in and around the airway. Decreasing the body mass index to 30 or less significantly reduces the frequency of obstructive sleep episodes. However, even small weight reductions can improve the patient's condition.

Supine isn't sublime

Sleeping on the side rather than in a supine (back-lying) position may reduce apnoeic episodes. Avoiding alcohol and sleeping pills can decrease the number and duration of these episodes.

Continuous positive airway pressure

CPAP therapy during sleep is the most common and effective treatment for OSAS. Positive pressure splints the airway open, preventing its collapse. The desired level of pressure varies with the type of CPAP device used. The patient wears either a full facial mask or a nasal mask.

Dental devices

Oral appliances worn during sleep may help to relieve airway obstruction. However, they may be uncomfortable for some patients and may cause excessive salivation.

Insomnia

Treatments for insomnia include relaxation, sleep hygiene, behavioural interventions, cognitive therapy, alternative and complementary therapies, and medications.

Relaxation techniques

Because many insomniacs display high levels of physiologic and cognitive arousal (both at night and during the day), relaxation-based interventions may provide relief. Techniques that help deactivate the arousal system include progressive muscle relaxation, abdominal or deep breathing, biofeedback and imagery training.

Sleep hygiene

For some patients, insomnia responds well to simple lifestyle changes, sometimes called *sleep hygiene*. Such changes include going to bed at the same time every night, optimising sleeping conditions and avoiding naps during the day. (See *Getting hygienic about sleep*.)

Behavioural interventions

Behavioural interventions aim to change maladaptive sleep habits, reduce autonomic arousal and alter dysfunctional beliefs and attitudes. A wide range of behavioural techniques may be used to treat chronic primary insomnia.

Stimulus control

Stimulus control centres on the theory that insomnia represents a learned response to bedtime and bedroom cues.

Paradoxical intention

In paradoxical intention, the patient does the opposite of what they want, sometimes taking it to an extreme. For instance, instead of going through activities that promote sleep, they prepare themselves for staying awake and doing something energetic. If worry is a factor in insomnia, they may deliberately intensify the worrying.

Biofeedback

In biofeedback, the patient is connected to a device that measures brain waves and other body functions. Then they are given feedback so that they can learn to recognise certain states of tension or sleep stages and either avoid or repeat these states voluntarily.

Sleep restriction

Sleep restriction creates a mild state of sleep deprivation, which may promote more rapid sleep onset and more 'efficient' sleep. The patient limits the amount of time spent in bed in order to increase the percentage of time spent asleep.

Getting hygienic about sleep

For most patients with insomnia, simple lifestyle measures, termed *sleep hygiene,* are used first. When teaching your patient about sleep hygiene, cover the following dos and don'ts.

Sleep-promoting measures

- Use the bed only for sleep and sex, not for reading, watching television or working.
- Establish a regular bedtime and a regular time for getting up in the morning. Stick to these times even on weekends and on holidays.
- Exercise in the evening. Energy levels bottom out a few hours after exercise, promoting sleep at that time.
- Take a warm bath 90 minutes to 2 hours before bedtime to alter core body temperature and help you fall asleep more easily.
- During the 30 minutes before bedtime, do something relaxing, such as reading, meditating or taking a leisurely walk.
- Keep the bedroom quiet, dark, relatively cool and well ventilated.
- Eat dinner 4 to 5 hours before bedtime. At bedtime, a light snack (low in sugar and calories) may promote sleep.
- Spend 30 minutes in the sun each day. (However, be sure to take precautions against overexposure.)
- If you don't fall asleep after 15 or 20 minutes, get up and go into another room. Read or perform a quiet activity, using dim lighting, until you feel sleepy.

- If your bed partner distracts you, consider moving to another bedroom or the sofa for a few nights. (One study showed that sleeping alone is more restful than sleeping with another person.)

What not to do

- Don't use the bedroom for work, reading or watching television.
- Avoid large meals before bedtime.
- Don't look at the clock. Obsessing over time makes it harder to sleep.
- Avoid naps, especially in the evening.
- Don't drink a large amount of fluid after dinner, or the need to urinate may disturb your sleep.
- Avoid exercising close to bedtime because this may make you more alert.
- Avoid alcohol and caffeine in the evening.
- Don't take a bath just before bedtime because this could increase your alertness.
- Don't engage in highly stimulating activities before bed, such as watching a frightening movie or playing competitive computer games.
- Quit smoking, because nicotine's effects may contribute to sleep loss.
- Avoid tossing and turning in bed. Instead, get up and read or listen to relaxing music. However, don't watch television because it emits too bright a light.

Bedtime amendments

To maintain a consistent sleep–awake pattern, the patients usually alter their bedtime rather than their rising time. However, time in bed shouldn't be reduced to fewer than 5 hours per day. Naps aren't allowed (except in elderly adults).

Cognitive therapy

Cognitive therapy helps the patients identify their dysfunctional beliefs and attitudes about sleep (such as 'I'll never fall asleep') and replace them with positive ones. Changing beliefs and attitudes can decrease the anticipatory anxiety that interferes with sleep. Cognitive therapy also focuses on actions intended to change behaviour.

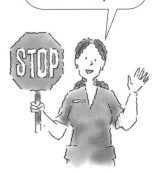

Unless the patient is elderly, sleep restriction means just say 'No!' to naps!

Alternative and complementary therapies

Alternative and complementary therapies that may be used to treat insomnia include acupressure, acupuncture, aromatherapy, massage, biofeedback, chiropractic, homoeopathy, light and dark therapy, meditation, reflexology, visualisation and yoga.

A mouthful of electromagnetic waves

Another technique, low-energy emission therapy, delivers electromagnetic waves through a mouthpiece and may benefit some patients.

Supplements to sleep by

Some patients use herbal preparations (such as St. John's wort and chamomile), nutritional substances and other non-prescription preparations to treat insomnia. However, few of such products have been demonstrated to be safe and effective.

Dietary supplements sometimes recommended for insomnia relief include vitamins B_6, B_{12} and D. Some practitioners also recommend calcium and magnesium. Tryptophan may relieve insomnia in some patients, but the patient must be monitored for adverse effects. Melatonin may increase sleepiness and is currently undergoing clinical studies.

Pharmacologic options

If insomnia persists despite other measures, the doctor may recommend drug therapy. The most commonly prescribed drugs are short-acting sedative-hypnotics (primarily benzodiazepines), anti-depressants and anti-histamines. (See *Pharmacologic therapy for sleep disorders*.)

Knockout pills

Sedative-hypnotics, usually temazepam and zolpidem are commonly prescribed for short-term management of insomnia.

Prescription and non-prescription anti-histamines can be used for short-term management of insomnia. Adverse effects include daytime sedation, cognitive impairment and anti-cholinergic effects (e.g., dry mouth, constipation and urine retention). Tolerance may also occur.

Anti-depressants may be given in low dosages, especially if the patient has a related psychiatric disorder or a history of substance abuse. However, some anti-depressants can exacerbate other disorders, such as mania and restless leg syndrome, so the patient should be monitored closely.

Pharmacologic therapy for sleep disorders

This chart highlights several drugs used to treat sleep disorders. A patient with insomnia may receive a benzodiazepine, such as temazepam or triazolam, a non-benzodiazepine, such as zopiclone or zolpidem.

Drug	Side effects	Contraindications	Nursing interventions
Temazepam	• Dizziness • Drowsiness • Lethargy • Orthostatic hypotension	• Pregnancy	• Teach the patient about the drug's action, dosage and adverse effects. • Instruct the patient not to take other medications unless the doctor approves. • Caution the patient not to drink alcohol, drive a motor vehicle or operate machinery while under the influence of this drug. • Advise the patient to change position slowly to avoid dizziness. • Inform the patient that prolonged use isn't recommended.
Zolpidem tartrate	• Abdominal pain • Daytime drowsiness • Dizziness • GI disturbances • Headache • Nightmares	• Breast feeding • Hepatic impairment • Pregnancy	• Teach the patient about the drug's action, dosage and adverse effects. • Advise the patient not to take the drug with or immediately after a meal. • Caution the patient against taking other medications unless the doctor approves. • Advise the patient not to drink alcohol, drive a motor vehicle or operate machinery while under the influence of this drug. • Inform the patient that tolerance may occur if this drug is taken for more than a few weeks.
Zopiclone	• Taste disturbance • Dizziness • Drowsiness • Nausea • Headache	• Respiratory failure • Breast feeding	• Teach the patient about the drug's action, dosage and adverse effects. • Inform the patient that this medication should be for short-term use only (up to 4 weeks) • Advise the patient that drowsiness may persist the next day and affect performance of skilled tasks, and that effects of alcohol are enhanced.

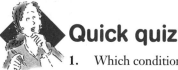

Quick quiz

1. Which condition is characteristic of REM sleep?
    A.   Light sleep
    B.   Paralysis of the muscles
    C.   Restricted eye movements
    D.   Non-vivid dreams

Answer: B. During REM sleep, many muscles are effectively paralyzed so the sleeping person won't act out dreams. Eye movements are rapid.

2. Which part of the brain regulates NREM sleep?
    A.   Pons
    B.   Hypothalamus
    C.   Basal forebrain
    D.   Amygdala

Answer: C. The basal forebrain controls NREM sleep. The pons and midbrain control REM sleep.

3. Which treatment is used to treat circadian rhythm sleep disorders?
    A.   Modafinil
    B.   Short-acting sedative-hypnotics
    C.   Relaxation techniques
    D.   Fluoxetine

Answer: B. Short-acting sedative-hypnotics are used to treat circadian rhythm sleep disorders.

4. Which treatment is most commonly used to treat delayed sleep phase sleep disorder?
    A.   Chronopharmacotherapy
    B.   Luminotherapy
    C.   Melatonin
    D.   Chronotherapy

Answer: D. Chronotherapy (progressively delaying bedtime by 1 or more hours each night) is most commonly used to treat delayed sleep phase sleep disorder.

Scoring

☆☆☆ If you answered all four questions correctly, way to go! You're no slouch when it comes to sleeping.

☆☆ If you answered three questions correctly, good job! You're waking up to good sleep habits.

☆ If you answered fewer than three questions correctly, don't lose sleep over it! Take a nap, review the chapter and try again.

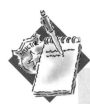

17 Pain management

Just the facts

In this chapter, you'll learn:

♦ types of pain and theories that explain them

♦ effective ways to document pain assessment findings

♦ history and examination techniques for the patient with pain

♦ psychological characteristics of pain

♦ specific uses of pain medications

♦ physiotherapies used in pain management

♦ roles of alternative and complementary therapies in relieving pain.

A look at pain

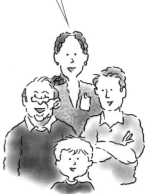

Reactions to pain vary from person to person and even within the same person at different times.

Pain is a complex, subjective phenomenon that involves biological, psychological, cultural and social factors. To put it succinctly, pain is whatever the patient says it is, and it occurs whenever they say it does. The only true authority on any given pain is the person experiencing it. Therefore, health-care professionals must understand and rely on the patient's description of their pain when developing a pain management plan.

Each patient reacts to pain differently because pain thresholds and tolerances vary from person to person. Pain threshold is a physiologic attribute that denotes the intensity of the stimulus needed to sense pain. Pain tolerance is a physiologic attribute that describes the amount of stimulus (duration and intensity) that the patient can endure before stating that they are in pain.

Theories about pain

Two theories attempt to explain the mechanisms of pain:

 specificity

 gate control.

Let's get specific

The specificity theory maintains that individual specialised peripheral nerve fibres are responsible for pain transmission. This biologically-oriented theory doesn't explain pain tolerance, nor does it allow for social, cultural or empirical factors that influence pain.

Opening the gate

The gate-control theory asserts that some sort of gate mechanism in the spinal cord allows nerve fibres to receive pain sensations. (See *Understanding the gate-control theory*). This theory has encouraged a more holistic approach to pain management and research by taking into account the non-biological components of pain. Pain management techniques, such as cutaneous stimulation, distraction and acupuncture are, in part, based on this theory.

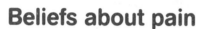

Hmmm. That's an interesting pattern. Deep, very deep . . .

Beliefs about pain

Patients' attitudes, beliefs, expectations of themselves, coping resources and beliefs about the health-care system affect the entire spectrum of their pain behaviours.

Behaviour and emotions are influenced by the interpretation as well as the facts of an event. This partly explains why patients may differ greatly in their beliefs about pain.

Carol, Alice, Bob and Ted

Take Carol and Alice, for instance. Both have lower back pain. Carol thinks her pain indicates a progressive disease, whereas Alice thinks her pain results from a stable, manageable problem. Who's likely to experience more suffering and behavioural dysfunction? You guessed it—Carol.

Let's peek in on their significant others, Bob and Ted. Both awaken with a headache. Bob assumes the headache is from a hangover, whereas Ted thinks he might have a brain tumour. Like Carol, Ted is setting himself up for more suffering than Bob.

Because of their beliefs, Bob and Alice will respond to their pain in markedly different ways from Ted and Carol. In essence, they're likely to experience less suffering and disability.

Coping

Patients' beliefs, judgments and expectations about an event's consequences—and belief in their ability to influence the outcome—can affect their ability to function. That's because such beliefs, judgments and expectations can influence mood directly and alter coping ability.

Patients with low back pain offer a good example. Many fail to comply with prescribed exercises. Their previous pain experience may foster a negative view of their abilities and an expectation of increased pain during exercise. These beliefs form a rationale for avoiding exercise.

Understanding the gate-control theory

Intensive research into the pathophysiology of pain has yielded several theories about pain perception, including the Melzack–Wall gate-control theory. According to this theory, pain and thermal impulses travel along small-diameter, slow-conducting afferent nerve fibres to the spinal cord's dorsal horns. There, they terminate in an area of grey matter called the substantia gelatinosa.

Open or close the gate

When sensory stimulation reaches a critical level, a theoretical 'gate' in the substantia gelatinosa opens, allowing nearby transmission cells to send the pain impulse to the brain along the interspinal neurons to the spinothalamic tract, and then to the thalamus and cerebral cortex (see illustration below, left). The small size of the fibres enhances pain transmission.

In contrast, large-diameter fibres inhibit pain transmission. Stimulation of these large, fast-conducting afferent nerve fibres counters the input of the smaller fibres; thereby closing the theoretical gate in the substantia gelatinosa and blocking the pain transmission (see illustration below, right).

Keys to the gate

Descending (efferent) impulses along various tracts from the brain and brain stem can enhance or reduce pain transmission at the gate. For example triggering specific brain processes, such as attention, emotions and memory of pain, can intensify pain by opening the gate.

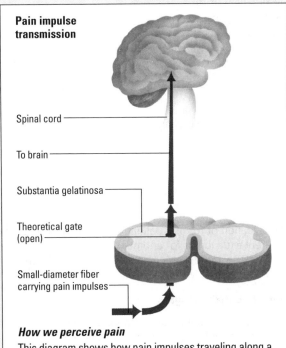

Pain impulse transmission

Spinal cord

To brain

Substantia gelatinosa

Theoretical gate (open)

Small-diameter fiber carrying pain impulses

How we perceive pain

This diagram shows how pain impulses traveling along a small-diameter nerve fiber pass through an open gate in the substantia gelatinosa, and then travel to the brain for interpretation.

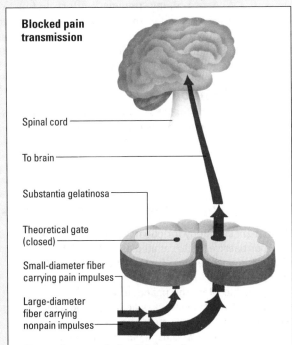

Blocked pain transmission

Spinal cord

To brain

Substantia gelatinosa

Theoretical gate (closed)

Small-diameter fiber carrying pain impulses

Large-diameter fiber carrying nonpain impulses

How pain transmission is blocked

Impulses carried by a large-diameter fiber can close the gate to small-fiber impulses, blocking the transmission of pain.

Helpless without feedback

The expectation of exercise-related pain reinforces patients' beliefs that their disability is pervasive. Patients who see disability as a necessary reaction to pain and view activity as dangerous are more likely to experience continued disability. Their failure to perform prescribed activities has negative effects:

- It robs them of the corrective feedback that could help counteract their beliefs.
- It reinforces the perception of helplessness and incapacity.

In contrast, developing positive coping strategies may alter the perception of pain intensity and promote the patient's ability to manage or tolerate pain and continue activities of daily living (ADLs).

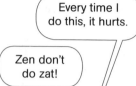

Every time I do this, it hurts.

Zen don't do zat!

Can you cope with these concepts?

Coping can be overt or covert; active or passive. Overt coping strategies include rest, drug therapy and use of relaxation techniques. Covert coping strategies include distraction, reassuring oneself that the pain will diminish, seeking information and solving problems.

Active coping strategies—efforts to function despite pain or to distract oneself from pain—lead to adaptive functioning. Passive coping strategies—restricting one's activities and depending on others for help in pain control—lead to greater pain and depression. (See *Encouraging active pain-coping strategies*.)

Attention

Pain can change the way the patient processes pain-related and other information by focusing attention on bodily signals. As these signals change,

---

Encouraging active pain-coping strategies

The patient's strategy for coping with pain may be active or passive. Active strategies include attempts to function despite pain. Passive strategies include relying on others for help in pain control.

If possible, steer the patient toward active coping strategies. A patient who uses active coping strategies tends to experience less pain and increased pain tolerance than one who uses passive strategies.

One strategy doesn't fit all

Even so, keep in mind that one particular active coping strategy isn't necessarily better than another. What's more, a given strategy may be helpful in one situation or for one patient, but not helpful in a different situation or for another patient.

Likewise, certain strategies may help at one time but prove ineffective in other situations.

Out-of-control thoughts

The most important feature of poor coping seems to be 'catastrophising'—thinking extremely negative thoughts about one's plight rather than choosing poorly among active coping strategies.

If the patient falls into this trap, teach them that imagining more positive outcomes may help reduce their pain.

they may assume that these changes mean that the underlying disease is getting worse and, as a result, may report increased pain.

In contrast, a patient who doesn't attribute symptoms to worsening disease tends to report less pain, even if their disease actually is progressing.

Too little feedback

Beliefs and expectations about a disease are hard to change. Patients tend to avoid experiences that might invalidate their beliefs and guide their behaviour in keeping with their beliefs. Commonly, health professionals refrain from challenging patients about irrational beliefs and excessively restrictive activities. In doing so, they fail to give patients valuable corrective feedback.

Successful rehabilitation

Beliefs about pain can influence the patient's disability level, response to treatment and compliance with prescribed activities. For rehabilitation to succeed, the patient must change from believing they are helpless and passive to believing in their ability to function regardless of pain.

A patient with chronic pain must learn to minimise the role of pain in determining their functioning level. Those patients who find successful ways to cope with pain tend to establish a balance between trying new activities despite persistent pain and respecting the physical limitations imposed by their condition.

Efficacy has its advantages

Being able to minimise the role of pain may stem in part from a personal conviction that one can successfully follow a course of action to produce a desired outcome. Known as self-efficacy, this concept is crucial to coping and successful rehabilitation.

A belief in self-efficacy grows from the patient's conviction that the demands of their situation won't exceed their ability to cope. A patient can build a sense of self-efficacy by performing increasingly difficult tasks to learn what physical sensations mean, and by using the relaxation and learning strategies that have helped others with similar conditions.

Pain beyond control?

What about pain that's hard to control? Commonly, patients with chronic pain—and limited success in controlling it—think of the pain as outside their control. They're unlikely to try new pain-management strategies.

Instead, they grow frustrated and demoralised by pain that interferes with their recreational, occupational and social activities. They may resort to passive coping strategies—inactivity, self-medication or alcohol abuse— to reduce emotional distress and pain.

It seems catastrophic

Patients who feel little control over pain are also more likely to 'catastrophise' the impact of a pain episode and any situations that tend to worsen pain. Depression and anxiety, common among patients with chronic pain, can influence pain perception.

In fact, anxiety about pain can change a person's pain threshold and tolerance level. Likewise, depression symptoms can reduce the capacity for successful coping.

Physical links to pain

Just as physical factors can affect a patient's psychological condition, psychological factors can affect their mood, coping ability and nociception (sensation of pain).

Cognitive interpretations and affective arousal may influence physiology by increasing autonomic sympathetic nervous system (SNS) arousal and promoting endogenous opioid (endorphin) production.

Autonomic arousal

Thinking about pain and stress can increase muscle tension, especially in already painful areas. Chronic and excessive SNS arousal is a precursor to increased skeletal muscle tone. It may set the stage for hyperactive and persistent muscle contractions, which promote muscle spasms and pain.

Arousing sympathy

Patients who exaggerate the significance of their problems or focus on them too closely may influence sympathetic arousal. This predisposes them to further injury and can complicate recovery in other ways.

A look at pain assessment

To ensure that the patient receives effective pain relief, you must conduct a thorough and accurate pain assessment. This can be difficult, because pain is so subjective.

Pain is influenced not just by physical pathology but also by cultural and social factors, expectations, mood, and perceptions of control. What's more, you and the patient may have dramatically different pain thresholds and tolerances, expectations about pain and ways of expressing pain.

You may even doubt the patient's complaints of pain, particularly if you think their behaviour doesn't match their report of pain. For instance, they may tell you they have moderate pain yet continue to chat and laugh with visitors. If no pathological cause for pain is found, you may even question the patient's report of pain.

The patient knows best

To keep your pain assessment on track, keep in mind the first principle of pain assessment: pain is whatever the patient says it is, occurring whenever they say it does. The patient's self-report of the presence and severity of pain is the most accurate, reliable means of pain assessment. If the patient reports pain, respect what they say and act promptly to assess and control it.

Pain threshold and tolerance

Pain threshold refers to the intensity of the stimulus a person needs to sense pain. Pain tolerance is the duration and intensity of pain that a person tolerates before openly expressing pain. Tolerance has a strong psychological component. Identifying pain threshold and tolerance are crucial to pain assessment and the development of a pain management plan.

Even so, remember that pain threshold and tolerance vary widely among patients. They may even fluctuate in the same patient as circumstances change.

Differentiating types of pain

Pain falls into three broad categories—acute pain, chronic pain (also called chronic persistent pain) and cancer pain.

Acute pain

Acute pain comes on suddenly, for instance after trauma, surgery or an acute disease, and can last for a few hours. Typically, it's sharp, intense and easily localised. It causes a withdrawal reflex and may trigger involuntary bodily reactions, such as sweating, fast heart and respiratory rates and elevated blood pressure. (See *Acute pain: A sympathetic response*, page 390.)

Acute pain may be constant (as in a burn), intermittent (as in a muscle strain that hurts only with activity), or both (as in an abdominal incision that hurts a little at rest and a lot with movement or coughing). It can also be prolonged or recurrent. (See *Differentiating acute and chronic pain*, page 390.)

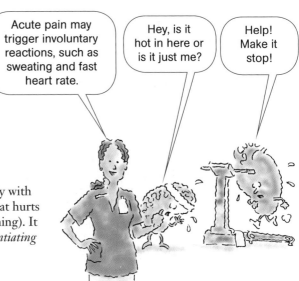

Acute pain may trigger involuntary reactions, such as sweating and fast heart rate.

Hey, is it hot in here or is it just me?

Help! Make it stop!

So long now

Prolonged acute pain usually results from tissue injury and inflammation (as from a sprain or surgery) and subsides gradually.

At the injury site, release or synthesis of chemicals heightens sensitivity in nearby tissues. This hypersensitivity, called hyperalgesia, is normal. In fact, tenderness and tissue hypersensitivity help protect the injury site and prevent further damage.

Differentiating acute and chronic pain

Acute pain may cause certain physiologic and behavioural changes that you won't observe in a patient with chronic pain.

Type of pain	Physiologic evidence	Behavioural evidence
Acute	• Increased respirations • Increased pulse • Increased blood pressure • Dilated pupils • Diaphoresis	• Restlessness • Distraction • Worry • Distress
Chronic	• Normal respirations, pulse, blood pressure and pupil size • No diaphoresis	• Reduced or absent physical activity • Despair, depression • Hopelessness

Acute pain: A sympathetic response

In acute pain, certain involuntary (autonomic) reflexes may occur. Acute pain causes the sympathetic branch of the autonomic nervous system (ANS) to trigger the release of epinephrine and other catecholamines. These substances, in turn, cause physiologic reactions such as those seen in the fight-or-flight response.

It'll get your attention

Sympathetic activation directs immediate attention to the injury site. This attention promotes reflexive withdrawal and fosters other actions that prevent further damage and enhance healing. For example if you place your hand on a hot stove, the ANS immediately generates a reflex withdrawal that jerks your hand away and minimises tissue damage.

Over and over again

Recurrent acute pain refers to brief painful episodes that recur at variable intervals. Examples include sickle cell vaso-occlusive crisis and migraine headache.

In migraine headache and some other recurrent conditions, pain serves no apparent useful purpose—no protective action can be taken and tissue damage can't be prevented. However, in others, such as sickle cell disease, acute pain encourages the person to seek medical treatment.

Chronic pain

Pain is considered chronic when it lasts beyond the normal time expected for an injury to heal or an illness to resolve. Many experts define chronic pain as pain lasting 6 months or longer that may continue during the patient's lifetime. Although it sometimes begins as acute pain, more typically it starts slowly and builds gradually. Unlike acute pain, chronic pain isn't protective and doesn't warn of significant tissue damage.

Causes of chronic pain include nerve damage, such as in brain injury, tumour growth or unexplained and abnormal responses to tissue injury by the central nervous system (CNS). It can cause serious disability (as in arthritis or avascular necrosis), or it may be related to poorly understood disorders such as fibromyalgia and complex regional pain syndrome. Neuropathic pain is one type of chronic pain. (See *Understanding neuropathic pain*.)

High cost of chronic pain

Chronic pain may be severe enough to limit a patient's ability and desire to participate in career, family life and even ADLs. If it's severe or intractable,

Understanding neuropathic pain

Commonly described as tingling, burning or shooting, neuropathic pain is a puzzling type of chronic pain generated by the nerves. It commonly has no apparent cause and responds poorly to standard pain treatment.

We don't know the precise mechanism of neuropathic pain. Possibly, the peripheral nervous system has experienced damage that injures sensory neurons, causing continuous depolarisation and pain transmission. Alternatively, it could result from repeated noxious stimuli that cause hypersensitivity and excitement in the spinal cord that results in chronic neuropathy in which a normally harmless stimuli causes pain.

The limb is gone, but the pain remains

Phantom pain syndrome is one example of neuropathic pain. This condition occurs when an arm or a leg has been removed but the brain still gets pain messages from the nerves that originally carried the limb's impulses. The nerves seem to misfire, causing pain.

Types of neuropathic pain

Neuropathic pain can involve peripheral or central pain.

Peripheral pain can occur as:

- polyneuropathy, which is pain felt along the peripheral nerves, as in diabetic neuropathy
- mononeuropathy, which is pain associated with an established injury and felt along the nerve, as in trigeminal neuralgia.

Central neuropathic pain also comes in two varieties:

- sympathetic pain, which results from dysfunction of the ANS
- de-afferentation pain, which is marked by elimination of sensory (afferent) impulses, as from damage to the central or peripheral nervous system (as in phantom limb pain).

the patient may experience decreased function, pain behaviours, depression, opioid dependence, 'doctor shopping' and suicide.

Assessment obstacles

You may find pain assessment especially difficult in a patient with chronic pain. Over time, the autonomic nervous system (ANS) adapts to pain, so the patient may lack typical autonomic responses, such as dilated pupils, increased blood pressure and fast heart and respiratory rates. Also, their facial expression may not suggest they are in pain. They may sleep periodically and shift their attention away from the pain. Regardless, don't let the lack of outward signs lead you to conclude that they aren't in pain.

Cancer pain

Cancer pain is a complex problem. It may result from the disease itself or from treatment. About 70% to 90% of patients with advanced cancer

Many experts define chronic pain as pain lasting 6 months or longer—it may continue during the patient's lifetime.

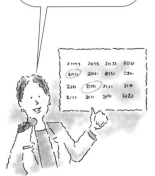

experience pain. Although cancer pain can be treated with medications, not everyone with cancer pain achieves satisfactory relief.

Sometimes pain results from the pressure of a tumour impinging on organs, bones, nerves or blood vessels. In other cases, limitations in ADLs may lead to muscle aches.

Don't treat me like that!

These cancer treatments may cause pain:
- chemotherapy, radiation or drugs used to offset the impact of these therapies on blood counts and infection risk (such as mouth ulcers, peripheral neuropathy and abdominal, bone or joint pain from chemotherapy agents)
- surgery
- biopsies
- blood withdrawal
- lumbar punctures.

The fifth vital sign

Pain is commonly called the fifth vital sign because pain assessment scores must be monitored and recorded regularly—and at least as vigilantly as you monitor and record vital signs.

Pain assessment tools

When a patient is admitted, ask them if they are currently in pain or have ongoing problems with pain. If it is ongoing pain, find out if they have an effective treatment plan. If so, continue with this plan if possible. If they don't, use a pain assessment tool assess their pain.

Pain rating scales

Pain rating scales quantify pain intensity—one of pain's most subjective aspects. These scales offer several advantages over semi-structured and unstructured patient interviews:
- They're easier to administer.
- They take less time.
- They can uncover concerns that warrant a more thorough investigation.
- When used before and after a pain control intervention, they can help determine if the intervention was effective.

All shapes and sizes

Pain rating scales come in many varieties. When choosing an appropriate scale for your patient, consider their visual acuity, age, reading ability and level of understanding.

Pain intensity rating scale

You can evaluate pain in a non-verbal manner for children age 3 and older or for adult patients with language difficulties. One common pain rating scale consists of six faces with expressions ranging from happy and smiling to sad and teary.

Putting a face on pain

To use a pain intensity rating scale, tell the patient that each face represents a person with progressively worse pain. Ask them to choose the face that best represents how they feel. Explain that although the last face has tears, they can choose this face even if they aren't crying. (See *Using a pain intensity rating scale*.)

Visual analogue scale

The visual analogue scale is a horizontal line, 10 cm long, with word descriptors at each end: 'no pain' on one end and 'pain as bad as it can be' on the other. The scale may also be used vertically.

Drawing the line on pain

Ask the patient to place a mark along the line to indicate the intensity of their pain. This measurement represents the patient's pain rating. Be aware that this scale may be too abstract for some patients to use. (See *Visual analogue scale*.)

Numerical rating scale

The numerical rating scale (NRS) is perhaps the most commonly used pain rating scale. Simply ask the patient to rate their pain on a scale from 0 to 10, with 0 representing no pain and 10 representing the worst pain imaginable. Instead of giving a verbal rating, the patient can use a horizontal or vertical line consisting of descriptive words and numbers.

Although most patients find the NRS quick and easy to use, it may be too abstract for some patients. (See *Using the numerical rating scale*, page 394.)

Verbal descriptor scale

With the verbal descriptor scale, the patient chooses a description of their pain from a list of adjectives, such as 'none', 'annoying' 'uncomfortable', 'dreadful', 'horrible' and 'agonising'.

Visual analogue scale

To use the visual analogue scale, ask the patient to place a line across the scale to indicate their current level of pain.

No pain   Pain as bad
as it can be

Using a pain intensity rating scale

A child or an adult patient with language difficulties may not be able to express the pain they're feeling. In such instances, use the pain intensity scale below. Ask your patient to choose the face that best represents the severity of their pain, on a scale from 0 to 5.

0

1

2

3

4

5

Like the NRS, the verbal descriptor scale is quick and easy, but it does have drawbacks:

- It limits the patient's choices.
- Patients tend to choose moderate rather than extreme descriptors.
- Some patients may not understand all the adjectives.

Overall pain assessment tools

Overall pain assessment tools evaluate pain in multiple dimensions, providing a wider range of information. These tools are time-consuming and may be more practical for outpatient use. Still, you might want to use one for a hospitalised patient with hard-to-control chronic pain. Be sure to document the patient's pain according to your local policy. (See *Documenting pain assessment findings*.)

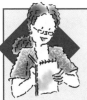

Take note!

Documenting pain assessment findings

Be sure to document baseline pain assessment findings so that you and other team members can use them for later comparison.

If the patient has unrelieved pain, you'll need to conduct frequent assessments. To make pain assessment findings more visible, they are now included on many vital sign or early warning system charts.

Analgesic infusion flow sheet

If the patient is receiving an analgesic infusion, you may use an analgesic infusion flow sheet to speed documentation and track their progress. Information to record on the flow sheet includes the:

* medication name and dosage
* date and time of each dose
* concentration of dose
* volume infused and volume remaining.

Pain assessment guide

Although lengthy, a pain assessment guide can help you collect important information about the patient's overall pain experience. These guides may vary from one area to the next.

Brief pain inventory

The brief pain inventory (BPI) focuses on the patient's pain during the last 24 hours. The patient or nurse can complete it in about 15 minutes. It's available in several languages.

Point to the pain, please

To use the BPI, have the patient rate the least and worst pain they have experienced over the last 24 hours and at the present time. Ask them to point to the location of the pain on a body map.

The BPI also asks questions that focus on:
* whether the patient has had pain other than common types (such as a headache or toothache)
* whether pain has interfered with their activities (such as walking, work and sleep) in the last 24 hours and, if so, to what extent
* whether the patient's current pain management plan is effective.

McGill pain questionnaire

The McGill's pain questionnaire assesses the multiple dimensions of neuropathic pain (a tingling, burning or shooting pain generated by nerves). It provides word descriptors to measure sensory, affective and evaluative pain domains.

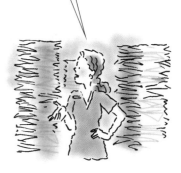

A pain assessment guide can help you collect important information. One drawback is that this assessment is lengthy. Okay, not this lengthy!

The long and the short of it

This tool is available in a short and long form. The short form has 15 word descriptors and takes less than 5 minutes. The long form consists of 78 word descriptors and takes about 20 minutes.

The McGill questionnaire can be used for baseline and periodic assessments. However, it doesn't quantify the patient's pain and isn't useful for frequent assessments.

Self-monitoring record

If your patient has chronic or recurrent pain, consider giving them a self-monitoring record (pain diary) to help them accurately describe pain occurrence and severity.

Assessing children

Assessing children's pain can be difficult, a suitable assessment tool should therefore be used. This will depend on the age and cognitive ability of the infant or child. Remember to note any changes in their vital signs together with alterations in their activity level, behaviour or appearance (RCN 2009). Many assessment tools designed for use with children are more visual, for example using faces, colours and chips.

Assessing people with dementia

Pain assessment for people with dementia may also prove difficult, they may not be able to fully understand or respond to the questions asked. You must therefore try different approaches in order to assess their pain. It may be helpful to ask a member of staff who knows the person well to undertake the assessment, where possible, and to ask the questions two or three times in a way the person understands. Using alternative words and closed questions may aid the process. Remember also to use a quiet room or area and keep the questions simple.

When the person is less able to communicate verbally it will be necessary to watch for any behavioural aspects that can indicate pain and the severity of it. For example these may include any changes in interpersonal interactions, facial expressions or body movements (Smith, 2007).

History and physical examination

Accurate pain assessment yields information that serves as the basis for an individualised pain management plan. For a patient with acute pain, a brief assessment may be adequate to formulate an appropriate plan.

However, a patient with chronic pain may require a thorough assessment that evaluates physical and psychosocial factors. Still, even the best history and examination techniques may not produce the definitive findings needed to make a precise diagnosis and clearly identify the origin of chronic pain. Usually, history and physical findings help the doctor interpret the results of diagnostic tests.

Patient history

Assessment begins with the patient interview. If they have acute pain from a traumatic injury, the interview may last for mere seconds. If they have chronic pain, it may be lengthy so try to pace the interview.

When interviewing a patient with chronic pain, try to gain information that sheds light on their thoughts, feelings, behaviours and physiologic responses to pain. Also find out about the environmental stimuli that can alter their response to pain.

During the interview, assess the cognitive, affective and behavioural components of the patient's pain experience. Doing so can help you later when working with the patient to develop pain management goals. Also ask questions to determine how the pain affects their mental state, relationships and work performance.

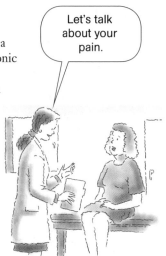

Let's talk about your pain.

Pain characteristics

Question the patient about these characteristics of their pain:
• onset and duration—When did the pain begin? Did it come on suddenly or gradually? Is it intermittent or continuous? How often does it occur? How long does it last? Is it prolonged or recurrent?
• location—Ask the patient to point to the painful parts of their body or to mark these areas on a diagram. Be sure to assess each pain site separately.
• intensity—Using a pain rating scale, ask the patient to quantify the intensity of the pain at its worst and at its best.
• quality—Ask the patient what the pain feels like, in their own words. Does it have a burning quality? Is it knife-like? Do they feel pressure? Throbbing? Soreness?
• relieving factors—Does anything help relieve the pain, such as a certain position or heat or cold applications? Besides helping to pinpoint the cause of the pain, their answers may aid in developing a pain management plan.
• aggravating factors—What seems to trigger the pain? What makes it worse? Does it get worse when the patient moves or changes position?

You may find the preview, question, read, state and test (PQRST) technique valuable when assessing pain. Each letter stands for a crucial aspect of pain to explore.

Medical and surgical history

The patient's medical history may offer clues to the source of pain or a condition that may exacerbate it. Ask them to list all of their past medical conditions, even those that have been resolved. Also question them about previous surgeries.

Past experience with pain

Explore the patient's experiences with pain. If they have experienced significant pain in the past, they may have anticipatory fear of future pain—especially if they received inadequate pain relief.

Play '20 Questions'

Ask the patient which previous treatments—pharmacological and otherwise—they have tried, and find out which treatments helped and which didn't. Keep in mind that non-pharmacological treatments include physical and occupational therapy, acupuncture, hypnosis, meditation, biofeedback, heat and cold therapy, transcutaneous nerve stimulation, and psychological counselling.

Medication history

Obtain a complete list of the patient's medications. (Many medications can alter the effectiveness of analgesics.) Besides prescribed drugs, ask if they take over-the-counter preparations, vitamins, nutritional supplements, or herbal or homemade remedies. Record the name, dose, frequency, administration route, and adverse effects of each agent they have used. Also ask them about drug allergies.

Find out if the patient currently takes or has previously taken medications to control pain and whether these were effective. If they currently receive analgesics, ask them exactly how they take them. If they haven't been taking them according to instructions, they may need additional teaching on proper administration.

Satisfaction survey

Ask the patient if they are satisfied with the level of pain relief their current medications bring. Find out how long these drugs take to work and whether the pain returns before the next dose is due.

Question the patient about adverse effects, such as nausea, constipation and drowsiness. If they are taking opioids for pain relief, note any worries they have about becoming drug-dependent. Listen carefully for concerns they may have about any medication.

Social history

Thorough pain assessment includes a social history. Many social factors can influence the patient's perception and reports of pain and vice versa. This information also helps guide interventions.

Chronic pain can have wide-ranging effects on a person's life. If your patient has chronic pain, explore the impact it has on their moods, emotions, expectations, coping efforts and resources. Also ask how their family responds to their condition.

A brave face

To provide culturally-sensitive care, you must determine the meaning of pain for each patient—particularly in the context of their culture and religion. Determine how their cultural background and religious beliefs may affect their pain experience. In some cultures, pain is openly expressed. Other cultures value stoicism and denial of pain. A patient who comes from a stoic culture may lead you to believe that they aren't in pain.

Be sure not to stereotype your patient. Keep in mind that, within each culture, the response to pain may vary from person to person. Also recognise your own cultural values and biases. Otherwise, you may end up evaluating the patient's response to pain according to your own beliefs instead of theirs.

Overt means observable

These overt behaviours may indicate that the patient is experiencing pain:
- verbal reports of pain
- vocalisations, such as sighs and moans
- altered motor activities (frequent position changes, guarded positioning, slow movements, rigidity)
- limping
- grimacing and other expressions
- functional limitations, including reclining for long periods
- actions to reduce pain such as taking medication.

Remember!

Acute pain may raise blood pressure, speed the heart and respiratory rates, and dilate pupils. Remember, however, that these autonomic responses may be absent in a patient with chronic pain because the body gradually adapts to pain. Don't assume lack of autonomic responses means lack of pain.

Psychological characteristics of pain

If diagnostic tests don't find a physical basis for the patient's pain, some health-care providers may label the pain psychogenic. Psychogenic pain refers to pain associated with psychological factors. A patient with psychogenic pain may have organic pathology, or a psychological disorder may be the pre-dominant influence on pain intensity.

Common psychogenic pain syndromes include chronic headache, muscle pain, back pain, and stomach or pelvic pain of unknown cause.

Keepin' it real

Keep in mind that psychogenic pain is real pain and doesn't mean that the patient is malingering. Remember, too, that although pain can cause emotional distress, such distress isn't necessarily the cause of the psychogenic pain.

Emotional by-products of pain

A patient with chronic pain may suffer significant emotional distress. Because pain is subjective, their suffering and disability are hard to prove, disprove or

---

Pain behaviour checklist

Pain behaviour is something a patient uses to communicate pain, distress, or suffering. Place a check in the box next to each behaviour you observe or infer while talking to your patient.
- ☐ Asking such questions as, 'Why did this happen to me?'
- ☐ Asking to be relieved from tasks or activities
- ☐ Avoiding physical activity
- ☐ Being irritable
- ☐ Clenching teeth
- ☐ Frequently shifting posture or position
- ☐ Grimacing
- ☐ Holding or supporting the painful body area
- ☐ Limping
- ☐ Lying down during the day
- ☐ Moaning
- ☐ Moving in a guarded or protective manner
- ☐ Moving very slowly
- ☐ Requesting help with walking
- ☐ Sighing
- ☐ Sitting rigidly
- ☐ Stopping frequently while walking
- ☐ Taking medication
- ☐ Using a cane, cervical collar, or other prosthetic device
- ☐ Walking with an abnormal gait

even quantify. So others may suspect they are faking or imagining the pain. What's more, if the patient is concerned that their pain may stem from an undiagnosed, possibly life-threatening condition, this belief will obviously add to their stress.

Shopping around

Some patients with chronic pain go from doctor to doctor and undergo exhausting procedures seeking a diagnosis and effective treatment. If their pain doesn't respond to treatment, they may feel health-care providers, employers and family are blaming—or doubting—them. In time, pain may become the central focus of their lives. They may withdraw from society, lose their jobs, and alienate family and friends.

Not surprisingly, many patients with chronic pain feel anxious, depressed, demoralised, helpless, hopeless, frustrated, angry and isolated. They may suffer from insomnia, disruption of usual activities, drug abuse and dependence, anger and violence. Some even attempt suicide.

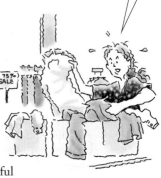

Patients with chronic pain may go from doctor to doctor trying to find someone who can give them effective treatment.

Road to success

For health-care providers, assessment and management of patients with pain—especially chronic pain—can be equally frustrating. However, that doesn't mean you should lose heart or blame the patient. Through careful assessment and regular re-evaluation, you can increase the odds for successful pain management—even in patients with seemingly intractable or chronic pain.

Treating pain successfully

When caring for a patient experiencing pain, you have three overall goals:

- reduce pain intensity

- improve the patient's ability to function

- improve the patient's quality of life.

To accomplish these goals, you must work with the patient to agree upon goals that are mutually desirable, realistic, measurable and achievable. In addition, you'll need to focus on the nociceptive and emotional aspects of pain. A patient responds to a painful physical condition based, in part, on their subjective interpretation of illness and symptoms. Their belief about the meaning of pain and their ability to function despite discomfort are important aspects of coping ability.

Harmful beliefs

Maladaptive responses to pain are more likely in a patient who believes that:
- they have a serious debilitating condition
- disability is a necessary aspect of pain
- activity is dangerous
- pain is an acceptable reason to reduce one's responsibilities.

Sometimes it pays to be a control freak

Many factors can promote or disrupt a patient's sense of control over the pain experience. These include:
- personal beliefs and expectations about pain
- coping ability
- social supports
- specific disorder that's causing the pain
- response of employers.

These factors also influence a patient's investment in treatment, acceptance of responsibility, perceptions of disability, adherence to treatment and support from significant others. To start the patient on the road to successful pain management, consider physical, psychosocial and behavioural factors—and the changes that occur in these relationships over time.

Making the effort

Treatment that increases perceived control over pain and reduces 'catastrophising' can decrease pain severity ratings and functional disability. Maintaining this sense of control—and the behavioural changes it fosters—depends on the patient's belief that successful pain control stems from one's own efforts.

Interdisciplinary pain-management team

An interdisciplinary team approach promotes effective pain management. Team members typically include an anaesthetist or pain specialist doctor, a nurse and pharmacist.

Treating types of pain

In addition to the three overall goals of treating pain, consider ways to treat specific types of pain.

Treating acute pain

The cause of acute pain can be diagnosed and treated, and the pain resolves when the cause is treated or analgesics are given. Drug regimens and invasive procedures that aren't reasonable for extended periods can be used more freely in acute pain.

Treating chronic pain

Medical treatment for chronic pain must be based on the patient's long-term benefit, not just on the current complaint of pain. Drug therapy and surgery, which typically provide only partial and temporary relief, should be individualised.

Medication alone almost never effectively relieves chronic pain. The patient must receive a combination of treatments. These may include drugs, non-drug therapies, temporary or permanent invasive therapies (such as nerve blocks or surgery), cognitive-behavioural therapy, alternative and complementary therapies and self-management techniques.

It pains me to say this

Even with medical management, however, chronic pain can be lifelong. Therefore, treatments that carry significant risks or aren't likely to prove effective over the long term may be inappropriate.

Rehab rewards

In many cases, treatment of chronic pain must focus on rehabilitation rather than a cure. Rehabilitation aims to:
• maximise physical and psychological functional abilities
• minimise pain experienced during rehabilitation and for the rest of the patient's life
• teach the patient how to manage residual pain and handle pain exacerbation caused by increased activity or unexplained reasons.

Treating cancer pain

Whether pain results from cancer or its treatment, it may cause the patient to become more anxious, especially if they think the pain means their illness is progressing. They may then feel helpless and become depressed. However, most types of cancer pain can be managed effectively, improving their quality of life.

Go for the goal

The success of a pain management plan hinges on having the patient choose an appropriate goal—a pain intensity rating that will reduce their discomfort to a tolerable level and let them engage comfortably in self-care activities. Team members should work together to choose a rating scale for measuring the patient's pain intensity and to develop appropriate pain management goals.

Thorough documentation and pain assessment tools communicate vital patient information to all team members. If the patient has chronic pain, periodic team meetings also may be crucial.

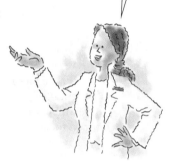

There's nothing cute about acute pain. Drug regimens and invasive procedures that aren't reasonable for extended periods can be used more freely in acute pain.

Pharmacological pain management

Pain management can be pharmacological or non-pharmacological. Pharmacological pain management includes non-opioid analgesics, opioids and adjuvant analgesics. In addition, non-pharmacological pain management can include alternative and complementary therapies.

Non-opioid analgesics

Non-opioid (non-narcotic) analgesics are used to treat pain that's nociceptive (caused by stimulation of injury-sensing receptors) or neuropathic (arising from nerves). These drugs are particularly effective against the somatic component of nociceptive pain such as joint and muscle pain. In addition to controlling pain, non-opioid analgesics reduce inflammation and fever.

Drug types in this category include:
- paracetamol
- non-steroidal anti-inflammatory drugs (NSAIDs)
- salicylates, such as aspirin.

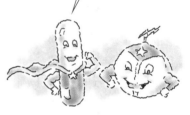

Additional analgesia and reduced risk of adverse effects.

Solo or combo

When used alone, paracetamol and NSAIDs provide relief from mild pain. NSAIDs can also relieve moderate pain; in high doses, they may help relieve severe pain. Given in combination with opioids, non-opioid analgesics provide additional analgesia, allowing a lower opioid dose and, thus, a lower risk of adverse effects.

Opioids

Opioids (narcotics) include derivatives of the opium (poppy) plant and synthetic drugs that imitate natural opioids. Unlike NSAIDs, which act peripherally, opioids produce their primary effects in the CNS. Opioids include opioid agonists, opioid antagonists and mixed agonist–antagonists.

Opioid agonists

Opioid agonists are used to treat moderate to severe pain without causing loss of consciousness. Opioid agonists include:
- codeine
- fentanyl
- methadone
- morphine (including sustained-release tablets and oral solution)
- oxycodone.

Opioid antagonists

Opioid antagonists aren't pain medications, but block the effects of opioid agonists. They're used to reverse adverse drug reactions, such as respiratory and CNS depression produced by opioid agonists. Unfortunately, by reversing analgesic effects, they may cause the patient's pain to recur.

Attached but not stimulating

Opioid antagonists attach to opiate receptors but don't stimulate them. As a result, they prevent other opioids, enkephalins and endorphins from producing their effects. Opioid antagonists include naloxone and naltrexone.

Mixed opioid agonist–antagonists

As their name implies, mixed opioid agonist–antagonists have agonist and antagonist properties. The agonist component relieves pain, while the antagonist component reduces the risk of toxicity and drug dependence. These agents also decrease the risk of respiratory depression and drug abuse. These agents include:
- buprenorphine
- pentazocine.

Potent potential

Originally, mixed agonist–antagonists seemed to have less addiction potential than pure opioid agonists as well as a lower risk of drug dependence.

Adjuvant analgesics

Adjuvant analgesics are drugs that have other primary indications but are used as analgesics in some circumstances. Adjuvants may be given in combination with opioids or used alone to treat chronic pain. Patients receiving adjuvant analgesics should be re-evaluated periodically to monitor their pain level and check for adverse reactions.

A real potpourri

Drugs used as adjuvant analgesics include certain anticonvulsants, local and topical anaesthetics, muscle relaxants, tricyclic antidepressants, serotonin 5-hydroxytryptamine agonists, selective serotonin re-uptake inhibitors, ergotamine alkaloids, benzodiazepines, psychostimulants, cholinergic blockers and corticosteroids.

Anticonvulsants

Anticonvulsants may be used to treat neuropathic pain (pain generated by peripheral nerves). These agents include:
- carbamazepine
- gabapentin
- phenytoin
- oxcarbazepine (unlicensed indication)
- amitriptyline (unlicensed indication).

  Carbamazepine and gabapentin are the anticonvulsants most commonly used as adjuvant analgesics.

Non-pharmacological pain management

Managing pain doesn't necessarily involve capsules, syringes, I.V. lines or medication pumps. Many non-pharmacological therapies are available too—and they're gaining popularity among the general public and health-care professionals alike.

What accounts for this trend? For one thing, many people are concerned about the overuse of drugs for conventional pain management. For another, some people simply prefer to self-manage their health problems.

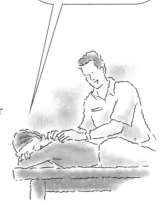

Non-pharmacologic approaches offer something for nearly everyone—from whirlpools to massage. Ahhh, I'm feeling better already!

Something for everyone

Collectively speaking, non-pharmacological approaches offer something for nearly everyone. They range from the relatively conventional (whirlpools, hot packs) to the electrifying (vibration, electrical nerve stimulation), sensual (aromatherapy, massage) and serene (meditation, yoga).

These therapies fall into three main categories:

 physical therapies

 alternative and complementary therapies

cognitive and behavioural therapies.

Many of these therapies can be used alone or combined with medication. A combination approach may improve pain relief by enhancing drug effects and allowing lower dosages.

Plenty of perks

Non-pharmacological approaches have other benefits in addition to pain management. For example they may help reduce stress, improve mood, promote sleep and give the patient a sense of control over pain.

More options

By understanding how these techniques work and how best to use them, you can provide additional options for patients who experience pain. Although the techniques discussed in this chapter can be effective for a wide range of patients, they should be administered by registered practitioners or experienced, credentialed lay people who are required to belong to either the Allied Health Proffesions Federation (AHPF) or the Federation of Holistic Therapists (FHT). Some require a doctor's referral.

Physical therapies

Physical therapies use physical agents and methods to aid rehabilitation and restore normal functioning after an illness or injury. With appropriate teaching, patients and their families can use them on their own, which helps them participate in pain management.

Physical therapies include:

- hydrotherapy
- heat
- cold
- massage
- transcutaneous electrical nerve stimulation (TENS).

Therapeutic goals

In addition to easing pain, physical therapies reduce inflammation, ease muscle spasms and promote relaxation. The goals of physical therapies are to:

- promote health
- prevent physical disability
- rehabilitate patients disabled by pain, disease or injury.

Hydrotherapy

Hydrotherapy uses water to treat pain and disease. Sometimes called the ultimate natural pain reliever, water comforts and soothes while providing support and buoyancy. Depending on the patient's problem, the water can be hot or cold, and liquid, solid (ice) or steam. It can be applied externally or internally.

Most commonly prescribed for burns, hydrotherapy relaxes muscles, raises or lowers tissue temperature (depending on water temperature), and eases joint stiffness (as in rheumatoid arthritis or osteoarthritis). In pain management, hydrotherapy is most commonly used to treat acute pain—for instance from muscle sprains or strains.

Jet set

Whirlpool baths—bathtubs with jets that force water to circulate—aid in rehabilitating injured muscles and joints. Depending on the desired effect, the water can be hot or cold. The water jets act to massage soothing muscles.

Whirlpools and certain other hydrotherapy treatments can be done at home. However, the more intensive forms are best done in a supervised clinical setting where the treatment and the patient's response can be monitored.

I don't need a medical book to tell me that baths are therapeutic!

Secrets revealed

Hydrotherapy's pain-relieving properties are related to the physics and mechanics of water and its effect on the human body. When a body is immersed in water, the resulting weightlessness reduces stress on joints, muscles and other connective tissues. This buoyancy may relieve some types of pain instantly.

Hot-water hydrotherapy eases pain through a sequence of events triggered by increased skin temperature. As skin temperature rises, blood vessels widen and skin circulation increases. As resistance to blood flow through veins and capillaries drops, blood pressure decreases. The heart rate then rises to maintain blood pressure. The result is a significant drop in pain and greater comfort.

Some restrictions apply

As with any treatment, be aware of these potential hazards of hydrotherapy. Below are a few measures to avoid these:
• Hydrotherapy may cause burns, falls or light-headedness, dizziness or faintness then stop the treatment session.
• Don't keep the patient in a heated whirlpool for more than 20 minutes.
• Know that hydrotherapy isn't recommended for pregnant women, children, elderly patients, or patients with diabetes, hypertension, hypotension or multiple sclerosis.

Heat

Heat is used to decrease pain, relieve stiff joints, ease muscle aches and spasms, improve circulation and increase the pain threshold. Heat can be applied with packs, paraffin wax or an electric heating pad. Moist heat can be applied with a hot pack, a warm compress or a special heating pad. Dry and moist heat involves conductive heating—heat transfer that occurs when the skin directly contacts a warm object.

What's the use?

Heat is used to treat pain caused by:
• headache
• muscle aches and spasms
• earache
• menstrual cramps
• temporomandibular joint disease
• fibromyalgia (syndrome of chronic pain in the muscles and soft tissues surrounding joints).
Heat enhances blood flow, increases tissue metabolism and decreases vasomotor tone. It produces analgesia by suppressing free nerve endings. It also may reduce the perception of pain in the cerebral cortex.

Regional heating, heat therapy of selected body areas, can bring immediate temporary pain relief. This method may have a systemic effect, too, resulting from autonomic reflex responses to localised heat application. The reflex-mediated responses may raise body temperature, enhance blood flow and cause other physiologic changes in areas distant from the heat application site.

Heat effects

Before administering heat, take these considerations into account:
• Determine the patient's awareness level and ability to communicate their response to the treatment.
• Follow manufacturers' instructions for the device.
• Be aware that some patients may prefer a slightly lower (or higher) temperature. Keep the heating agent at a temperature that's comfortable for the patient.
• Wrap the heating agent so it doesn't directly contact the patient's skin.
• Regularly assess skin at the heat application site for irritation and redness.
• Frequently evaluate the patient's response to treatment and their pain level.
• Stop the treatment if the patient's pain increases.
• Don't apply heat to an area that's infected, bleeding or receiving radiation therapy or where oil or menthol has been applied.
• Know that heat is contraindicated in patients with vascular insufficiency, neuropathy, skin desensitisation or neoplasms.

Cold

Applying an ice pack to a specific body area can reduce fever, and this technique can also provide immediate pain relief and help reduce or prevent oedema and swelling. Methods include cold packs and ice bags. The cold blocks the nerve fibre activity causing numbness reducing the stimulation in the CNS.

Hot and cold

Another technique, known as contrast therapy, involves cold and heat application being applied alternately during the same session. Contrast therapy may benefit patients with rheumatoid arthritis and certain other conditions.

Freezing out pain

Cold is commonly used for acute pain—especially when caused by a sports injury (such as a muscle sprain). It may also be indicated for pain resulting from:
• acute trauma
• joint disorders such as rheumatoid arthritis
• headache such as migraine
• muscle aches and spasms
• incisions
• surgery.

Constrict and reduce

Cold constricts blood vessels at the injury site, reducing blood flow to the site. This, in turn, thickens the blood, resulting in decreased bleeding and increased blood clotting.

Applying cold to a muscle sprain

Ice packs help reduce pain and oedema when used during the first 24 to 72 hours after an injury. For best results, follow these guidelines.

Method and materials

- Apply cold to the painful area four times daily for 20 to 30 minutes each time.
- Use enough crushed ice to cover the area.
- Place the ice in a plastic bag, and place the bag inside a pillowcase or a large piece of cloth, as shown here. Then apply the bag over the painful area for the specified treatment time.

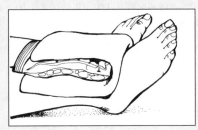

Switch over!

- After 24 to 72 hours, when swelling has subsided or when cold can no longer help, switch to heat therapy.

Wise words

- Inform the patient that ice eases pain in a joint that has begun to stiffen—but caution them not to let the analgesic effect lull them into overusing the joint.

Cold application also slows oedema development, prevents further tissue damage and minimises bruising.

Cooler endings

Cold also decreases sensitivity to pain by cooling nerve endings. It eases muscle spasms by cooling muscle spindles—the part of the muscle tissue responsible for the stretch reflex. (See *Applying cold to a muscle sprain*.) Contrast therapy is thought to stimulate endocrine function, reduce inflammation, decrease congestion and improve organ function.

Remember this

When administering ice packs, remember these points:
- As appropriate, encourage your patient to try cold application. Many patients aren't aware that cold relieves pain.
- Before applying cold, assess the pain or injury site and the patient's pain level. Assess them for impaired circulation (such as from Raynaud's disease), inability to sense temperature (as from neuropathy), extreme skin sensitivity and inability to report the response to treatment (for instance a young child or a confused elderly patient).
- If the patient has a cognitive impairment, measure the temperature of the cooling agent. It should be no colder than 15°C.
- Wrap cold packs so they don't directly contact the patient's skin. Keep them at a comfortable temperature.
- Stop the treatment if the patient's skin becomes numb.
- Use caution when applying ice to the elbow, wrist or outer part of the knee. These sites are more susceptible to cold-induced nerve injury.
- Be aware that re-freezable gel packs and chemical packs may be colder than ice. Also, they may leak.

Explaining the benefits of using ice packs to a patient may be a bit more of a challenge. I can understand why! Brrrrr…

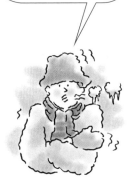

• Regularly assess the patient for adverse effects, such as skin irritation, joint stiffness, numbness, frostbite and nerve injury.
• Don't apply cold to areas that have poor circulation or have received radiation.

TENS

In TENS therapy, a portable, battery-powered device transmits painless alternating electric current to peripheral nerves or directly to a painful area. Used post-operatively and for patients with chronic pain, TENS reduces the need for analgesic drugs and helps the patient resume normal activities.

Belt it on

The patient usually wears the TENS unit on a belt. Units have several channels and lead placements. The settings allow adjustment of wave frequency, duration and intensity.

Typically, a course of TENS therapy lasts 3 to 5 days. Some conditions (such as phantom limb pain) may require continuous simulation. Others, such as a painful arthritic joint, call for shorter treatment periods—perhaps 3 to 4 hours.

Top TENS list

TENS can provide temporary relief of acute pain (such as post-operative pain) and ongoing relief of chronic pain (such as in sciatica). Specific pain problems that have responded to TENS include:
• chronic pain
• cancer pain
• bone fracture pain
• low back pain
• sports injuries
• myofascial pain
• neurogenic pain (as in neuralgia and neuropathy)
• phantom limb pain
• arthritis
• menstrual pain.

Still a mystery

Although TENS has existed for about 30 years, experts still aren't sure exactly how it relieves pain. Some believe that it works according to the gate-control theory, which proposes that painful impulses pass through a 'gate' in the brain. According to this theory, TENS alters the patient's perception of pain by closing the gate to painful stimuli. More research is needed in this area.

TENS to-do list

Consider these points when administering TENS therapy:
• To ensure that your patient is a willing and active participant in TENS therapy, provide complete instructions on using and caring for the TENS unit as well as expected results of treatment.
• Before TENS therapy begins, assess the patient's pain level and evaluate for skin irritation at the sites where electrodes will be placed.
• Don't use TENS if the patient has undiagnosed pain, uses a pacemaker, or has a history of heart arrhythmias.
• Don't apply a TENS unit over the carotid sinus, an open wound or anesthetised skin.
• Don't place the unit on the head or neck of a patient who has a vascular disorder or seizure disorder.

Massage

Massage is a relaxing experience using the unspoken communication based on touch. It can be used for relaxation, psychological or physical reasons. Massage involves kneading, stroking, rolling, warming and pressing of the skin and muscles thus reducing muscle tension, thereby easing muscle spasm. Different types of massage are available depending upon the effect that is wanted such as relaxation or to improve a physical condition. Massage increases blood and lymph circulation and can encourage the production of endorphins and can reduce pain and create a feeling of well-being.

Alternative and complementary therapies

Alternative and complementary therapies greatly expand the range of therapeutic choices for patients suffering pain. Today, patients are increasingly seeking these therapies—not just to treat pain but also to address many other common health conditions. Various theories have been offered to explain the increased interest in alternative and complementary therapies. (See *Understanding the alternative trend*, page 412.)

Wholly holistic

Regardless of the problem for which they're used, alternative and complementary therapies address the whole person—body, mind and spirit—rather than just signs and symptoms.

Defining the terms

Although alternative and complementary therapies are usually discussed together, they aren't exactly the same:
• Alternative therapies are those used instead of conventional or mainstream therapies—for example the use of acupuncture rather than analgesics to relieve pain.

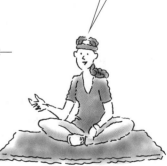

Alternative and complementary therapies address the whole person, rather than just symptoms…and who doesn't want to be treated like a person?!

Understanding the alternative trend

Why are more people turning to alternative and complementary therapies to treat health problems? One reason is that most therapies are non-invasive and cause few adverse reactions.

People with certain chronic conditions may be drawn to these therapies because conventional medicine has few, if any, effective treatments for them. Also, people are encouraged by reports that document their effectiveness.

Holistic

Conventional medicine tends to treat only signs and symptoms, whereas alternative and complementary therapies focus on the whole person, thus holism.

Time—the healer?

Many people also value the extra time alternative practitioners spend with the patient and the attention they pay to the patient's temperament, behavioural patterns and perceived needs. In an increasingly stressful world, people are searching for someone who will take the time to listen to them and treat them as people, not just bodies displaying signs and symptoms.

Spiritual hunger

Some people view modern society as spiritually malnourished and hungry for meaning. Alternative practitioners seem to be more responsive to this need.

Cultural connections

Lastly, in a culturally diverse country, such as the United Kingdom, a wide variety of traditional healing practices and beliefs exist. Some are based on the same principles that underlie alternative and complementary therapies.

• Complementary therapies are those used in conjunction with conventional therapies—such as meditation used as an adjunct to analgesic drugs.

East meets West

Some of the alternative and complementary therapies practiced today have been used since ancient times and come from the traditional healing practices of many cultures, particularly in the Eastern part of the world.

Many mainstream Western doctors have become more open-minded about these therapies. In fact, some medical doctors even administer them. However, others still object to them on the grounds that they aren't based solely on empirical science.

Pain relief prospects

Nonetheless, alternative and complementary therapies commonly relieve some types of pain that don't respond to Western techniques. They may prove especially valuable when a precise cause evades Western medicine, as typically occurs in chronic low back pain.

Cognitive and behavioural approaches

Cognitive approaches to pain management focus on influencing the patient's interpretation of the pain experience. Behavioural approaches help the patient develop skills for managing pain and changing their reaction to it.

Cognitive and behavioural approaches to managing pain include meditation, biofeedback and hypnosis. These techniques improve the patient's sense of control over pain and allow them to participate actively in pain management.

Meditation

Meditation is thought to relieve stress and reduce pain through an effect called the relaxation response, a natural protective mechanism against overstress. Learning to activate the relaxation response through meditation may offset some of the negative physiologic effects of stress.

Biofeedback

Biofeedback uses electronic monitors to teach patients how to exert conscious control over autonomic functions. By watching the fluctuations of various body functions on a monitor, patients learn how to change a particular body function by adjusting thoughts, breathing pattern, posture or muscle tension.

As they modify vital functions, patients may develop the ability to control pain without using conventional treatments.

Hypnosis

Hypnosis harnesses the power of suggestion and altered levels of consciousness to produce positive behaviour changes and treat various conditions. Under hypnosis, a patient typically relaxes and experiences changes in respiration, which may lead to a positive shift in behaviour and a greater sense of well-being.

Quick quiz

1. Which pain medication is an opioid agonist?
   A. Carbamazepine
   B. Butorphanol
   C. Fentanyl
   D. Buprenorphine

Answer: C. Fentanyl is an opioid agonist; all the other medications are mixed opioid agonist–antagonists.

2. Applying heat causes which effect?
   A. Vasodilation
   B. Paresthesia
   C. Vasoconstriction
   D. Vasocompression

Answer: A. Heat causes vasodilation, which enhances blood flow to the affected area.

3. Massage promotes increased circulation and softening of connective tissues. It also has which effect?
   A. Narrows blood vessels
   B. Eases muscle spasms
   C. Causes hyperventilation
   D. Widens blood vessels

Answer: B. Massage decreases muscle tension, thereby easing muscle spasms.

Scoring

☆☆☆ If you answered all three questions correctly, wow! You must be feelin' great!

☆☆ If you answered two questions correctly, good job! You sure don't have any opioids clouding your brain.

☆ If you answered fewer than two questions correctly, feel no pain! Review the chapter and try again.

(18) Nutrition

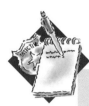

Just the facts

In this chapter, you'll learn:

♦ role nutrients play in health promotion

♦ ways to differentiate between good nutrition and poor nutrition

♦ about applying policies, initiatives and guidelines

♦ purpose of digestion and absorption

♦ structures of the GI tract wall, digestive organs, and accessory organs as well as their functions in digestion and absorption

♦ ways to promote proper diet.

A look at nutrition

Nutrition refers to the processes by which a living organism ingests, digests, absorbs, transports, uses and excretes *nutrients* (food and other nourishing material). Nutrition as a clinical area is primarily concerned with the properties of food that build sound bodies and promote health.

More than just a pretty process

Because good nutrition is essential to good health and disease prevention, any person involved in health care needs a thorough knowledge of nutrition and the body's nutritional requirements throughout the life span. What's more, the study of nutrition must focus on health promotion.

> Understanding and practising good nutrition can make you and your patients healthier throughout your life spans!

Nutrients

There are two types of nutrients:

Non-essential nutrients are nutrients that aren't needed in the diet because they're manufactured by the body.

Essential nutrients are nutrients that must be acquired through food because the body can't produce them on its own in adequate quantities.

Certain and essential

For nutrition to be adequate, a person must receive certain essential nutrients—carbohydrates, fats, proteins, vitamins, minerals and water. These nutrients must be present for proper growth and functioning. In addition, the digestive system must function properly to make use of these nutrients.

No lone nutrients

Each nutrient has several specific metabolic functions, but no nutrient works alone. Close metabolic relationships exist among all of the basic nutrients as well as among their metabolic products.

Nutrient breakdown dance

Nutrients can be used by the body for its immediate needs, or they can be stored for later use. The body breaks down nutrients into simpler compounds for absorption in the stomach and intestines in two ways:

mechanical breakdown, which begins in the GI tract with chewing

chemical breakdown, which starts with salivary enzymes in the mouth and continues with acid and enzyme action through the rest of the GI tract.

Role of a lifeline

Nutrients play a vital role in maintaining health and wellness. They have several important functions:
• providing energy, which can be stored in the body or transformed for vital activities
• building and maintaining body tissue
• controlling metabolic processes, such as growth, cell activity, enzyme production and temperature regulation.

Metabolism

Regulated mostly by hormones, metabolism is a combination of several processes by which energy is extracted from certain nutrients (carbohydrates, proteins and fats) and then used by the body. Vitamins and minerals don't directly provide us with energy, but they're an important part of the metabolic process. Metabolism can be broken down into two parts:

Catabolism is the breakdown of complex substances into simpler ones, resulting in the release of energy.

Anabolism is the synthesis of simple substances into more complex substances. This process provides the energy necessary for tissue growth, maintenance and repair.

Energy

Energy, in the form of adenosine triphosphate, is produced as a by-product of carbohydrate, fat and protein metabolism. The amount of energy in food products is measured in kilocalories (kcal), which are commonly referred to as *calories*.

Through the processes of digestion and absorption, energy is released from food into the body. Small amounts of energy are stored within cells for immediate use. Larger amounts of energy are stored in glycogen and fat tissue to fuel long-duration activities.

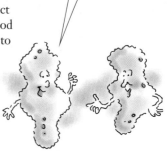

Metabolism, regulated mostly by hormones like us, is a combination of several processes by which energy is extracted from certain nutrients and then used by the body.

Balancing act

In a healthy adult, the rate of anabolism equals the rate of catabolism, and energy balance is obtained. In other words, energy balance occurs when the caloric intake from food equals the number of calories expended. These calories may be used for voluntary activities (such as physical activity) or involuntary activities (such as basal metabolism).

Nutrition and health promotion

Many patients may consider themselves healthy because they don't feel sick. However, you must be concerned about a more holistic meaning of the term *health*, one that incorporates aspects of the patient's internal and external environments, in order to best care for your patients.

For you, health promotion must consider all of a patient's needs, including physical, emotional, mental and social needs. Only when these needs are met can it be said that a person is healthy, or well. Furthermore, wellness implies a state of balance between a person's activities and goals. Maintaining this balance allows the patient to maintain their vitality and ability to function productively in society. A nutritious diet provides the basis for health promotion and disease prevention, making it an important part of caring for any patient.

Health policies, initiatives, recommendations and guidelines all have an influence upon patients' nutritional status and the provision of nutritious meals. *The Essence of Care* (DH, 2001) has a nutrition section, which includes benchmarks for good practice, along with core standards in *Standards for Better Health* (DH, 2004). The Nursing and Midwifery Council (2007) identify skills relating to nutrition and fluid management which students must develop at different stages of their pre-registration programme. Many of these skills are covered in this chapter, such as assisting patients to eat and drink, taking part in the nutritional screening of patients, providing an environment conducive to eating and drinking and participating in the provision of alternative nutrition when a patient is unable to take food orally.

Nutrition and a balanced diet

You're part of a health-care team that's responsible for making sure the patient maintains optimal nutritional health, even though they may be battling illness or recovering from surgery. It's also your job to stress to the patient the importance of good nutrition in maintaining health and recovering from illness, so that they can continue sound nutritional practices when they're no longer in your care.

Nutritional status

You must use your knowledge of nutrition to promote health through education and of sick and healthy patients. This includes encouraging patients to consume appropriate types and amounts of food. It also means considering poor food habits as a contributing factor in a patient with chronic illness. Therefore, assessing nutritional status and identifying nutritional needs to meet the requirements of a balanced diet are primary activities in planning patient care. Within The NHS Institute for Innovation and Improvement (2007) *Releasing Time to Care: The Productive Ward*, there is a module titled '*Meals*' which 'gives guidance on how to ensure the best experience for patients while making the delivery quick and easy for staff. This results in less wasted time in meal delivery and re-investing it to make sure patients get the correct nutritional assessment and staff have time to feed patients who require support'.

Assessing nutritional status

A patient's nutritional status can influence the body's response to illness and treatment. Regardless of your patient's overall condition, an evaluation of their nutritional health is an essential part of your assessment. Assessment of the patient's nutritional status includes determining nutritional risk factors as well as individual needs.

The NICE (2006) issued clinical guidelines to help identify patients who are malnourished or at risk of malnutrition. The guidelines recommend that on admission to hospital or a first visit to outpatients, all patients should be screened for malnourishment or at risk of malnutrition. These patients should be weighed, measured and have their body mass index (BMI)

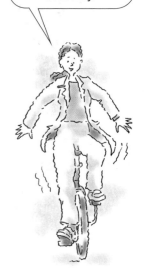

Wellness implies a state of balance between a person's activities and goals. Maintaining this balance allows the patient to maintain his vitality and ability to function productively in society.

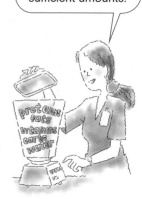

Optimal nutrition requires a varied diet of carbs, proteins, fats, vitamins, minerals, water and fibre in sufficient amounts.

calculated. This screening should then be repeated weekly and there should be a process to follow if the patient is assessed as being at risk of malnutrition or as being malnourished.

Calculating a patient's BMI forms an important part of the assessment in a range of nutritional screening tools. The British Association for Parenteral and Enteral Nutrition (BAPEN) and its Malnutrition Advisory Group (MAG) developed the 'Malnutrition Universal Screening Tool' (MUST), which is used in some clinical areas. For further information on 'MUST', see www.bapen.org.uk.

Good nutrition

Good nutrition, or *optimal nutrition*, is essential in promoting health, preventing illness and restoring health after an injury or illness. To achieve optimal nutrition, a person must eat a varied diet containing carbohydrates, proteins, fats, vitamins, minerals, water and fibre in sufficient amounts. Although excesses of certain nutrients can be detrimental to a patient's health, intake of essential nutrients should be greater than minimum requirements to allow for variations in health and disease and to provide stores for later use.

Poor nutrition

Poor nutrition, or *malnutrition*, is a state of inadequate or excess nutritional intake. It's most common among people living in poverty, especially those with greater nutritional requirements, such as elderly people, pregnant women, children and infants. It also occurs in hospitals and long-term care, because the patients in these situations have illnesses that place added stress on their bodies, raising nutritional requirements. A publication by Age Concern (2006), *Hungry to be heard: The scandal of malnourished older people in hospital*, provides case studies of patients' nutritional requirements not being met. The publication identifies seven steps that can be implemented, such as protected mealtimes, where non-urgent clinical activity ceases so that patients can eat their meal or be assisted to eat without being interrupted; patients then eat more improving their nutritional status. Another step is the introduction of the 'red tray' system, which helps alert staff to the patients that require assistance with eating.

Don't underestimate undernourishment

Undernutrition occurs when a patient consumes fewer daily nutrients than their body requires, resulting in a nutritional deficit. Typically, an undernourished patient is at greater risk for physical illnesses. They may also suffer from limitations in cognitive and physical status.

Undernutrition can result from:
- inability to metabolise nutrients
- inability to obtain the appropriate nutrients from food
- accelerated excretion of nutrients from the body
- illness or disease that increases the body's need for nutrients.

Don't overdo it

In contrast, overnutrition occurs when a patient consumes an excessive amount of nutrients. For example, overnutrition may occur in patients who self-prescribe megadoses of vitamins and mineral supplements and in those who overeat. These practices can result in damage to body tissue or obesity.

Nutrient standards

To maintain healthy populations, most developed countries have established nutrition standards for major nutrients. These standards serve as guidelines for nutrient intake based on the nutritional needs of most healthy population groups.

Other standards

In impoverished countries, where quality of food and nutrition are lacking, standards are set by the Food and Agriculture Organization and the World Health Organization. No matter who sets forth the standards, the goal is the same: to promote good health and prevent disease through sound nutrition.

Dietary guidelines

The Government's prevention strategy to reduce early deaths from cancer and coronary heart disease is to improve the nation's diet and nutrition. Diet and nutrition are key areas highlighted in The NHS Plan, National Service Frameworks for Coronary Heart Disease, the National Service Frameworks for Coronary Heart Disease and Diabetes and Older People, aiming to reduce fat, sugar and salt content in our diet and increase the amount of fruit and vegetable eaten. The government led programme '5 A DAY' recommends that everyone should aim to eat at least 5 portions of fruit or vegetables daily, in an attempt to reduce the risk of certain cancers, heart disease and other chronic conditions. Local Education Authority (LEA)-maintained schools are now involved in offering a free piece of fruit or vegetable each day to all 4- to 6-year-olds. Resources are available to help educate those groups of people with the lowest intakes of fruit and vegetables.

A look at digestion and absorption

The basic purpose of digestion and absorption is to deliver essential nutrients to the cells in order to sustain life. To break food down into these essential nutrients, the body sends it through various mechanical and chemical processes in the GI tract, or *alimentary canal*. Successful digestion and absorption depend on the coordinated function of the GI tract wall's muscles and nerves, the GI tract organs and the accessory organs of digestion. (See *Structures of the GI system*.)

Structures of the GI system

The GI system includes the alimentary canal (pharynx, oesophagus, stomach, and small and large intestines) and the accessory organs (liver, biliary duct system and pancreas).

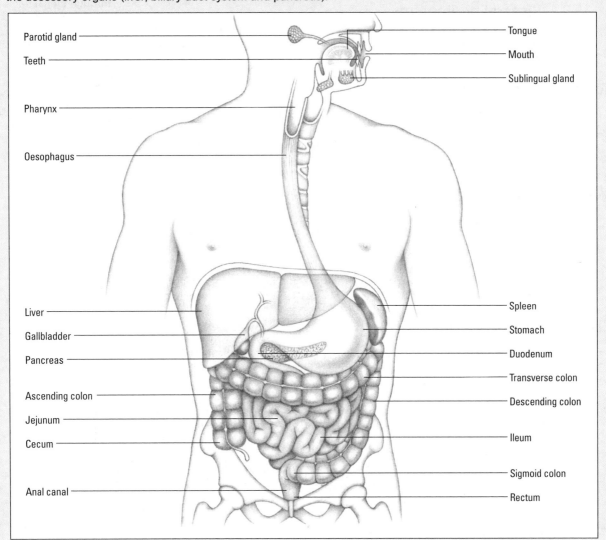

Parotid gland

Teeth

Pharynx

Oesophagus

Liver

Gallbladder

Pancreas

Ascending colon

Jejunum

Cecum

Anal canal

Tongue

Mouth

Sublingual gland

Spleen

Stomach

Duodenum

Transverse colon

Descending colon

Ileum

Sigmoid colon

Rectum

GI tract wall structures

The wall of the GI tract consists of four major layers:

 visceral peritoneum

 tunica muscularis

submucosa

 mucosa.

Visceral peritoneum

The *visceral peritoneum* is the GI tract's outer covering. It covers most of the abdominal organs and lies next to an identical layer, the *parietal peritoneum*, which lines the abdominal cavity.

To serve and protect

The main job of this outer layer of the GI tract wall is to protect the blood vessels, nerves and lymphatics. It also attaches the jejunum, ileum and transverse colon to the posterior abdominal wall to prevent twisting.

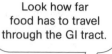

Look how far food has to travel through the GI tract.

Many names, one layer

The visceral peritoneum has many names. In the oesophagus and rectum, it's called the *tunica adventitia*. Elsewhere, in the GI tract, it's called the *tunica serosa*.

Tunica muscularis

The *tunica muscularis*, which lies within the visceral peritoneum, is a layer composed of skeletal muscle in the mouth, pharynx and upper oesophagus.

Elsewhere in the tract…

The tunica muscularis is made up of longitudinal and circular smooth-muscle fibres. At points along the tract, the circular fibres thicken to form sphincters.

Pucker pouches

In the large intestine, these fibres gather into three narrow bands (*taeniae coli*) down the middle of the colon and pucker the intestine into characteristic pouches (*haustra*).

Between the two muscle layers lies a nerve network—the *myenteric plexus*, also known as *Auerbach's plexus*. The stomach wall contains a third muscle layer made up of oblique fibres.

Submucosa

The *submucosa*, also called the *tunica submucosa*, lies under the tunica muscularis. It's composed of loose connective tissue, blood and lymphatic vessels and another nerve network called the *submucosal plexus*, or *Meissner's plexus*.

Mucosa

The *mucosa*, the innermost layer of the GI tract wall, is also called the *tunica mucosa*. This layer consists of epithelial and surface cells and loose connective tissue. Villi, from surface cells, secrete gastric and protective juices and absorb nutrients.

GI tract wall functions

The nerves and muscles of the GI tract wall work jointly to ensure that food moves spontaneously through the digestive system (motility). GI tract functions include innervation and secretion.

GI tract innervation

Distention of the submucosal plexus in the submucosa or myenteric plexus in the tunica muscularis stimulates transmission of nerve signals to the smooth muscle, which initiates contraction and relaxation of these muscles, called *peristalsis*. During peristalsis, longitudinal fibres of the tunica muscularis shorten the lumen length and circular fibres reduce the lumen diameter.

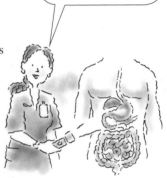

> Look how far food has to travel through the GI tract.

GI tract secretion

Five major substances secreted by the GI tract contribute to the chemical process of digestion:

Mucus protects the lining of the GI tract and aids in motility.

Enzymes are proteins that break down nutrients.

Acid and various buffer ions contribute to the level of alkalinity or acidity (pH) needed to activate digestive enzymes.

Electrolytes and water carry nutrients through the GI tract and aid in the absorption process.

Bile emulsifies fat to promote intestinal absorption of fatty acids, cholesterol and other lipids.

How digestion and absorption work

The organs of the GI tract play the major role in mechanical and chemical digestion and absorption of food and fluid. (See *Functions of the digestive system organs*.) Aided by the GI tract wall and accessory organs, the organs of the GI tract process nutrients in three phases of digestion:

cephalic

gastric

intestinal.

Functions of the digestive system organs

This chart lists the digestive system organs and their primary functions.

Organ	Function
Mouth	• breaks down food into smaller particles • releases saliva to promote chewing and swallowing • secretes amylase (ptyalin)
Oesophagus	• propels food downward into the stomach
Stomach	• acts as a food reservoir • mixes food with gastric secretions (hydrochloric acid, pepsin, mucus, intrinsic factor) • begins protein digestion • absorbs water, alcohol and some drugs
Liver	• produces bile • metabolises carbohydrates, protein and fat • stores nutrients • detoxifies drugs and waste products
Gall bladder	• concentrates and stores bile • releases bile into the duodenum
Pancreas	• produces and secretes insulin and glucagon • produces and secretes digestive enzymes: proteases, lipase and amylase
Small intestine	• secretes hormones to stimulate the secretion of pancreatic juices, bile and intestinal enzymes • secretes digestive enzymes: peptidases, disaccharidases • absorbs iron, magnesium, and calcium (duodenum) • absorbs water-soluble vitamins and simple sugars (jejunum) • absorbs amino acids, peptides, fat-soluble vitamins, fats, cholesterol, bile salts and vitamin B_{12} (ileum)
Large intestine	• absorbs water, sodium, potassium and vitamin K formed by colonic bacteria • eliminates solid waste

Cephalic phase

The cephalic phase of digestion uses the GI tract organs of the mouth, pharynx and oesophagus to begin the mechanical processes of digestion. Mechanical digestion breaks down food into smaller particles, which increases the surface area on which digestive enzymes can work.

Mouth

Digestion begins in the mouth (also called the *buccal cavity* or *oral cavity*). Ducts connect the mouth with the three major pairs of salivary glands:
* parotid
* sub-mandibular
* sub-lingual.

These glands secrete the enzyme *ptyalin* (a salivary amylase) to moisten food during chewing (mastication) and begin breaking down starch into maltose. (See *Causes of dry mouth in older adults*.)

Pharynx

The *pharynx* is a cavity extending from the base of the skull to the oesophagus. The pharynx aids swallowing by grasping food and propelling it towards the oesophagus.

Oesophagus

A muscular tube, the oesophagus extends from the pharynx through the mediastinum to the stomach.

Down the hatch

When a person swallows, the cricopharyngeal sphincter in the upper oesophagus relaxes, allowing food to enter. In the oesophagus, the glossopharyngeal nerve activates peristalsis, which moves the food bolus down towards the stomach.

One slippery bolus

As food passes through the oesophagus, glands in the oesophageal mucosal layer secrete mucus, which lubricates the bolus and protects the mucosal membrane from damage caused by poorly chewed foods.

Stomach express

Because food is in the mouth only for a short time, digestion of starch is limited. The salivary amylase that's swallowed continues to work for another 15 to 30 minutes in the stomach before it's inactivated by gastric acids. By the time the food bolus is travelling towards the stomach, the stomach has begun secreting digestive juices (hydrochloric acid [HCl] and pepsin).

Gastric phase

When food enters the stomach, the gastric phase of digestion begins. (See *Sites and mechanisms of gastric secretion*, page 426.)

Ages and stages

Causes of dry mouth in older adults

As people age, salivation decreases, leading to dry mouth and a reduced sense of taste. Certain drugs, such as anticholinergics, antihistamines, tricyclic antidepressants, phenothiazines, clonidine and opioid analgesics, can also decrease salivation. Be sure to take a drug history for older adults. Other causes of dry mouth in older adults include facial nerve paralysis, salivary duct obstruction, Sjögren's syndrome and radiation of the mouth or face.

Sites and mechanisms of gastric secretion

The body of the stomach lies between the lower oesophageal, or *cardiac*, sphincter and the pyloric sphincter. Between these sphincters lie the fundus, body, antrum and pylorus. These areas have a rich variety of mucosal cells that help the stomach carry out its tasks.

Glands and gastric secretions

Cardiac glands, pyloric glands and gastric glands secrete 2 to 3 L of gastric juice daily through the stomach's gastric pits.

- The *cardiac gland* (near the lower oesophageal sphincter [LES]) and the *pyloric gland* (near the pylorus) secrete thin mucus.
- The *gastric gland* (in the body and fundus) secretes HCl, pepsinogen, intrinsic factor and mucus.

Protection from self-digestion

Specialised cells line the gastric glands, gastric pits and surface epithelium. Mucous cells in the necks of the gastric glands produce thin mucus. Mucous cells in the surface epithelium produce an alkaline mucus. Both substances lubricate food and protect the stomach from self-digestion by corrosive enzymes.

Other secretions

Argentaffin cells produce gastrin, which stimulates gastric secretion and motility. *Chief cells* produce pepsinogen, which breaks proteins down into polypeptides.

Large parietal cells scattered throughout the fundus secrete HCl and intrinsic factor. HCl degrades pepsinogen, maintains an acid environment, and inhibits excess bacteria growth. Intrinsic factor promotes vitamin B_{12} absorption in the small intestine.

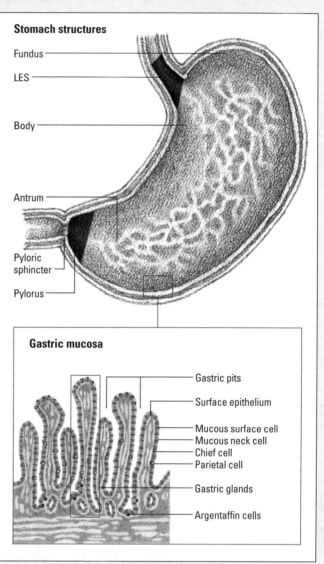

Stomach structures

Fundus
LES
Body
Antrum
Pyloric sphincter
Pylorus

Gastric mucosa

Gastric pits
Surface epithelium
Mucous surface cell
Mucous neck cell
Chief cell
Parietal cell
Gastric glands
Argentaffin cells

Stomach

Chemical digestion, which occurs as food mixes with digestive enzymes, begins in the stomach. The stomach acts, in part, as a temporary storage area for food and has four main regions:

 cardia

 fundus

body

 antrum.

Cardia

The *cardia* lies near the junction of the stomach and oesophagus. Relaxation of the cardiac sphincter in this region allows food to pass from the oesophagus to the stomach.

Fundus

The *fundus* is an enlarged portion above and to the left of the oesophageal opening into the stomach. Continued peristaltic activity in this region propels the intact food bolus towards the stomach body.

Body

The *body* is the middle portion of the stomach. In this region, distention of the stomach wall due to the food bolus stimulates secretion of gastrin.

Gassing up with gastrin

Gastrin, in turn, stimulates the stomach's motor functions and release of digestive secretions by the gastric glands. Highly acidic (pH of 0.9 to 1.5), these secretions consist mainly of HCl, intrinsic factor (which helps the body absorb vitamin B_{12}) and proteolytic enzymes (which help the body use proteins). (See *GI system changes in older adults*, page 428.)

HCl helps absorb calcium and iron and activates gastric enzymes that kill most food-borne bacteria. HCl is also needed to convert the enzyme pepsinogen into pepsin.

Enzyme with pep

Pepsin becomes the major protein-splitting enzyme and, in turn, activates the secretion of the gastric mucus that protects the gastric lining. The mucus also helps move the food bolus along the path to the small intestine.

Not much at all but alcohol

Normally, except for alcohol, little food absorption occurs in the stomach. Peristaltic contractions in the stomach body churn the food into tiny particles and mix it with gastric juices, forming chyme.

Antrum

The *antrum* is the lower portion of the stomach, lying near the junction of the stomach and duodenum. Stronger peristaltic waves move the chyme from the stomach body into the antrum. Here, the chyme backs up against the pyloric sphincter before being released into the small intestine and triggering the intestinal phase of digestion. (See *Stomach emptying*, page 428.)

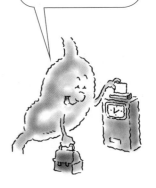

I punch the clock for chemical digestion. Yep, it all starts with me!

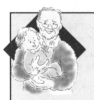

Ages and stages

GI system changes in older adults

Age-related changes in the GI system can lead to conditions that impact nutrition. Reduced gastric acid secretion in older adults can result in pernicious anaemia, iron-deficiency anaemia and reduced calcium absorption. Reduced production of bile acid, enlargement of the common bile duct and increased output of cholecystokinin can lead to biliary stasis, cholelithiasis and reduced appetite.

Intestinal phase

Most absorption occurs during the intestinal phase of digestion, which involves the small and large intestines.

Small intestine

The longest organ of the GI tract, the *small intestine* is a tube measuring about 6.1 m long. It performs most of the work of digestion and absorption. (See *Digestion and absorption in the small intestine*.)

The small intestine has three major divisions:

The duodenum is the longest and most superior division.

The *jejunum*, the middle portion, is the shortest segment.

The *ileum* is the most inferior portion.

Break it down, please

In the small intestine, intestinal wall contractions and digestive enzymes break down carbohydrates, proteins and fats so the intestinal mucosa can facilitate absorption of these nutrients into the bloodstream (along with water and electrolytes). These nutrients are then available for use by the body.

The great intestinal wall

The intestinal wall has structural features that significantly increase its absorptive surface area. These features include:
* *plicae circulares*—circular folds of the intestinal mucosa, or mucous membrane lining
* *villi*—finger-like projections on the mucosa
* *microvilli*—tiny cytoplasmic projections on the surface of epithelial cells.

Secretion police

The small intestine also releases hormones that help control the secretion of bile, pancreatic juice and intestinal juice.

Stomach emptying

The rate of stomach emptying depends on several factors, including gastrin release; neural signals generated when the stomach wall distends, and the enterogastric reflex.

Enterogastric reflex

The *enterogastric reflex* is a response in which the duodenum releases secretin and gastricinhibitory peptide, and the jejunum secretes cholecystokinin. Both reactions decrease gastric motility.

Digestion and absorption in the small intestine

The small intestine performs most of the work of digestion and absorption. Here's a summary of the small intestine's major tasks.

Mechanical digestion

- Small muscles mix chyme.
- Peristaltic motions propel the food mass over the length of the intestine.
- Surface villi mix chyme at the intestinal wall, enhancing absorption.
- Long muscle moves the food mass in a circular motion, providing new surface sites for absorption.
- Segmentation rings from circular muscle mix the food into soft masses and then mix it with secretions.

Chemical digestion

- Lipase breaks fats into fatty acids and glycerides.
- Amylase converts starch to the disaccharides maltose and sucrose.
- Enterokinase activates trypsinogens, which become trypsin.
- Trypsin and chymotrypsin split protein molecules into small peptides and then into individual amino acids.
- Disaccharidases convert their respective disaccharides to monosaccharides.
- Bile from the liver helps to digest and absorb fat.
- Carbohydrate foods are changed into simple sugars.
- Fats are changed into fatty acids and glycerides.
- Proteins are changed into amino acids.
- Vitamins and minerals are also released.

Absorption

- Microvilli, villi and mucus absorb essential nutrients.
- Absorption is controlled by diffusion, passive for the small materials and carrier-assisted for larger items.
- Digestive contents are mostly water-soluble and can be absorbed directly into the circulation.
- Fatty contents aren't water-soluble; they must pass through the villi, then into the lymph system, and finally into the bloodstream.

Large intestine

The main tasks of the large intestine are absorption of body water and elimination of digestive waste. In addition, the large intestine harbours the bacteria *Escherichia coli*, *Enterobacter aerogenes*, *Clostridium perfringens* and *Lactobacillus bifidus*. All of these bacteria help synthesise vitamin K and break down cellulose into usable carbohydrates. Bacterial action also produces *flatus*, which helps propel stools towards the rectum.

Protection from bacterial action

The mucosa of the large intestine also produces alkaline secretions from tubular glands composed of goblet cells. This alkaline mucus lubricates the intestinal walls as food pushes through, protecting the mucosa from acidic bacterial action.

From start to finish

The large intestine extends from the ileocaecal valve (the valve between the ileum of the small intestine and the first segment of the large intestine) to the anus. The large intestine has five segments:

 caecum

 ascending colon

transverse colon

 descending and sigmoid colons

rectum.

Caecum

The *caecum*, a sac-like structure, makes up the first few inches of the large intestine. The caecum is connected to the ileum of the small intestine by the ileocaecal pouch.

Ascending colon

The ascending colon rises on the right posterior abdominal wall, and then turns under the liver at the hepatic flexure. By the time chyme passes through the ileocaecal valve and enters the ascending colon of the large intestine, it has been reduced to mostly indigestible substances.

Transverse colon

The transverse colon is located above the small intestine, passing horizontally across the abdomen and below the liver, stomach and spleen. It proceeds to turn downwards at the left colic flexure. Through blood and lymph vessels, the large intestine has absorbed all but about 100 ml of water from the chyme by the time it leaves the transverse colon. It also absorbs large amounts of sodium and chloride at this point.

Got to have your fibre

Because dietary fibre isn't digested, it travels through the large intestine unabsorbed and contributes to the formation of faeces.

Descending and sigmoid colons

The descending colon starts near the spleen and extends down the left side of the abdomen into the pelvic cavity. The sigmoid colon descends through the pelvic cavity, where it becomes the rectum. The descending and sigmoid colons are responsible for evacuation. Contents move slowly along the tract, enabling water and electrolytes to be absorbed.

Rectum

The *rectum*, the last few inches of the large intestine, terminates at the anus.

Mass movement

In the lower colon, long and relatively sluggish contractions cause propulsive waves, or *mass movements*. Normally occurring several times per day, these movements propel intestinal contents into the rectum and produce the urge to defecate.

Accessory organs of digestion and absorption

Accessory organs of the digestive system—the liver, biliary duct system and pancreas—contribute hormones, enzymes and bile vital to digestion and absorption.

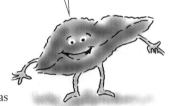

Hey, I don't mean to brag, but it says right here I'm the body's largest gland and highly vascular at that!

Liver

The body's largest gland, the highly vascular liver is enclosed in a fibrous capsule in the right upper quadrant of the abdomen. The *lesser omentum*, a fold of peritoneum, covers most of the liver and anchors it to the lesser curvature of the stomach. The *hepatic artery* and *hepatic portal vein* as well as the common bile duct and hepatic veins pass through the lesser omentum.

Functioning features

The liver's functional unit, the *lobule*, consists of a plate of hepatic cells, or *hepatocytes*, that encircle a central vein and radiate outwards. Separating the hepatocyte plates from each other are *sinusoids*, the liver's capillary system. Reticuloendothelial macrophages (*Kupffer's cells*) lining the sinusoids remove bacteria and toxins that have entered the blood through the intestinal capillaries.

Go with the blood flow

The sinusoids carry oxygenated blood from the hepatic artery and nutrient-rich blood from the portal vein. Unoxygenated blood leaves through the central vein and flows through hepatic veins to the inferior vena cava.

All that and a bag of chips

The liver performs many important functions in the processes of digestion and absorption. The liver:
- aids in carbohydrate metabolism
- detoxifies various endogenous and exogenous toxins, such as drugs and alcohol
- synthesises plasma proteins, non-essential amino acids and vitamin A
- stores essential nutrients, such as vitamins K, D, B_{12} and iron
- removes ammonia from body fluids, converting it to urea for excretion in urine
- converts glucose to glycogen and stores it as fuel for the muscles
- produces and secretes bile to aid in digestion
- stores fats and converts the excess sugars to fats to store in other parts of the body.

Biliary duct system

The biliary duct system consists of a network of ducts and includes the gall bladder.

Ducts

Think of ducts as a subway system transporting bile through the GI tract. *Bile* is a greenish liquid composed of water, cholesterol, bile salts and phospholipids. From the liver, bile travels via the common bile duct to the small intestine, entering through the duodenum.

Bile salts

When bile salts are absent from the intestinal tract, lipids are excreted and fat-soluble vitamins are absorbed poorly.

Report on bile production

The liver recycles about 80% of bile salts into bile, combining them with bile pigments (biliverdin and bilirubin, the breakdown products of red blood cells) and cholesterol. The liver secretes this alkaline bile continuously. Bile production may increase from stimulation of the vagus nerve, release of the hormone secretin, increased blood flow in the liver and the presence of fat in the intestine. (See *GI hormones: Production and function.*)

Gall bladder

The *gall bladder* is a pear-shaped organ joined to the ventral surface of the liver by the cystic duct. The gall bladder:
- stores and concentrates bile produced by the liver
- releases bile into the common bile duct for delivery to the duodenum in response to the contraction and relaxation of the sphincter of Oddi.

Cholecystokinin contraction

The secretion of the hormone cholecystokinin causes the gall bladder to contract. This contraction allows the release of bile into the common bile duct for delivery to the duodenum.

Pancreas

The *pancreas* is a somewhat flat organ that lies behind the stomach. Its head and neck extend into the curve of the duodenum and its tail lies against the spleen. The pancreas performs exocrine and endocrine functions.

Exocrine function

The pancreas's exocrine function involves scattered cells that secrete more than 1,000 ml of digestive enzymes every day. Lobules and lobes of the clusters (*acini*) of enzyme-producing cells release their secretions into ducts

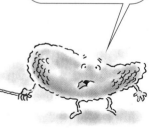

I may not be as large as the liver, but I perform important exocrine and endocrine functions.

GI hormones: production and function

When stimulated, GI structures secrete four hormones. Each hormone plays a different part in digestion.

Hormone and production site	Stimulating factor or agent	Function
Gastrin Produced in pyloric antrum and duodenal mucosa	• Pyloric antrum distention • Vagal stimulation • Protein digestion products • Alcohol	Stimulates gastric secretion and motility
Gastric inhibitory peptides Produced in duodenal and jejunal mucosa	• Gastric acid • Fats • Fat digestion products	Inhibits gastric secretion and motility
Secretin Produced in duodenal and jejunal mucosa	• Gastric acid • Fat digestion products • Protein digestion products	Stimulates secretion of bile and alkaline pancreatic fluid
Cholecystokinin Produced in duodenal and jejunal mucosa	• Fat digestion products • Protein digestion products	Stimulates gallbladder contraction and secretion of enzyme-rich pancreatic fluid

that merge into the pancreatic duct. The pancreatic duct runs the length of the pancreas and joins the bile duct from the gall bladder before entering the duodenum. The vagus nerve stimulates the production and release of secretin and cholecystokinin, which are the two hormones responsible for regulating the rate and amount of pancreatic secretions.

Endocrine function
The endocrine function of the pancreas involves the islets of Langerhans. Two types of cells formulate the islets of Langerhans: alpha and beta cells.

The ABC's of alpha and beta cells

There are over 1 million of these alpha and beta cells in the islets. Alpha cells secrete *glucagon*, a hormone that stimulates glycogenolysis in the liver; beta cells secrete insulin to promote carbohydrate metabolism. Both hormones flow directly into the blood. Their release is stimulated by blood glucose levels.

Pancreatic duct

Running the length of the pancreas, the *pancreatic duct* joins the bile duct from the gall bladder before entering the duodenum. Vagal stimulation and release of the hormones secretin and cholecystokinin control the rate and amount of pancreatic secretion.

> Remember that patients hospitalised for more than 2 weeks risk developing a nutritional disorder.

A look at altered nutrition

Patients with nutritional problems may experience such signs and symptoms as excessive weight loss or gain, anorexia or muscle wasting. Lifestyle habits, culture and economic resources can also affect a person's nutritional status. Remember that clinical signs of nutritional deficiencies appear late. Also, be aware that patients hospitalised for more than 2 weeks risk developing a nutritional disorder. (See *Evaluation of nutritional findings*.)

Excessive weight loss

Patients with nutritional deficiencies usually experience weight loss. Weight loss may result from decreased food intake, decreased food absorption, increased metabolic requirements or a combination of the three. Other possible causes include endocrine, neoplastic, GI and psychiatric disorders; chronic disease; infection; and neurologic lesions that cause paralysis and dysphagia.

Consumption conundrums

Excessive weight loss may also occur if the patient has a condition that prevents them from consuming a sufficient amount of food, such as painful oral lesions, ill-fitting dentures or a loss of teeth. In addition, poverty, fad diets, excessive exercise or certain drugs may contribute to excessive weight loss.

Excessive weight gain

When a person consumes more calories than their body requires for energy, their body stores excess adipose tissue, resulting in weight gain. Emotional factors (such as anxiety, guilt and depression) as well as social factors can trigger overeating, resulting in excessive weight gain. Excessive weight gain is also a primary sign of many endocrine disorders. In addition, patients with conditions that limit activity, such as cardiovascular or respiratory disorders, may also experience excessive weight gain. (See *Overweight children*.)

Evaluation of nutritional findings

This chart will help you interpret your nutritional assessment findings.

Body system or region	Sign or symptom	Implications
General	• Weakness and fatigue	• Anaemia or electrolyte imbalance
	• Weight loss	• Decreased calorie intake, increased calorie use or inadequate nutrient intake or absorption
Skin, hair and nails	• Dry, flaky skin	• Vitamin A, vitamin B-complex or linoleic acid deficiency
	• Dry skin with poor turgor	• Dehydration
	• Rough, scaly skin with bumps	• Vitamin A or essential fatty acid deficiency
	• Petechiae or ecchymoses	• Vitamin C or K deficiency
	• Sore that won't heal	• Protein, vitamin C or zinc deficiency
	• Thinning, dry hair	• Protein or zinc deficiency
	• Spoon-shaped, brittle or ridged nails	• Iron deficiency
Eyes	• Night blindness; corneal swelling, softening, or dryness; Bitot's spots (grey triangular patches on the conjunctiva)	• Vitamin A deficiency
	• Red conjunctiva	• Riboflavin deficiency
Throat and mouth	• Cracks at corner of mouth	• Riboflavin or niacin deficiency
	• Magenta tongue	• Riboflavin deficiency
	• Beefy, red tongue	• Vitamin B_{12} deficiency
	• Soft, spongy, bleeding gums	• Vitamin C deficiency
	• Swollen neck (goitre)	• Iodine deficiency
Cardiovascular	• Oedema	• Protein deficiency
	• Tachycardia and hypotension	• Fluid volume deficit
GI	• Ascites	• Protein deficiency
Musculoskeletal	• Bone pain and bow leg	• Vitamin D or calcium deficiency
	• Muscle wasting	• Protein, carbohydrate and fat deficiency
	• Pain in calves and thighs	• Thiamine deficiency
Neurologic	• Altered mental state	• Dehydration and thiamine or vitamin B_{12} deficiency
	• Paresthesia	• Vitamin B_{12}, pyridoxine or thiamine deficiency

Ages and stages

Overweight children

Like adults, the number of children considered overweight has dramatically increased in recent years. An estimated 15% of children and teens are overweight (as determined by their body mass index); another 15% risk becoming overweight. Most overweight children become overweight or obese adults.

More weight, more risks

Children who are overweight are more likely to have high cholesterol and high blood pressure (risk factors for heart disease) as well as type 2 diabetes. They also tend to suffer from poor self-esteem and depression because of their weight.

Counting causes

During your nutritional assessment, look for these common causes of excessive weight gain in children:

* lack of exercise
* sedentary lifestyle (involving an excessive amount of watching television, using computers or playing video games)
* unhealthy eating habits.

Healthy habits

Help the child develop an exercise plan and suggest nutritious eating habits to prevent weight gain and promote a healthy lifestyle.

Anorexia

Defined as a lack of appetite despite a physiologic need for food, *anorexia* commonly occurs with GI and endocrine disorders. It can also result from anxiety, chronic pain, poor oral hygiene and changes in taste or smell that normally accompany aging. Short-term anorexia rarely jeopardises health, but chronic anorexia can lead to life-threatening malnutrition. *Anorexia nervosa* is a psychological condition in which the patient severely restricts food intake, resulting in excessive weight loss.

Muscle wasting

Usually a result of chronic protein deficiency, muscle wasting, or *atrophy*, results when muscle fibres lose bulk and length. The muscles involved shrink and lose their normal contour, appearing emaciated or even deformed. Associated signs and symptoms include chronic fatigue, apathy, anorexia, dry skin, peripheral oedema and dull, sparse, dry hair.

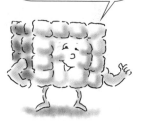

You need me to avoid atrophy, which can lead to lots of other undesirable conditions!

Lifestyle habits

Eating habits are usually set in childhood and can vary greatly from one person to another. Peer pressure and gender-role stereotypes can affect a person's eating patterns. Food fads can also affect dietary patterns and may interfere with a healthy eating pattern. Nutritional supplements may not always have a scientific basis for their claims of better nutrition.

Today's fast-paced lives place families in tough situations when trying to provide well-balanced meals while maintaining busy schedules. The availability of pre-packaged foods and fast food options is tempting.

Culture and beliefs

Culture plays a large role in the type of food eaten and dietary habits and patterns. Asians may eat rice with most meals, whereas Mexican Americans may have spicy, hot foods and Italians may prefer pasta.

Religious beliefs also play a large role in dietary habits. Certain religions restrict a particular food during a religious holiday whereas others may encourage fasting. Still others restrict the kinds of foods that can be eaten in the same meal. (See *Religious practices and dietary restrictions*.)

Economic resources

A person's economic resources or lack of resources can severely alter their eating patterns and food choices. The lower a person's income, the less likely they'll be to have good nutrition. Low-income families, especially the elderly, may have to sacrifice their food money to buy much needed prescriptions or to pay other bills, such as for heat and electricity. Because their income is lower, they may make poorer food choices because of their budgets. These choices may result in meals that are low in protein and high in starch.

Religious practices and dietary restrictions

Religious beliefs can greatly impact dietary practices and, therefore, dietary nursing considerations. For example:

- Orthodox Jews who follow Kosher laws don't consume milk and other dairy products with meat or poultry.
- Many Seventh-Day Adventists are lacto-ovo vegetarians. Among those who do eat meat, pork is avoided.
- Hindus and Buddhists may also avoid consuming meat.

Preventing altered nutrition

The most important role a nurse can provide to prevent altered nutrition is to teach the patient about proper diet and health promotion. To accomplish this goal, try to increase the patient's understanding of what a healthy diet includes. Knowledge doesn't always guarantee that the patient will follow the healthy diet, but the odds are greater if they have an understanding of what they should or shouldn't eat.

Promoting optimal intake

Illness greatly affects a person's eating habits and desire for food. Food should be served in an attractive, appetising manner and be at the right temperature.

The room should be pleasant and void of distractions. The patient's food preferences should be considered.

Pain medications and medications given to control nausea and pain should be timed to help the patient achieve optimal relief at mealtimes. Providing oral care before meals promotes taste and comfort. If possible and the patient's condition permits, the patient should receive meals sitting upright and out of bed in a chair. This position facilitates chewing and prevents choking and reflux of stomach contents.

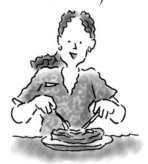

Now this looks mighty appetising!

Assisting an adult with feeding

Confusion, arm or hand immobility, injury, weakness or restrictions on activities or positions may prevent a patient from feeding themselves. Feeding the patient then becomes a key nursing responsibility. An injured or debilitated patient may experience depression and subsequent anorexia. Meeting such a patient's nutritional needs requires determining food preferences; conducting the feeding in a friendly, unhurried manner; encouraging self-feeding to promote independence and dignity; and documenting intake and output.

What you need

Meal tray ✳ overbed table ✳ napkin or protection for clothes if patient would prefer ✳ condiments ✳ assistive feeding devices if necessary

Getting ready

• Raise the head of the bed if allowed or assist patient to sit in a chair. An upright position of 90 degrees makes swallowing easier and reduces the risk of aspiration and choking.
• Before the meal tray arrives, offer the patient a chance to use the toilet or wash hands. If necessary, you may wash their hands for them.
• Wipe the overbed table with soap and water or alcohol, especially if a urinal or bedpan was on it.
• Ensure that the patient has a clean mouth and dentures if required.
• When the meal tray arrives, make sure it contains foods appropriate for the patient's condition. (See *Special diets*.)

How you do it

• *Because many adults consider being fed demeaning*, allow the patient some control over mealtime, such as letting them set the pace of the meal or decide the order in which they eat various foods.
• Encourage the patient to feed themself if they can. If the patient is restricted to the prone or the supine position but can use their arms and hands, encourage them to try foods they can pick up, such as sandwiches. If they can assume a sitting position but has limited use of their arms or hands, teach them how to use assistive feeding devices. (See *Using assistive feeding devices*, page 440.)

Special diets

Patients who are hospitalised may have different diets according to the reason for their hospitalisation. Dietary intake is commonly changed to promote healing or to prevent complications such as a nil-by-mouth status before surgery. Always check, before giving patients their meals, that they're receiving the correct diet.

Nil by mouth

The term nil by mouth is actually the withholding of food or liquids. It may be indicated to:

- clear the GI tract of contents before surgery or a diagnostic procedure
- prevent aspiration in high-risk patients
- treat severe nausea and vomiting
- prevent aspiration during surgery
- rest the GI tract to promote healing
- treat medical problems such as a bowel obstruction.

Clear liquid

A clear-liquid diet includes only liquids that don't contain residue. It includes juices without pulp (such as apple or cranberry), tea, clear soup and jelly. It's commonly used prior to GI surgery or before some diagnostic tests.

Full liquid

A full-liquid diet includes all foods and fluids that become a liquid at room temperature, such as ice cream or sherbet. This diet is commonly ordered for post-operative patients after free fluids (coffee/tea/squash/milk) have been tolerated. It's also used for patients who can't chew properly such as after a stroke.

Soft

A soft diet includes foods that are soft with reduced fibre. They may be further chopped or pureed for patients who have difficulty chewing or have no teeth.

Diet as tolerated

A diet classified as *tolerated* can change as the patient's tolerance changes. For instance a post-operative patient may start out with clear liquids but may progress to a regular diet if they hasn't had nausea or vomiting.

Restrictive diets

A restrictive diet is a diet that limits certain foods or a particular nutrient, such as sodium, potassium and fat, or calorie content, depending on the patient's disease or metabolic status. For example, a patient who's obese may need to limit calorie intake and a cardiac patient may need to limit sodium intake.

- Offer a napkin or something to protect the patient's clothes if they prefer.
- Position a chair next to the patient's bed or chair, so you can sit comfortably if you need to feed them yourself.
- Set up the patient's tray, remove the plate from the tray warmer, and discard all plastic wrappings. Then cut the food into bite-size pieces.

Peas at 12, corns at 3

- To help the blind or visually impaired patient feed themselves, tell them that placement of various foods on their plate corresponds to the hours on a clock face. Maintain consistent placement for subsequent meals.

Using assistive feeding devices

Various feeding devices, available through occupational therapy, can help the patient who has limited arm mobility, grasp, range of movement (ROM) or coordination. Before introducing your patient to an assistive feeding device, assess their ability to master it. Don't introduce a device they can't manage. If their condition is progressively disabling, encourage them to use the device only until their mastery of it falters.

Introduce the assistive device before mealtime, with the patient seated in a natural position. Explain its purpose, show the patient how to use it, and encourage them to practice. After meals, wash the device thoroughly and store it in the patient's bedside locker. Document the patient's progress and share it with staff and family members to help reinforce the patient's independence. Specific devices are discussed here.

Plate guard

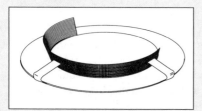

A plate guard blocks food from spilling off the plate. Attach the guard to the side of the plate opposite the hand the patient uses to feed with. Guiding the patient's hand, show them how to push food against the guard to secure it on the utensil. Ask them to try again with food of a different consistency. When the patient tires, feed them the rest of the meal. At subsequent meals, encourage the patient to feed themself for progressively longer periods until they can feed themselves an entire meal.

Swivel spoon

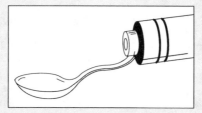

A swivel spoon helps the patient with limited ROM in their forearm and will fit in universal cuffs.

Universal cuffs

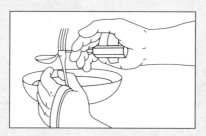

Universal cuffs are flexible bands that help the patient with flail hands or diminished grasp. Each cuff contains a slot that holds a fork or spoon. Attach the cuff to the hand the patient uses to feed themselves. Then place the fork or spoon in the cuff slot. Bend the utensil to facilitate feeding.

Long-handled utensils

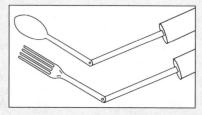

Long-handled utensils have jointed stems to help the patient with limited ROM in their elbow and shoulder.

Utensils with built-up handles

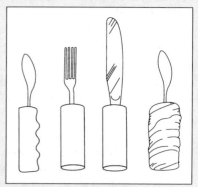

Utensils with built-up handles can help the patient with diminished grasp. They can be purchased or improvised by wrapping tape around the handles.

- Ask the patient which food they prefer to eat first *to promote their sense of control over the meal.* Some patients prefer to eat one food at a time, whereas others prefer to alternate foods.
- If the patient has difficulty swallowing, offer liquids carefully with a spoon. Pureed or soft foods, such as custard or jelly, may be easier to swallow than liquids.

We now pause for a break

- Ask the patient to indicate when they're ready for another mouthful. Pause between courses and whenever the patient wants to rest. During the meal, wipe the patient's mouth and chin as needed.
- When the patient finishes eating, remove the tray. If necessary, clean up spills and change the bed linen. Provide mouth care.

Practice pointers

- Don't feed the patient too quickly *because this can upset them and impair digestion.*
- If the patient is restricted to the supine position, provide foods that they can chew easily. If they're restricted to the prone position, feed them liquids carefully and only after they have swallowed their food *to reduce the risk of aspiration.*
- If the patient won't eat, try to find out why. For example, confirm their food preferences. Also, make sure the patient isn't in pain at mealtimes or that they haven't received any treatments immediately before a meal that could upset or nauseate them. Find out if any medications cause anorexia, nausea or sedation. Of course, clear the bedside of inappropriate items at mealtimes.

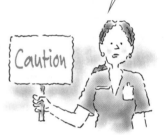

Don't feed a patient too quickly or you might upset him and impair digestion.

Caution

A plausible pattern

- Establish a pattern for feeding the patient, and share this information with the rest of the staff *so the patient doesn't need to repeatedly instruct staff members about the best way to feed them.*
- If the patient and their family are willing, suggest that family members assist with feeding. *Involving the family may make the patient feel more comfortable at mealtimes and ease discharge planning.*
- If the patient has a swallowing difficulty (such as in stroke or head injury), consult with speech therapy before feeding *to best determine the type of foods the patient requires (thickened and so forth).*
- Document the patient's progress. (See *Recording fluid intake and output,* page 442.)

Feeding tube insertion and removal

Inserting a feeding tube into the stomach or duodenum allows patients who can't or won't eat to receive nourishment. The feeding tube also permits administration of supplemental feedings to patients who have high nutritional requirements, such as unconscious patients or those with extensive burns.

Recording fluid intake and output

Accurate intake and output records help evaluate a patient's fluid and electrolyte balance, suggest various diagnoses and influence the choice of fluid therapy. These records are mandatory for patients with burns, renal failure, electrolyte imbalance, recent surgical procedures, heart failure or severe vomiting and diarrhoea, and for patients receiving diuretics or corticosteroids. Intake and output records are also significant in monitoring patients with nasogastric (NG) tubes or drainage collection devices, and those receiving intravenous (I.V.) therapy.

Fluid intake consists of all fluid entering the patient's body, including beverages, fluids contained in solid foods taken by mouth, and foods that are liquid at room temperature, such as jelly, custard, ice cream and some beverages. Additional intake includes GI feeds, bladder irrigations and I.V. fluids.

Fluid output consists of all fluids that leaves the patient's body, including urine, loose stools, vomit, aspirated fluid loss, and drainage from surgical drains, NG tubes and chest tubes.

When recording fluid intake and output, enlist the patient's help if possible. Record amount in millilitres (ml). Measure; don't estimate. For a small child, weigh nappies if appropriate. Monitor intake and output during each shift, and notify the doctor if amounts differ significantly over a 24-hour period. Document your findings in the appropriate location; describe any fluid restrictions and the patient's compliance.

Can't stomach this

The doctor may order duodenal feeding when the patient can't tolerate gastric feeding or when they expect gastric feeding to produce aspiration. Absence of bowel sounds or possible intestinal obstruction contraindicates using a feeding tube.

Flexibility rules!

Feeding tubes are made of silicone, rubber or polyurethane and have small diameters and great flexibility. To ease passage, some feeding tubes are weighted with tungsten, and some need a guide wire to keep them from curling in the back of the throat. These small-bore tubes usually have radiopaque markings and a water-activated coating, which provides a lubricated surface.

What you need

For enteral feeding
Enteral feed * graduated container * water for flushing feed out of tubing * plastic bottle or PVC bag if feed needs decanting * feed administration tubing appropriate for continuous infusion via a pump, gravity or bolus feeding * 50-ml feeding syringe for bolus feeding * pH test strip.

Getting ready
- Be sure to refrigerate formulas prepared in the pharmacy. Refrigerate commercial formulas only after opening them.
- Check the date on all formula containers.
- Discard expired commercial formula.
- Use powdered formula within 24 hours of mixing.

Shake...

- Always shake the container well to mix the solution thoroughly.
- Allow the formula to warm to room temperature before administration. *Cold formula can increase the chance of diarrhoea.*
- Never warm it over direct heat or in a microwave *because heat may curdle the formula or change its chemical composition. Also, hot formula may injure the patient.*

...and pour

- Pour 60 ml of water into the graduated container.
- After closing the flow clamp on the administration set, pour the appropriate amount of formula into the bag.
- For a feed that has been decanted, hang no more than a 4 hour supply at one time *to prevent bacterial growth.*
- Open the flow clamp on the administration set *to remove air from the lines and prevent air from entering the patient's stomach, causing distention and discomfort.*

How you do it
- Provide privacy and wash your hands.
- Inform the patient that they'll receive nourishment through the tube, and explain the procedure to them. If possible, give them a schedule of subsequent feedings.

Delivering a gastric feeding
- Elevate the bed to a semi-upright position *to prevent aspiration by gastroesophageal reflux and to promote digestion.*
- Check placement of the feeding tube *to make sure it hasn't slipped out since the last feeding.*
- Never give a tube feed until you're sure the tube is properly positioned in the patient's stomach. *Administering a feed through a misplaced tube can cause formula to enter the patient's lungs.*
- *To check tube patency and position,* remove the cap or plug from the feeding tube, and use the syringe to aspirate gastric secretions gently.

Proper pH please!

- Examine the aspirate and place a small amount on the pH test strip. Proper placement of the gastric tube is likely if the aspirate has a typical

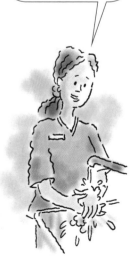

This is an important first step.

gastric fluid appearance (grassy-green, clear and colourless with mucus shreds or brown) and the pH is 5.0 or less.

• Connect the bag to the feeding tube. Depending on the type of tube used, you may need to use an adaptor to connect the two.

• If you're using a catheter-tip syringe, remove the plunger and attach the syringe to the pinched-off feeding tube *to prevent excess air from entering the patient's stomach, causing distention.*

• If you're using an infusion controller, thread the tube from the formula container through the controller according to the manufacturer's directions.

• Purge the tubing of air and attach it to the feeding tube.

• Open the regulator clamp on the tubing and adjust the flow rate appropriately.

• When using a bulb syringe, fill the syringe with formula and release the feeding tube *to allow formula to flow through it.* The height at which you hold the syringe will determine flow rate. When the syringe is three-quarters empty, pour more formula into it.

• *To prevent air from entering the tube and the patient's stomach,* never allow the syringe to empty completely.

• If you're using an infusion controller, set the flow rate according to the manufacturer's directions.

Slowly please!

• Always administer a tube feeding slowly—typically 200 to 350 ml over 15 to 30 minutes, depending on the patient's tolerance and directions from the nutrition team—*to prevent sudden stomach distention, which can cause nausea, vomiting, cramps or diarrhoea.*

• After administering the appropriate amount of formula, flush the tubing by adding about 60 ml of water to the bag or syringe. *Flushing maintains the tube's patency by removing excess formula, which could occlude the tube.*

• If you're administering a continuous feeding, flush the feeding tube every 4 hours *to help prevent tube occlusion.*

We're all done

• To discontinue gastric feeding (depending on the equipment you're using), close the regulator clamp on the tubing, disconnect the syringe from the feeding tube, or turn off the infusion controller.

• Cover the end of the feeding tube with its plug or cap *to prevent leakage and contamination of the tube.*

• Leave the patient in semi-upright position for at least 30 minutes.

• Rinse all reusable equipment with warm water.

• Dry it and store it in a convenient place for the next feeding. Change equipment every 24 hours or according to local policy.

Practice pointers

- If the patient becomes nauseated or vomits, stop the feeding immediately. *The patient may vomit if the stomach becomes distended from overfeeding or delayed gastric emptying.*
- *To reduce oropharyngeal discomfort from the tube*, allow the patient to brush their teeth or care for their dentures regularly, and encourage frequent gargling.
- If the patient is unconscious, administer oral and lip care as required.

I'm parched

- Dry mucous membranes may indicate dehydration, which requires increased fluid intake.
- Clean the patient's nostrils with cotton-tipped applicators, apply lubricant along the mucosa, and assess the skin for signs of breakdown.
- During continuous feedings, assess the patient frequently for abdominal distention. Flush the tubing by adding about 50 ml of water to the bag or syringe. *Flushing the tubing maintains the tube's patency by removing excess formula, which could occlude the tube.*
- If the patient develops diarrhoea, administer small, frequent, less-concentrated feedings, or administer bolus feedings over a longer time.
- Make sure that the formula isn't cold and that proper storage and sanitation practices have been followed. The loose stools associated with tube feedings make extra perineal and skin care necessary. Changing to a formula with more fibre may eliminate liquid stools.

More fruits and veggies

- If the patient becomes constipated, the doctor may increase the fruit, vegetable or sugar content of the formula.
- Assess the patient's hydration status *because dehydration may produce constipation.* Increase fluid intake as necessary. If the condition persists, administer an appropriate drug or enema, as prescribed.
- Drugs can be administered through the feeding tube, preferably in liquid form. Do not crush tablets without speaking to the pharmacist first.

Hold the wire

- Small-bore feeding tubes may kink, making instillation impossible. If you suspect this problem, try changing the patient's position, or withdraw the tube a few centimetres and restart. Never use a guide wire to reposition the tube.
- Constantly monitor the flow rate of a blended or high-residue formula *to determine if the formula is clogging the tubing as it settles.* To prevent such clogging, squeeze the bag frequently *to agitate the solution.*
- The patient's blood glucose should be performed regularly as per local policy.
- The patient's full blood count, urea and electrolytes, blood glucose, fluid balance and body weight will be monitored closely by the nutrition team.

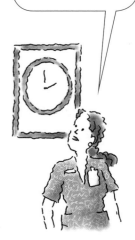

Check the flow rate hourly to ensure correct infusion.

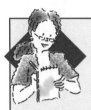

Take note!

Documenting tube feedings

When documenting tube feedings be sure to include the details listed below:

- On the intake and output sheet, record the date, volume of formula and volume of water.
- In your notes, include verification of tube placement; amount, type and time of feeding; and tube patency.

- Discuss the patient's tolerance of the feeding, including nausea, vomiting, cramping, diarrhoea and distention.
- Include the date and time of administration set changes, oral and nasal hygiene.

Check the flow, Flo!

- Check the flow rate hourly *to ensure correct infusion*.
- For duodenal or jejunal feeding, most patients tolerate a continuous drip better than bolus feedings. *Bolus feedings can cause such complications as hyperglycaemia and diarrhoea.*
- Until the patient acquires a tolerance for the formula, you may need to dilute it to one-half or three-quarters strength to start, and increase it gradually.
- Document the procedure and the feeding according to your local policy. (See *Documenting tube feedings*.)

Quick quiz

1. Through metabolism, energy is extracted from which nutrients?
    A. Carbohydrates, proteins and fats
    B. Carbohydrates, fats and sodium
    C. Fats, adenosine triphosphate and minerals
    D. Vitamins, minerals and electrolytes

Answer: A. Energy is produced through the metabolism of carbohydrates, proteins and fats.

2. Essential nutrients are supplied to the body by:
    A. vitamin or mineral supplements.
    B. certain food combinations.
    C. body functions.
    D. food in many different combinations.

Answer: D. Essential nutrients are supplied by the many combinations of food consumed.

3. Which GI hormone stimulates gastric secretion and motility?
  A. Gastric inhibitory peptides
  B. Gastrin
  C. Secretin
  D. Pepsinogen

Answer: B. Gastrin is produced in the pyloric antrum and duodenal end mucosa and stimulates gastric secretion and motility.

4. In which phase of digestion does the stomach secrete the digestive juices HCl and pepsin?
  A. Cephalic
  B. Gastric
  C. Intestinal
  D. Mastication

Answer: A. By the time the food is travelling towards the stomach, the cephalic phase—during which the stomach secretes digestive juices—has begun.

Scoring

☆☆☆ If you answered all four questions correctly, gee whiz! Your nutritional knowledge is optimal.

☆☆ If you answered three questions correctly, great! Your ingestion of nutrition facts is quite sufficient.

☆ If you answered fewer than three questions correctly, no worries! Review the chapter, absorb some more facts and start over.

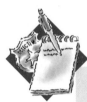

Just the facts

In this chapter, you'll learn:

♦ process of urine formation

♦ factors that affect urinary elimination

♦ common urinary abnormalities

♦ proper methods for obtaining urine specimens

♦ steps for insertion, care and removal of an indwelling urinary catheter

♦ proper method for applying a condom catheter.

A look at the urinary system

The urinary system consists of the kidneys, ureters, bladder and urethra.

Kidneys

The essential functions of the urinary system—such as forming and excreting urine to maintain the proper balance of fluids and electrolytes, minerals and organic substances for homoeostasis—take place in the highly vascular kidneys. These bean-shaped organs are 11.4 to 12.7 cm long and 6.4 cm wide.

Located retroperitoneally on either side of the lumbar vertebrae, the kidneys lie posterior to the abdominal organs and are protected by the contents of the abdomen. The right kidney extends slightly lower than the

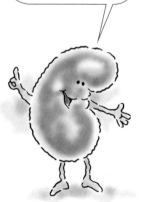

I'm essential to a well-balanced urinary system.

left kidney. A layer of fat surrounds each kidney, offering further protection. Each kidney consists of three regions:

 renal cortex (outer region)

 renal medulla (middle region)

 renal pelvis (inner region). (See *A close look at the kidneys*.)

A close look at the kidneys

The kidneys are located in the lumbar area, with the right kidney situated slightly lower than the left to make room for the liver, which is just above it. The position of the kidneys shifts somewhat with changes in body position. Covering the kidneys are the fibrous capsule, perirenal fat and renal fasciae.

Blood's cleansing journey

The kidneys receive waste-filled blood from the renal artery, which branches off the abdominal aorta. After passing through a complicated network of smaller blood vessels and nephrons, the filtered blood returns to the circulation by way of the renal vein, which empties into the inferior vena cava.

Continuing the clean-up

The kidneys excrete waste products that the nephrons remove from the blood. These excretions combine with other waste fluids (such as urea, creatinine, phosphates and sulphates) to form urine. An action called peristalsis (the circular contraction and relaxation of a tube-shaped structure) passes the urine through the ureters and into the urinary bladder. When the bladder has filled, nerves in the bladder wall relax the sphincter. In conjunction with a voluntary stimulus, this relaxation causes urine to pass into the urethra for elimination from the body.

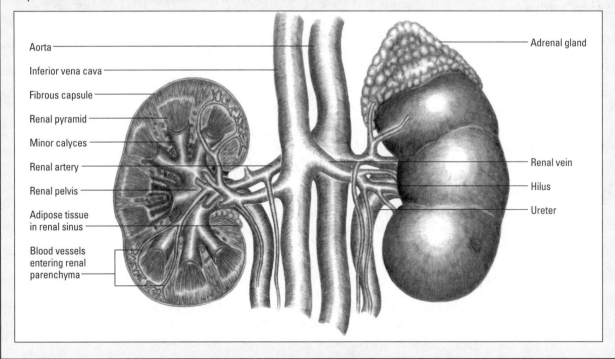

Aorta

Inferior vena cava

Fibrous capsule

Renal pyramid

Minor calyces

Renal artery

Renal pelvis

Adipose tissue in renal sinus

Blood vessels entering renal parenchyma

Adrenal gland

Renal vein

Hilus

Ureter

Filtering station

The outer portion of the kidney is called the renal cortex. It contains blood-filtering mechanisms called nephrons and is protected by a fibrous capsule and layers of fat.

Renal wonder

The renal medulla contains 8 to 12 renal pyramids—striated wedges that are composed mostly of tubular structures. The tapered portion of each pyramid empties into a cup-like calyx that channels formed urine from the pyramids into the renal pelvis. The renal pelvis receives urine through the major calyces and then urine moves into the ureters and lastly to the bladder.

All in a day's work

Kidney functions include:
- elimination of wastes and excess ions (in the form of urine)
- blood filtration (by regulating chemical composition and blood volume)
- maintenance of fluid-electrolyte and acid-base balances
- production and release of renin to promote angiotensin II activation and aldosterone production in the adrenal gland
- promotion of erythropoietin (a hormone that stimulates red blood cell production and such enzymes as renin, which governs blood pressure and kidney function)
- conversion of vitamin D to a more active form.

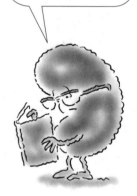

Hmm . . . It appears that I'm responsible for several important functions.

Makin' urine

The nephron is the functional unit of the kidneys. Each kidney contains roughly 1 million nephrons. Urine gathers in the collecting tubules and ducts of the nephrons and then drains into the ureters, down into the bladder and out through the urethra.

A wealth of minerals

Formed urine consists of water, sodium, chloride, potassium, calcium, magnesium, sulphates, phosphates, bicarbonates, uric acid, ammonium ions, creatinine and urobilinogen (a derivative of bilirubin).

Go with the flow

Approximately 250 to 400 ml of urine is expressed when someone voids. All but 5 to 10 ml of urine is typically emptied from the bladder. Daily urine output averages 720 to 2,400 ml, varying with fluid intake and climate.

Ureters

The ureters are a pair of muscular tubes that extend 25.5 to 30.5 cm from the urinary bladder. The left ureter is slightly longer than the right because of the left kidney's higher position. The diameter of each ureter varies from 3 to 6 mm, with the narrowest part at the ureteropelvic junction.

Where the action is

Located along the posterior abdominal wall, the ureters enter the bladder anteromedially. They carry urine from the kidneys to the bladder by peristaltic contractions that occur one to five times per minute.

Colour clues

Normal urine colour ranges from straw yellow to dark yellow. Certain medications and reduced or increased fluid intake can alter its colour. Rifampicin may produce orange-red urine. Very dilute urine is almost colourless, and concentrated urine can be dark amber or orange-brown. Some foods also alter the colour of urine, for example beetroot if eaten in large quantities.

Clear is cool

Freshly voided urine should appear clear with no sediment. Urine collected from an indwelling urinary catheter bag may contain mucus shreds, but urine in the tubing should still be clear.

Odour alert

The more dilute urine is, the fainter the odour. Concentrated urine will have a strong odour, and collected urine that's long-standing may develop a strong ammonia smell. Certain infections may also cause urine to have a foul or offensive odour.

Bladder

Located in the pelvis, the bladder is a hollow, muscular organ that serves as a temporary storage reservoir for urine collection. When the bladder is empty, it lies behind the pelvic bone; when it's full, it becomes displaced under the peritoneal cavity. Bladder capacity ranges from 500 to 700 ml in healthy adults and is lower in children and the elderly.

Urethra

The urethra is a small duct that carries urine from the bladder and out of the body. A woman's urethra is only 2.5 to 5 cm long and is anterior to the vaginal opening. Because a man's urethra must pass through the erectile tissue of the penis, it's about 15.2 cm longer than a woman's.

Dual role

In men, the urethra is part of the reproductive system because it also transports semen.

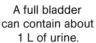

A full bladder can contain about 1 L of urine.

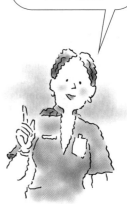

Factors affecting urinary elimination

Several factors can affect how urine is eliminated, including body position, decreased muscle tone, fluid intake, hypotension, infection, loss of body fluid, medications, neurologic injury, nutrition, obstruction of urinary flow, psychological problems and surgery.

Body position

The ability to empty the bladder during each voiding is dependent on proper body positioning, which is normally standing for men and sitting for women.

Up or down

Offering a urinal to a male patient who's flat in bed will affect his ability to initiate a urine stream and empty his bladder completely. Conversely, placing a female patient on a bedpan while she's lying flat in bed will affect her ability to urinate and empty her bladder completely.

Decreased muscle tone

A voluntary contraction and relaxation of the abdominal and perineal muscles controls urination. Weakened perineal detrusor or abdominal muscles can result from trauma, surgery, obesity, multiple pregnancies, stretching during childbirth and chronic constipation. When these muscles become weak and muscle tone is decreased, it becomes more difficult for the patient to control the urge to void, which results in incontinence.

A cystocele is a protrusion of the bladder into the vaginal canal that occurs when the vaginal wall musculature weakens as a result of muscle straining during childbirth or other straining such as heavy lifting. It can cause stress incontinence, dribbling, frequency and an inability to empty the bladder completely.

Stretch and tone

A patient who has had a long-standing indwelling urinary catheter may have trouble regaining bladder control when the catheter is removed. The continuous drainage caused by the indwelling catheter doesn't allow the bladder to fill or stretch to capacity. Because the bladder wall doesn't stretch, atrophy can develop. Dribbling after the catheter is removed is usually temporary until bladder tone returns.

Fluid intake

A patient's fluid intake is directly related to urinary volume and frequency. Urine output will decrease if fluid intake decreases. Similarly, urine output will increase if fluid intake increases. If fluid intake increases significantly, frequency of urination will also increase.

When abdominal and perineal muscles become weak and muscle tone is decreased, it becomes more difficult for the patient to control the urge to void.

Yin and yang

The correlation of intake affecting output is regulated by several hormones, such as angiotensin I and II, aldosterone, erythropoietin and anti-diuretic hormone (ADH). The most important hormone is ADH, which regulates the amount of re-absorption that occurs in the nephrons of the kidney and conserves body water by reducing urine output. ADH is released when fluid intake is decreased. The kidney then reabsorbs more water and produces more highly concentrated urine. When fluid intake increases, ADH suppression is reduced.

Hypotension

Hypotension (low arterial blood pressure) reduces blood flow to the kidneys. Adequate blood flow to the kidneys is necessary for urine production. Thus, hypotension prevents filtration from occurring. Surgery, trauma or a severe fluid loss from vomiting or diarrhoea can cause hypotension, which results in a decrease in circulating blood volume and decreased filtration and urinary excretion.

Infection

The urinary tract is sterile, except at the urinary meatus, and microorganisms there usually get washed away during urination. Urinary tract infections (UTIs) occur when microorganisms from the perineal or anal area come in contact with the urinary meatus and ascend into the urethra. This contact is usually the result of sexual intercourse, poor hygiene after bowel movements or insertion of a urinary catheter or a diagnostic instrument. UTIs can cause urgency, frequency and dysuria.

Infection protection

Lower UTIs are more common and occur in the urethra or bladder. Upper UTIs occur in the ureters, kidneys, pelvis or renal tubule system. They're more serious and can lead to kidney damage and renal failure. If left untreated, however, lower UTIs can progress to the kidneys and result in renal damage and renal failure (and become upper UTIs).

Women are particularly susceptible to UTIs due to the proximity of the urinary meatus to the vagina and rectum and because their urethra is much shorter.

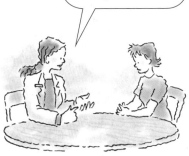

Women are particularly susceptible to UTIs.

Loss of body fluids

Loss of body fluids can result from excessive diuresis caused by fever, exercise, vomiting, diarrhoea and excessive wound drainage or blood loss from surgery or trauma. The kidneys respond to this loss by increasing water absorption to conserve water, causing a decrease in urine output.

Medications

Diuretics are used to promote the excretion of water and electrolytes by the kidneys.

To go . . .

Commonly used diuretics include furosemide (frusemide), bendroflumethiazide (bendrofluazide), amiloride and spironolactone (Aldactone).

Cholinergic medications, such as bethanechol chloride, may be prescribed because they stimulate contraction of the detrusor muscle, which promotes voiding.

Urinary frequency or urgency may be treated with oxybutynin (Ditropan) because of its anti-spasmodic effect on the detrusor muscle.

. . . or not to go.

Other medications can also affect urinary output. Opioids can decrease the glomerular filtration rate and the sensation of a full bladder. Phenothiazines, belladonna alkaloids, tricyclic anti-depressants and anti-histamines have anti-muscarinics effects and can increase urine retention.

Neurologic injury

The frontal lobe of the brain controls voluntary urination. Haemorrhage, trauma or a tumour in this lobe can result in urinary incontinence. A spinal cord injury or a stroke also can interfere with normal urinary elimination.

Reflex control

Injury to the sacral area of the spinal cord, which controls the urination reflex, can change urinary elimination patterns. When the bladder becomes full and stretched to capacity, it contracts and urination occurs. This is called reflex neurogenic bladder. An autonomous neurogenic bladder that can occur as a result of neurologic injury results in urine retention because the bladder fills without the bladder stretch mechanism in place.

Nutrition

A diet consisting of foods high in water content, such as soups, vegetables and fruits, will increase urine output. Salty foods can decrease urine output, especially if water intake doesn't increase. Food and drinks containing caffeine (chocolate, coffee, tea and cola), which is a diuretic, and alcohol can increase urine output.

Obstruction of urine flow

Obstruction of urine flow can lead to decreased urinary elimination. Structural abnormalities in the urinary system can cause obstructions, such as urinary tumours, renal stones and an enlarged prostate gland. Obstruction can also result from clogs or kinks in an indwelling catheter. Unrelieved obstruction causes increased resistance to urine flow and can lead to hydronephrosis (distension of the renal pelvis).

An infection connection

Prolonged obstruction can lead to urinary stasis, a condition that provides a breeding ground for microorganisms and resulting UTIs.

Psychological factors

Urination is a voluntary function that's affected by internal and external factors.

Into the void

Stress and anxiety can cause a patient to contract their muscles involuntarily, making urination impossible or making the urge to urinate uncontrollable. In addition, asking a patient for a urine sample or to urinate 'on demand' can make them unable to urinate.

Babbling brook

The sound or feel of running water can intensify the need to urinate. If a patient has difficulty voiding, try a warm bath to initiate urination.

Privacy, please

Always consider a patient's need for privacy, especially when a bedpan or urinal must be used.

Surgery

Most patients should be able to urinate within 6 to 8 hours after surgery. If a patient can't urinate following surgery, limited fluid intake and fluid and blood loss during surgery with a resulting depletion in fluid volume may be the cause. The stress that accompanies surgery can cause the release of ADH, which also decreases urinary output. Urine retention is also an adverse effect of some pain medications such as opioids.

Oedema dilemma

Urinary, intestinal or reproductive surgery also predisposes a patient to post-operative urinary retention. Trauma to the tissues causes oedema and can obstruct urinary flow.

How dry am I?

Medications used for spinal anaesthesia or regional blocks can cause temporary urinary problems because they impair sensory and motor impulses

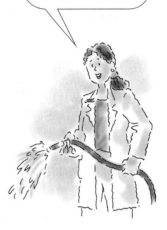

The sound or feel of running water can intensify the need to urinate.

that control urination. When the anaesthetic wears off, the patient should be able to resume their normal voiding pattern.

Common urinary abnormalities

Common abnormalities in the urinary system include dysuria; haematuria; nocturia; polyuria; urinary frequency, urgency, and hesitancy; and urinary incontinence.

Dysuria

Pain during urination, or dysuria, commonly signals a lower UTI. The onset of the pain signifies the cause. Pain immediately before urination indicates bladder irritation or distension, whereas pain at the onset usually signals a bladder outlet obstruction. Bladder spasm can cause pain at the end of the stream. Pain throughout urination may indicate pyelonephrosis, especially when accompanied by fever, chills, haematuria and flank pain.

Haematuria

Brown or bright red urine is a sign of haematuria, or blood in the urine. When the bleeding occurs during elimination, it can indicate the location of the underlying problem. For example a urethral disorder will cause bleeding at the onset of urination. Bleeding at the end of the stream suggests a disorder of the bladder neck or prostate gland.

From the neck up

Bleeding throughout urination indicates a disorder located above the bladder neck. Haematuria can also be caused by gastrointestinal (GI), vaginal or some coagulation disorders or cancer.

Only temporary

In addition, males may experience haematuria temporarily following urinary tract or prostate surgery or after a urethral catheterisation.

Nocturia

Excessive urination at night, known as nocturia, is a common sign of kidney or lower urinary tract disorders. It can result from a disruption of normal urine patterns or overstimulation of the nerves and muscles that control urination. Cardiovascular, endocrine or metabolic disorders; diuretics; and increased fluid intake can also produce nocturia.

In men, nocturia can result from benign prostatic hyperplasia (BPH), when significant urethral obstruction develops, or from prostate cancer.

Polyuria

Polyuria is the production and excretion of more than 2,500 ml of urine per day. It's a fairly common condition that's usually a result of diabetes insipidus, diabetes mellitus or diuretic use. Other causes of polyuria include urologic disorders, such as pyelonephritis and post-obstructive uropathy, and some psychological, neurologic and renal disorders. Patients with polyuria are at risk for developing hypovolaemia.

Urinary frequency, urgency and hesitancy

Urinary frequency commonly results from decreased bladder capacity and is a classic symptom of a UTI. Frequency also occurs with urethral stricture, neurologic disorders, pregnancy and uterine tumours.

In men, urinary frequency also occurs with BPH, urethral stricture or a prostate tumour, all of which can put pressure on the bladder.

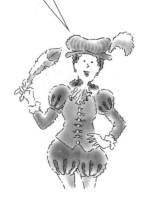

It's a classic! Urinary frequency is a classic symptom of a UTI.

Pain picture

The sudden urge to urinate, or urinary urgency, when accompanied by bladder pain is another symptom of a UTI. Even small amounts of urine in the bladder can cause pain because inflammation decreases bladder capacity. Urgency without pain may be a symptom of an upper motor neuron lesion.

Start 'er up?

Difficulty starting a urine stream, or urinary hesitancy, can occur with a UTI, a partial obstruction of the lower urinary tract, neuromuscular disorders or the use of certain drugs.

Stalling

Urinary hesitancy is most common in older male patients with an enlarged prostate gland, which can cause partial obstruction of the urethra.

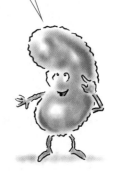

What to do, what to do! I just can't decide if I want to go or not.

Urinary incontinence

Urinary incontinence is a common condition that may be transient or permanent with a minimal or significant release of urine. Possible causes include stress incontinence, tumour, bladder cancer and calculi, and such neurologic disorders as Guillain–Barré syndrome, multiple sclerosis and spinal cord injury.

In men, urinary incontinence may also be a symptom of BPH, prostate infection, or prostate cancer.

Nursing interventions for altered urinary elimination

Nursing interventions for altered urinary elimination include bedpan and urinal use, collecting urine specimens, applying a penile sheath, and insertion, care and removal of an indwelling urinary catheter.

Bedpan and urinal use

Patients should always be taken to the toilet where possible; this will afford them privacy and maintain their dignity. Some patients may need to stay by the bedside but they can still use a commode, as this is a more natural position. However, bedpans and urinals permit elimination by a bedridden patient and provide a way to accurately observe and measure urine and stool. A female patient can use a bedpan for urination and defecation. A male patient normally uses a urinal for urination and a bedpan for defecation. Be sure to offer these devices frequently, before meals, visiting hours, morning and evening care and treatments or procedures. Always allow the patient their privacy and offer them hand-washing facilities afterwards.

What you need
Regular bedpan or 'slipper' pan, or urinal with cover ✳ toilet tissue ✳ gloves ✳ apron ✳ towel ✳ absorbent pad ✳ pillow ✳ hand-washing facilities

Big and little
Bedpans are available in adult and paediatric sizes, disposable and reusable (must be sterilised) models. The slipper pan, a type of bedpan, is used when spinal injuries, body or leg casts, or other conditions prohibit or restrict turning the patient.

Getting ready
- Obtain the appropriate bedpan or urinal.
- If you're using a metal bedpan, warm it under running water to avoid startling the patient and stimulating muscle contraction, which hinders elimination.
- Dry the bedpan thoroughly and test its temperature.
- If necessary, sprinkle talcum powder on the edge of the bedpan to reduce friction during placement and removal.
- For a thin patient, place a pad at the edge of the bedpan or use a slipper pan to minimise pressure on the coccyx.

How you do it
- Always provide privacy.
- Put on gloves and apron to prevent contact with body fluids and comply with standard precautions.

Placing a bedpan
• If allowed, elevate the head of the bed slightly to prevent hyperextension of the spine when the s raise their buttocks.
• Rest the bedpan on the edge of the bed. Then turn down the corner of the bedclothes and draw up the patient's gown. Ask them to raise their buttocks by flexing the knees and pushing down on the heels. While supporting the patient's lower back with one hand, centre the curved, smooth edge of the bedpan beneath their buttocks.
• If the patient can't raise their buttocks, lower the head of the bed to the horizontal position and help the patient roll onto one side with the buttocks towards you. Position the bedpan properly against the buttocks, and then help the patient roll back onto the bedpan. When the patient is positioned comfortably, raise the head of the bed as indicated.

Position is everything

• After positioning the bedpan, elevate the head of the bed further, if allowed, until the patient is sitting erect. This position aids in defecation and urination.
• If elevation of the head of the bed is contraindicated, tuck a small pillow or folded bath blanket under the patient's back to cushion the sacrum against the edge of the bedpan and support the lumbar region.
• If the patient can be left alone, place the bed in a low position and raise the side rails to ensure their safety. Place toilet tissue and the call button within the patient's reach, and instruct them to press the call bell after elimination. If the patient is weak or disoriented, remain with them.
• Before removing the bedpan, lower the head of the bed slightly. Then ask the patient to raise their buttocks off the bed. Support the lower back with one hand, and gently remove the bedpan with the other to avoid skin injury caused by friction. If the patient can't raise their buttocks, ask them to roll off the pan while you assist with one hand. Hold the pan firmly with the other hand to avoid spills. Cover the bedpan and place it on the chair.
• Help clean the anal and perineal area, as necessary, to prevent irritation and infection. Turn the patient on their side, wipe carefully with toilet tissue, clean the area with a damp washcloth and soap, and dry with a towel. Clean a female patient from front to back to avoid introducing rectal contaminants into the vaginal or urethral openings.

Placing a urinal
• Give the urinal to the patient and allow them to position it.
• If the patient can't position the urinal themselves, spread their legs slightly and hold the urinal in place to prevent spills.
• After the patient voids, carefully withdraw the urinal.

After use of a bedpan or urinal
• Provide hand-washing facilities. Check the bed linen for wetness or soiling, and straighten or change them, if needed. Make the patient comfortable. Place the bed in the low position and raise the side rails if required.

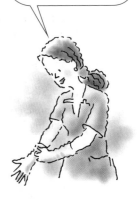

Be sure to put on gloves before performing a procedure where there's a risk of contact with body fluids.

- Observe the colour, odour and consistency of its contents. Measure and record the amount of urine on the fluid balance chart (if required).
- Dispose of the disposable bedpan or urinal following local policy. If using non-disposable equipment, empty the bedpan or urinal into the toilet. Rinse with cold water and clean it thoroughly, following local infection prevention and control policies.
- Remove and discard your gloves and apron. Wash your hands.

Practice pointers

- Explain to the patient that drug treatment and changes in environment, diet, and activities may disrupt their usual elimination schedule. Try to anticipate elimination needs, and offer the bedpan or urinal frequently to help reduce embarrassment and minimise incontinence.
- Avoid placing a bedpan or urinal on top of the bedside locker or bed table to avoid contamination of clean equipment and food trays. Similarly, avoid placing it on the floor to prevent the spread of microorganisms from the floor to the patient's bed linen when the device is used.
- If the patient experiences pain or discomfort on a standard bedpan, use a slipper pan. The slipper pan is slipped under the buttocks from the front rather than the side. It's also shallower than a standard bedpan, so you need to lift the patient only slightly to position it. Ask a colleague to help if the patient is unable to lift onto the bedpan.
- If the patient has an indwelling urinary catheter, carefully position and remove the bedpan to avoid tension on the catheter, which could dislodge it or irritate the urethra. After the patient defecates, wipe, clean and dry the anal region, taking care to avoid catheter contamination. If necessary, clean the urinary meatus with soap and water.
- Avoid leaving the urinal, slipper pan or bedpan in place for extended periods to prevent skin breakdown.

Collecting a random urine specimen

A routine urine specimen is collected as part of the nursing assessment or at various times during hospitalisation. It is a quick test which can detect urinary and systemic disorders, it helps to determine whether a more detailed laboratory screening is needed.

What you need

Bedpan ✳ fracture pan or urinal with cover

Getting ready

- Tell the patient that a urine specimen is needed for analysis.
- Explain the procedure to the patient to promote cooperation and prevent accidental disposal of specimens.

How you do it

- Provide privacy. Instruct the patient on bed rest to void into a clean bedpan or urinal, or ask the ambulatory patient to void into either one in the bathroom.

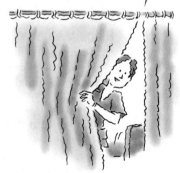

It's important to maintain a patient's dignity by providing them with as much privacy as their condition allows.

Pour, record, discard

- Put on gloves and apron.
- Observe urine for smell, colour and clarity.
- Immerse all pads on the reagent strip and remove immediately.
- Remove any excess urine by running the strip along the side of the container.
- Hold the strip horizontally to prevent the colours running, and compare the colours against the colour chart on the bottle.
- Dispose off urine; remove gloves and apron.
- Wash hands to prevent cross-contamination.
- Record the results in the patient's records. (See *Documenting urine specimen collection*.)

Practice pointers

- Be sure to test the specimen immediately, or within 4 hours, because delays may alter test results.
- The specimen can be placed in a refrigerator, but it is important to let it reach room temperature before testing it.

Urine specific gravity

Urine specific gravity is determined by comparing the weight of a urine specimen with the weight of an equivalent volume of distilled water, which is 1.000. Because urine contains dissolved salts and other substances, it's heavier than 1.000. Urine specific gravity ranges from 1.003 (very dilute) to 1.035 (highly concentrated); normal values range from 1.010 to 1.025.

High and low

Elevated specific gravity reflects an increased concentration of urine solutes, which occurs in conditions that cause renal hypoperfusion, and may indicate heart failure, dehydration, hepatic disorders or nephrosis. Low specific gravity reflects failure to reabsorb water and concentrate urine. It may indicate hypercalcemia, hypokalemia, alkalosis, acute renal failure, pyelonephritis, glomerulonephritis or diabetes insipidus.

Applying a penile sheath

Many patients don't require an indwelling urinary catheter to manage incontinence. For male patients, a penile sheath reduces the risk of a UTI associated with catheterisation. It also promotes bladder retraining when possible, helps prevent skin breakdown and maintains the patient's self-image.

A penile sheath is secured to the shaft of the penis and connected to a leg bag or drainage bag. It can cause skin irritation and oedema.

What you need

Penile sheath ✳ urinary drainage bag ✳ adhesive strip ✳ gloves ✳ apron ✳ bowl ✳ warm water ✳ towel or wipes

Take note!

Documenting urine specimen collection

Be sure to record the times of urine specimen collection. Record abnormal results as well as the specific gravity, pH, odour, colour and unusual characteristics of the specimen. If necessary, record urine volume in the intake and output record.

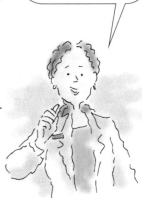

A urinary sheath reduces the risk of a UTI associated with catheterisation.

Getting ready
- Explain the procedure to the patient and gain consent.
- Bring the equipment to the bedside.
- Ensure privacy and dignity is maintained.

How you do it
- Wash your hands thoroughly; put on gloves and apron.

Applying the device
- If the patient is circumcised, wash the penis with soap and water, rinse well and pat dry with a towel. If the patient isn't circumcised, gently retract the foreskin, and clean beneath it. Rinse well and dry. Replace the foreskin to avoid penile constriction.
- If necessary, trim the pubic hair at the base and shaft of the penis to prevent the adhesive strip from pulling pubic hair.

Making it stick
- If you're using a pre-cut commercial adhesive strip, insert the glans penis through its opening, and position the strip 2.5 cm from the scrotal area. If you're using uncut adhesive, cut a strip to fit around the shaft of the penis. Remove the protective covering from one side of the adhesive strip and press this side firmly to the penis to enhance adhesion. Remove the covering from the other side of the strip.

Positioning the catheter
- Position the rolled condom catheter at the tip of the penis, with its drainage opening at the urinary meatus. Allow 2.5 to 5 cm of space at the tip of the penis to prevent erosion and to allow for expansion when the patient voids.
- Unroll the catheter upwards, past the adhesive strip on the shaft of the penis. Then gently press the sheath against the strip until it adheres. (See *How to apply a penile sheath*.)
- After the penile sheath is in place, secure it with hypoallergenic tape or an incontinence sheath holder.
- Connect the penile sheath to the leg bag or drainage bag. Remove and discard your gloves. Wash your hands.
- Change the penile sheath every day to protect the patient's skin and prevent UTIs.

Removing the device
- Put on gloves and apron. Simultaneously roll the penile sheath and adhesive strip off the penis and discard them.
- Clean the penis with lukewarm water, rinse thoroughly and dry. Check for swelling or signs of skin breakdown.
- Remove the urinary drainage bag closing the drain clamp.
- Discard your gloves and wash your hands.

How to apply a penile sheath

Apply an adhesive strip to the shaft of the penis about 2.5 cm from the scrotal area.

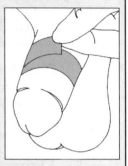

Then roll the penile sheath on to the penis past the adhesive strip, leaving about 1.3 cm clearance at the end. Press the sheath gently against the strip until it adheres.

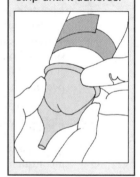

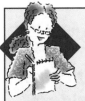

Male catheterisation

Important!

Catheterisation is a skilled procedure and should only be undertaken by trained and competent health-care workers.

Male catheterisation requires additional training.

Practice pointers

- Select the correct size sheath; different lengths and diameters are available. Too small will cause discomfort and too large will allow urine to leak out.
- Apply the adhesive strip snugly; however, make sure that it isn't too tight to avoid circulatory constriction.
- Inspect the penile sheath for twists and the tubing for kinks to prevent obstruction of urine flow, which could cause the sheath to balloon and eventually dislodge.

Inserting an indwelling urinary catheter

An indwelling urinary catheter, also called a Foley, or retention, catheter, provides the patient with continuous urine drainage. It's inserted into the bladder and a balloon is inflated at the catheter's distal end to prevent it from slipping out. Insert the catheter with extreme care to prevent injury and infection.

What you need

Catheterisation pack ✳ sterile indwelling catheter (latex or silicone, Ch6 to Ch8 for children up to Ch30 [average adult size: Ch12 to Ch14]) ✳ syringe filled with 10 ml of sterile water (normally included with the catheter) ✳ sterile 0.9% sodium chloride solution ✳ absorbent pad ✳ sterile gloves ✳ gloves ✳ sterile anaesthetic gel ✳ sterile drainage collection bag ✳ fluid balance chart ✳ light source ✳ catheter stand

In case of contamination

Have an extra pair of sterile gloves and two appropriate-size catheters available at the bedside in case of contamination during insertion.

Getting ready

- Check the patient's identity.
- Explain the procedure to the patient and gain consent.

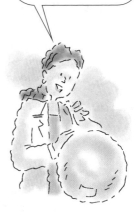

A Foley catheter has a balloon at the distal end to prevent it from slipping out. That's handy!

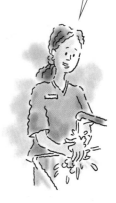

It's important to wash your hands before and after performing a procedure.

- Wash your hands.
- Select the appropriate equipment and assemble it at the patient's bedside.

How you do it
- Strict aseptic technique is needed.
- Provide privacy. Check the patient's chart and ask when they voided last. Percuss and palpate the bladder to establish baseline data. (Some areas now use a bladder scan, you must be trained and assessed as competent to use these.)
- Have a second nurse to hold a light so you can see the urinary meatus clearly.

Assume the position

- Place the female patient in the supine position, with her knees flexed and separated and her feet flat on the bed, about 61 cm apart. If this position is uncomfortable, have her flex one knee and keep the other leg flat on the bed. (See *Positioning the elderly female*.)

Sterile fieldwork

- Put on apron.
- Place the absorbent pad on the bed between the patient's legs and under the hips.
- Open the catheterisation pack careful not to touch the sterile field.
- Carefully tip onto the sterile field the anaesthetic gel, catheter (do not remove this from the inner package), and sterile gloves.
- Open the urinary drainage bag, make sure that all tubing ends remain sterile and that the clamp at the emptying port of the drainage bag is closed to prevent urine leakage from the bag.
- Pour in the sterile sodium chloride solution into the galipot.
- Put on the sterile gloves.
- Separate the labia majora and labia minora as widely as possible with the thumb, middle and index fingers of your non-dominant hand so you have a full view of the urinary meatus. Keep the labia well separated throughout the

Ages and stages

Positioning the elderly female

The elderly female patient may need pillows or rolled towels or blankets for positioning support. If necessary, ask her to lie on her side with one knee drawn up to her chest during catheterisation (as shown here). This position may also be helpful for a disabled patient.

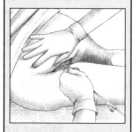

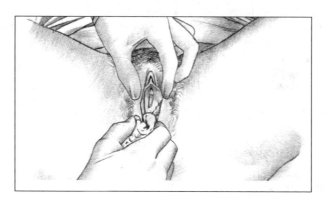

Preventing indwelling catheter problems

These precautions can help prevent problems with an indwelling urinary catheter:

- Never force the catheter during insertion. Instead, manoeuvre it gently as the patient bears down or coughs. If you still meet resistance, stop and notify the doctor. Sphincter spasms, strictures, misplacement in the vagina (in females) or an enlarged prostate (in males) may cause resistance.
- Establish urine flow, and then inflate the balloon to ensure that the catheter is in the bladder.

More helpful hints

Observe the patient carefully for hypovolemic shock and other adverse reactions caused by removing excessive volumes of residual urine. Check your Trust's policy in advance to determine the maximum amount of urine that may be drained at one time; some facilities limit the amount to 1,000 ml. (Be aware, however, that controversy exists over the wisdom of limiting the amount of urine drainage.) Clamp the catheter at the first sign of an adverse reaction, and notify the doctor.

---

procedure so they don't obscure the urinary meatus or contaminate the area when it's cleaned.
- With your dominant hand, wipe one side of the urinary meatus with a single downward motion (as shown here). Similarly, wipe the other side with another cotton ball. Then wipe directly over the meatus with still another cotton ball.
- Where local policy indicates use of anaesthetic gel, insert the gel into the urethra and allow time for the anaesthetic properties to work (as per manufacturer's advice.)

Advanced class

- For the female patient, advance the catheter 5.1 to 7.5 cm—while continuing to hold the labia apart—until urine begins to flow (as shown in this illustration). If the catheter is inadvertently inserted into the vagina, leave it there as a landmark. Then begin the procedure again using new supplies.

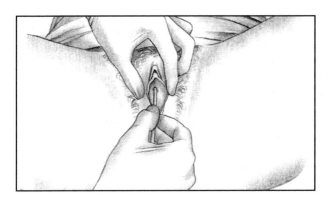

Inflate, hang and secure

- When urine stops flowing, attach the filled syringe to the luer-lock.
- Push the plunger and inflate the balloon to keep the catheter in place in the bladder.
- Hang the collection bag below bladder level to prevent urine reflux into the bladder, which can cause infection, and to promote gravity drainage of the bladder. Make sure that the tubing doesn't get tangled in the bed's side rails.
- Secure catheter to prevent it from causing trauma to the urethra.
- Dispose of all used supplies properly. Remove apron and wash your hands.

Practice pointers

- The balloon size determines the amount of solution needed for inflation. The exact amount is usually printed on the distal extension of the catheter used for inflating the balloon.
- Empty the collection bag to prevent excessive fluid volume to prevent traction on the catheter wall. (See *Documenting indwelling catheter insertion*.)
- Most drainage bags have a plastic clamp on the tubing to attach them to the sheet; this will help prevent pulling of the tube.

Indwelling catheter care and removal

When performed, catheter care is completed after the patient's morning bath, immediately after perineal care. When the patient's condition warrants catheter removal, you must also remove the indwelling catheter.

Catheter care

NICE (2003) recommend that the daily washing of the genital area with soap and water is all that is required, this will ensure any secretions will be removed, therefore lessen the risk of infection. Many patients will be able to do this for themselves but for patients who cannot, care must be undertaken in a sensitive way so not to embarrass the patient.

Wipe away

- Put on gloves and apron. Use disposable wipes, soap and water to clean the outside of the catheter and the tissue around the meatus. To avoid contaminating the urinary tract, always clean by wiping away from—never towards—the urinary meatus. Remove encrusted material. Don't pull on the catheter while you're cleaning it. Doing so can injure the urethra and the bladder wall. What's more, it can expose a section of the catheter that was inside the urethra and, when you release the catheter, the newly contaminated section will re-enter the urethra, introducing potentially infectious organisms.
- Remove your gloves and apron. Wash your hands.

 Take note!

Documenting indwelling catheter insertion

If your patient has an indwelling catheter, be sure to record:

- date and time of catheter insertion
- size and type of catheter used
- amount, colour and other characteristics of urine drainage
- patient's tolerance of the procedure (if large volumes of urine were drained)
- whether a urine specimen was sent for laboratory analysis
- output on the fluid balance chart.

For catheter removal
Gloves ✳ apron ✳ 10-ml syringe, or larger if necessary ✳ absorbent pad ✳ receiver ✳ clinical waste bag

Getting ready
- Explain the procedure to the patient and provide privacy.
- Put on apron and wash your hands and bring all equipment to the patient's bedside.

How you do it
Catheter removal
- Place absorbent pad underneath the buttocks.
- Position the patient with legs apart to allow easier of removal of the catheter.
- Place receiver between the legs.
- Attach the syringe into the port of the catheter and allow the water from the balloon to fill the syringe.
- Gently pull the catheter out and place in the receiver.
- Dispose of all equipment; remove gloves and apron; and wash your hands.
- Ensure patient is comfortable.
- Record time of removal and amount of urine in the drainage bag. (See *Documenting indwelling catheter care and removal*.)

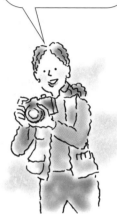

Adequate lighting isn't just important for photography. It's also essential for proper indwelling catheter care.

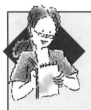

Take note!

Documenting indwelling catheter care and removal

When providing care for a patient with an indwelling catheter, be sure to record:

- care you performed
- patient comfort
- condition of the perineum and urinary meatus
- characteristics of urine in the drainage bag
- whether a specimen was sent for laboratory analysis
- fluid intake and output. (Usually, an hourly record is required for critically ill patients and haemodynamically unstable patients with renal insufficiency.)

Catheter removal

When removing a catheter, be sure to record:

- date and time of catheter removal
- patient's tolerance of the procedure
- when and how much the patient voided after removal (usually for first 24 hours)
- associated problems.

Stay low

Practice pointers

• Avoid raising the drainage bag above bladder level to prevent urine reflux, which may contain bacteria.
• If the patient will be discharged with an indwelling catheter, teach them how to care for the catheter and how to empty the drainage bag.

Collecting urine from an indwelling catheter

Obtain an indwelling catheter specimen of urine (CSU) by aspirating a specimen of urine from the port on the drainage bag, this can be done with a needle and syringe or just a syringe, depending upon the manufacturer. Both procedures require sterile collection technique to prevent catheter contamination and risk of a UTI.

What you need

Gloves ✳ apron ✳ alcohol swab ✳ 10-ml syringe ✳ 21G needle ✳ sterile specimen container with lid ✳ label ✳ laboratory request form

How you do it

• Put on gloves and apron. The drainage tube has a built-in sampling port near the connection to the catheter, wipe the port with an alcohol pad and allow to dry. Some ports require a needle to be used to draw out the urine while newer ones have needleless ports, which only need the syringe to be attached. If a needle is required, attach the needle on the syringe and insert the needle into the sampling port at a 45-degree angle to the tubing. Aspirate the specimen into the syringe. (See *Aspirating a urine specimen.*)

> Please note! Specimens must not be collected directly from the drainage bag as this will be contaminated.

> Don't forget to unclamp the drainage tube after collecting urine.

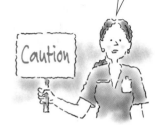

Aspirating a urine specimen

To aspirate a urine specimen when the patient has an indwelling urinary catheter in place, if there is no urine present in the tube, a clamp can be used. Clamp the tube distal to the aspiration port until sufficient urine is collected. Wipe the port with an alcohol pad, and insert a needle attached to a 10-ml syringe into the port perpendicular to the tube. Aspirate the required amount of urine, and expel it into the specimen container. Follow the same procedure for a needleless port by attaching the syringe directly into the port. Remove the clamp on the drainage tube.

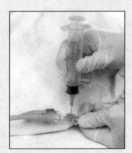

Practice pointers
- Never clamp the catheter because doing so may cause damage to it.
- Make sure that you unclamp the drainage tube after collecting the specimen to prevent urine backflow, which may cause bladder distension and infection.
- Never disconnect the catheter from the drainage bag to obtain a urine sample, this will increase the risk of urine infection.
- Never take a urine sample from the drainage bag.
- Transfer the specimen to a sterile container, label it with patient's full details, and send it to the laboratory immediately. If a urine culture is ordered, include a list of current antibiotic therapy on the laboratory request form.

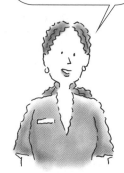

Collecting urine can be easy and safe if you follow the proper steps!

Quick quiz

1. A patient complains of lower abdominal pressure, and you note a firm mass extending above the symphysis pubis. You suspect:
    A. distended bladder.
    B. enlarged kidney.
    C. UTI.
    D. inflamed ovary.

Answer: A. The bladder is usually non-palpable unless it's distended. The feeling of pressure is usually relieved with urination.

2. Although the male and female urinary systems function in the same way, there's a difference in the length of the:
    A. bladder neck.
    B. ureter.
    C. epididymis.
    D. urethra.

Answer: D. Because a man's urethra passes through the erectile tissue of the penis, it's about 15.2 cm longer than a woman's urethra.

3. In a healthy adult, what's the normal range of bladder capacity?
    A. 50 to 100 ml
    B. 200 to 300 ml
    C. 500 to 600 ml
    D. 700 to 900 ml

Answer: C. In a healthy adult, bladder capacity ranges from 500 to 600 ml.

4. The left ureter is slightly longer than the right ureter because the:
    A. left kidney is higher than the right.
    B. right kidney is higher than the left.
    C. left kidney performs more functions.
    D. left ureter has a three-layered wall.

Answer: A. The left kidney is slighter higher than the right kidney. Therefore, the left ureter needs to be longer to reach the bladder.

Scoring

☆☆☆ If you answered all four questions correctly, sensational! You're as smooth as a perfect indwelling catheter removal.

☆☆ If you answered three questions correctly, great! You've got a great capacity for knowledge.

☆ If you answered fewer than three questions correctly, don't worry. Review the chapter, and you'll begin to filter all the important facts!

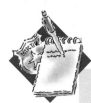

20 Bowel elimination

Just the facts

In this chapter, you'll learn:

♦ organs and structures that make up the gastro-intestinal (GI) system

♦ causes and characteristics of abnormalities in the GI system

♦ factors that affect bowel elimination

♦ abnormalities of bowel elimination

♦ methods for obtaining a stool specimen

♦ proper way to administer an enema

♦ proper colostomy and ileostomy care.

A look at the GI system

The GI system consists of two major divisions: the GI tract and the accessory organs.

GI tract

The GI tract, also called the *alimentary canal*, is a hollow tube that begins at the mouth and ends at the anus. It consists of smooth muscle alternating with blood vessels and nerve tissues. About 7.5 m long, the GI tract includes the pharynx, oesophagus, stomach, small intestine and large intestine.

Open wide

Digestion begins in the mouth with chewing, salivating and swallowing. Three pairs of glands, the parotid, sub-mandibular and sub-lingual, produce saliva. The tongue provides the sense of taste.

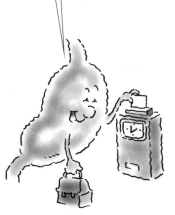

I couldn't do my job without my colleagues—the pharynx, the oesophagus and the small and large intestines.

Proceed to the pharynx

The pharynx, or throat, allows the passage of food from the mouth to the oesophagus. It assists in swallowing and secretes mucus that aids in digestion. The epiglottis, a thin, leaf-shaped structure made of fibrocartilage, is directly behind the root of the tongue. When food is swallowed, the epiglottis closes over the larynx and the soft palate lifts to block the nasal cavity, preventing food and fluid from aspirating into the airway.

Down the oesophagus

The oesophagus is a muscular, hollow tube about 25.5 cm long that moves food from the pharynx to the stomach. When food is swallowed, the upper oesophageal sphincter relaxes and the food moves into the oesophagus. Specialised circular and longitudinal fibres contract, causing peristalsis, which propels food through the GI tract towards the stomach. The gastroesophageal sphincter at the lower end of the oesophagus remains closed to prevent the reflux of gastric contents.

Sitting in the stomach

The stomach is a dilated, saclike structure that serves as a reservoir for food. It lies obliquely in the left upper quadrant below the oesophagus and diaphragm, to the right of the spleen, and partially under the liver. The stomach contains two important sphincters: the cardiac sphincter, which protects the entrance to the stomach, and the pyloric sphincter, which guards the exit.

The stomach has three major functions:

stores food

mixes food with gastric juices (hydrochloric acid [HCl])

passes chyme—a watery mixture of partly digested food and digestive juices—into the small intestine for further digestion and absorption.

Expands to size

Accordion-like folds in the stomach lining, called *rugae*, allow the stomach to expand when large amounts of food and fluid are ingested.

Slipping through the small intestine

The small intestine is about 6.1 m long. Named for its diameter, not its length, it consists of the duodenum, the jejunum and the ileum. As chyme passes into the small intestine, the end products of digestion are absorbed through its thin mucous membrane lining into the bloodstream.

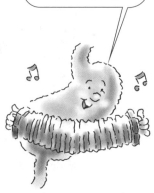

Large amounts of food are like music to my rugae!

Leaping through the large intestine

The large intestine, or colon, is about 1.5 m long. Its main functions are:
- absorbing excess water and electrolytes
- storing food residue
- eliminating waste products in the form of faeces.

The large intestine includes the caecum; the ascending, transverse, descending and sigmoid colons; the rectum; and the anus—in that order. The appendix, a finger-like projection, is attached to the caecum. Bacteria in the colon produce gas, or flatus.

Accessory organs

Accessory GI organs include the liver, pancreas, gall bladder and bile ducts. The abdominal aorta and the gastric and splenic veins also aid the GI system.

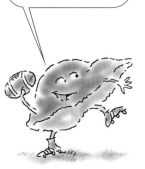

I'm a key player when it comes to digesting fats and absorbing fatty acids.

Spotting the liver

The liver is located in the right upper quadrant under the diaphragm, and is the heaviest organ in the body, weighing about 1.4 kg in a healthy adult. It's divided into two major lobes by the falciform ligament.

The liver's functions include:
- metabolising carbohydrates, fats and proteins
- detoxifying blood
- converting ammonia to urea for excretion
- synthesising plasma proteins, non-essential amino acids, vitamin A and essential nutrients, such as iron and vitamins D, K and B$_{12}$.

Believe in bile

The liver also secretes bile, a greenish fluid that helps digest fats and absorb fatty acids, cholesterol and other lipids.

Gaping at the gall bladder

The gall bladder is a small, pear-shaped organ about 10 cm long that lies halfway under the right lobe of the liver. Its main function is to store bile. The small intestine initiates chemical impulses that cause the gall bladder to contract and empty bile into the duodenum.

Probing the pancreas

The pancreas, which measures 15 to 20.5 cm in length, lies horizontally in the abdomen, behind the stomach. It consists of a head, tail and body. The body of the pancreas is located in the right upper quadrant and the tail is in the left upper quadrant, attached to the duodenum.

The pancreas releases insulin and glycogen into the bloodstream and produces pancreatic enzymes that are released into the duodenum for digestion.

Beholding the bile ducts

The bile ducts provide passageways for bile to travel from the liver to the intestines. Two hepatic ducts drain the liver and the cystic duct drains the gall bladder. These ducts converge into the common bile duct, which then empties into the duodenum.

Visualising the vascular structures

The abdominal aorta supplies blood to the GI tract. It enters the abdomen, separates into the common iliac arteries and branches into many arteries that extend the length of the GI tract.

The gastric and splenic veins drain absorbed nutrients into the portal vein of the liver. After entering the liver, the venous blood circulates and exits the liver through the hepatic vein, emptying into the inferior vena cava.

Digestion and elimination

Digestion starts in the oral cavity, where chewing (mastication), salivation (the beginning of starch digestion) and swallowing (deglutition) all take place. When a patient swallows, the hypopharyngeal sphincter in the upper oesophagus relaxes, allowing food to enter the oesophagus.

Long day's journey into the stomach

In the oesophagus, the glossopharyngeal nerve activates peristalsis, which moves food down—towards the stomach. As food passes through the oesophagus, glands in the oesophageal mucosa layer secrete mucus, which lubricates the bolus and protects the mucosal membrane from damage caused by poorly chewed food.

> Fill and empty. Fill and empty. Do I ever get a break?

Stomach emptying

Food can remain in the stomach for 3 to 4 hours. The rate of stomach emptying depends on gastrin release; neural signals generated when the stomach wall distends, and the enterogastric reflex. This reflex causes the duodenum to release secretin and gastric-inhibiting peptide and the jejunum to secrete cholecystokinin, both of which decrease gastric motility.

Small intestine

Nearly all digestion and absorption takes place in the small intestine. (See *Small intestine: How form affects absorption.*)

Small but mighty

In the small intestine, intestinal contractions and various digestive secretions break down carbohydrates, proteins and fats, actions that enable the

Small intestine: How form affects absorption

Nearly all digestion and absorption take place in the 6.1 m of small intestine. The structure of the small intestine, as shown here, is key to digestion and absorption.

Specialised mucosa

Multiple projections of the intestinal mucosa increase the surface area for absorption several hundredfold, as shown in the enlarged views.

Circular projections (Kerckring's folds) are covered by villi. Each villus contains a lymphatic vessel (lacteal), a venule, capillaries, an arteriole, nerve fibres and smooth muscle.

Each villus is densely fringed with about 2,000 microvilli, making it resemble a fine brush. The villi are lined with columnar epithelial cells, which dip into the lamina propria between the villi to form intestinal glands (crypts of Lieberkühn).

Types of epithelial cells

The type of epithelial cell dictates its function:
- Mucus-secreting *goblet cells* are found on and between the villi on the crypt mucosa.
- Specialised *Brunner's glands* in the proximal duodenum also secrete large amounts of mucus to lubricate and protect the duodenum from potentially corrosive acidic chyme and gastric juices.
- Duodenal *argentaffin cells* produce the hormones secretin and cholecystokinin.
- *Undifferentiated cells* deep within the intestinal glands replace the epithelium.
- *Absorptive cells* consist of large numbers of tightly packed microvilli over a plasma membrane that contains transport mechanisms for absorption and produces enzymes for the final step in digestion.

Intestinal glands

The intestinal glands primarily secrete a watery fluid that bathes the villi with chyme particles. Fluid production results from local irritation of nerve cells and, possibly, from hormonal stimulation by secretin and cholecystokinin. The microvillous brush border secretes various hormones and digestive enzymes that catalyse final nutrient breakdown.

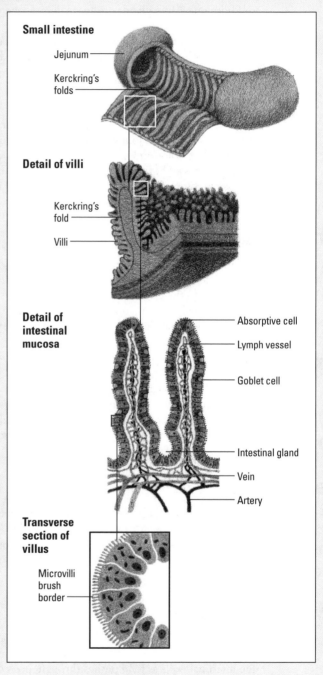

Small intestine
Jejunum
Kerckring's folds

Detail of villi
Kerckring's fold
Villi

Detail of intestinal mucosa
Absorptive cell
Lymph vessel
Goblet cell
Intestinal gland
Vein
Artery

Transverse section of villus
Microvilli brush border

intestinal mucosa to absorb these nutrients into the bloodstream (along with water and electrolytes) for use by the body. Pancreatic enzymes, bile and hormones from glands of the small intestine mix with chyme and aid in digestion.

By the time the chyme passes through the small intestine and enters the ascending colon of the large intestine, it's reduced to mostly indigestible substances.

Large intestine

The food bolus begins its journey through the large intestine where the ileum and the caecum join with the ileocaecal pouch. The bolus moves up the ascending colon and past the right abdominal cavity to the liver's lower border. It crosses horizontally below the liver and stomach, by way of the transverse colon and descends the left abdominal cavity to the iliac fossa through the descending colon.

The journey continues

From there, the bolus travels through the sigmoid colon to the lower midline of the abdominal cavity, then to the rectum and finally to the anal canal. The anus opens to the exterior through two sphincters. The internal sphincter contains thick, circular smooth muscle under autonomic control; the external sphincter contains skeletal muscle under voluntary control.

Super absorption

The large intestine doesn't produce hormones or enzymes. It continues the absorption process through blood and lymph vessels in its sub-mucosa. The proximal half of the large intestine absorbs all but about 100 ml of the remaining water in the colon. It also absorbs large amounts of sodium and chloride.

Bacteria in action

The large intestine harbours the bacteria *Escherichia coli*, *Enterobacter aerogenes*, *Clostridium perfringens* and *Lactobacillus bifidus*. These bacteria help synthesise vitamin K and break down cellulose into usable carbohydrates. Bacterial action also produces flatus, which helps propel stool towards the rectum.

Mucosa on a mission

In addition, the mucosa of the large intestine produces alkaline secretions from tubular glands composed of goblet cells. This alkaline mucus lubricates the intestinal walls as food pushes through, protecting the mucosa from acidic bacterial action.

Mass movement

In the lower colon, long and relatively sluggish contractions cause propulsive waves, or mass movements. These movements occur several times per day and propel intestinal contents into the rectum, producing the urge to defecate.

Defecation normally results from the defecation reflex, a sensory and parasympathetic nerve-mediated response, along with voluntary relaxation of the external anal sphincter. (See *GI changes with aging*.)

> Watch out for those propulsive waves.

Characteristics of normal stool

Stool is 25% solids and 75% water. The solids consist of bacteria, undigested fibre, fat, inorganic matter and some protein.

Bili Brown

The chemical conversion of bilirubin produces the brown colour of stool. Certain foods and medications can alter stool's colour. Beets will turn stool to a reddish colour, and medications, such as iron taken orally, can discolour stool. Stool colour can also be indicative of certain medical conditions. White or clay-coloured stools, for example, can signal a malabsorption disorder or a blockage in the liver or biliary system.

Pardon my odour!

Bacterial decomposition of protein in the solids produces stool's characteristic, unpleasant odour.

Ages and stages

GI changes with aging

The physiologic changes that accompany aging usually prove less debilitating in the GI system than in most other body systems. Normal changes include diminished mucosal elasticity and reduced GI secretions that, in turn, modify some processes, for example digestion and absorption. GI tract motility, bowel wall and anal sphincter tone and abdominal muscle strength may also decrease with age. Any of these changes may cause complaints in an older patient, ranging from loss of appetite to constipation.

Changes in the oral cavity also occur. Tooth enamel wears away, leaving the teeth prone to cavities.

Periodontal disease increases and the number of taste buds declines. The sense of smell diminishes and salivary gland secretion decreases, leading to appetite loss.

Liver changes

Normal physiologic changes in the liver include decreased liver weight, reduced regenerative capacity, and decreased blood flow to the liver. Because liver enzymes involved in oxidation and reduction markedly decline with age, the liver metabolises drugs and detoxifies substances less efficiently.

Let's get in shape

Stool normally has a soft consistency and a cylindrical form that mimics the shape of the rectum. Thin and ribbon-like stools may be a result of internal haemorrhoids or are a warning sign of colorectal cancer.

Different strokes for different folks

Each patient's elimination pattern differs. The frequency of bowel movements can range from one or two bowel movements per day to one bowel movement every 2 or 3 days. If dietary fibre intake is reduced, fewer stools will be produced.

Bacterial decomposition of protein in the solids produces stool's characteristic, unpleasant odour.

Factors affecting bowel elimination

Many factors affect bowel elimination including body position, exercise and activity, faecal diversion, fluid intake, ignoring the urge to defecate, lifestyle, medications, nutrition and surgery.

Body position

Semi-squatting or sitting is the most conducive position for having a bowel movement because it allows gravity to aid in stool movement. It also promotes contraction of the abdominal and pelvic muscles that are used during bowel elimination. A patient who uses a bedpan while they are flat in bed may have difficulty having a bowel movement.

Exercise and activity

Good muscle tone and regular exercise facilitates peristalsis and aids in bowel elimination. Abdominal and pelvic muscles create the intra-abdominal pressure needed to have a bowel movement. Lack of or reduced physical activity can increase the chances of developing constipation. Also, loss of neurologic control due to illness or trauma will impair muscle tone.

Faecal diversion

Faecal diversion is the creation of an alternate route for bowel elimination. This procedure removes all or part of the colon, rectum and anus. An alternative exit site, called a *stoma*, is created that redirects a portion of the remaining bowel through the abdominal wall to a spot on the abdomen. Faecal diversions may be temporary or permanent and are sometimes performed in a patient with bowel cancer or a bowel obstruction, or to rest the bowel in disorders such as Crohn's disease.

All those ostomies

When a part of the small intestine is redirected through the abdominal wall, it's called an *ileostomy*. *Colostomy* refers to a faecal diversion that brings a portion of the large intestine or colon through the abdominal wall. (See *Reviewing types of ostomies*.)

Fluid intake

Stool is 75% water. If the body doesn't take in enough fluid, the bowel will conserve more water by absorbing it from the stool. Stools then become hard and difficult to pass.

A storage problem

The longer stool remains in the colon, the greater the amount of water absorbed, resulting in hard, dry stool. Conversely, stool that doesn't remain in the colon long enough for water to be absorbed will be watery, resulting in fluid loss.

Reviewing types of ostomies

The appropriate type of ostomy for a patient depends on the patient's condition. Temporary ostomies, such as a double-barrel or loop colostomy, help treat perforated sigmoid diverticulitis and other conditions in which intestinal healing is expected. Permanent colostomy or ileostomy accompanies extensive abdominal surgery such as the removal of a malignant tumour.

Double-barrel colostomy

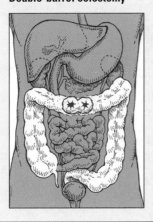

Loop colostomy

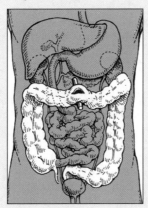

Permanent colostomy

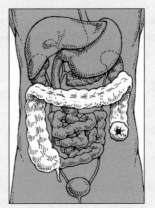

Ileostomy

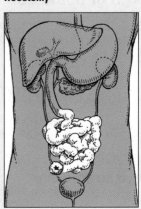

Ignoring the urge to defecate

If the initial reflex urge to defecate is ignored, it subsides in a few minutes. Stool remains in the rectum until another mass movement propels more stool into the rectum, creating another urge. A patient with a chronic condition, such as haemorrhoids, may ignore the urge because of painful bowel movements. Lack of privacy may also cause a patient to ignore the urge to defecate. Ignoring the urge to have a bowel movement can lead to constipation.

Lifestyle

Bowel elimination patterns are commonly part of patients' daily routines and are convenient for their lifestyle. Some patients may be used to waiting until they have the urge to defecate. An early riser may consistently have a bowel movement in the morning, while a patient who works the night shift may have their daily bowel movements in the late afternoon.

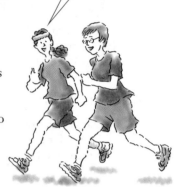

A person's bowel elimination pattern is commonly part of their daily routine and is convenient for their lifestyle.

Here we go—or not

Holidays, changing jobs and strong emotions such as anxiety, anger, fear, depression or excitement can alter bowel habits. Hospitalisation or a disruption in personal relationships can also be stressful enough to alter bowel habits.

Medications

Medications, such as opioids and iron preparations, can cause constipation. Antibiotics can cause diarrhoea. Antacids can cause constipation or diarrhoea.

To go or not to go

Stool softeners and laxatives are normally prescribed to increase stool consistency or bowel elimination. Other medications, such as antidiarrhoeals, are given to decrease stool frequency.

Nutrition

A high fibre diet (20 to 30 g of dietary fibre per day) should produce enough bulk to assist in bowel elimination. Foods high in fibre include fruits, vegetables and cereal grains.

Hard to tolerate

Certain patients may not be able to tolerate lactose (a sugar contained in milk products) or gluten (a protein found in barley, rye, oats and wheat) and should avoid foods containing these substances. If a lactose-intolerant patient eats or drinks milk products, it may cause abdominal distension, gas formation, abdominal cramping and diarrhoea. If a gluten-intolerant patient ingests foods containing gluten, bulky greasy stools, abdominal distension and bloating will likely result.

Surgery

Surgery can significantly impact bowel elimination patterns. A patient who's scheduled for operative procedures is commonly required to restrict food and water intake pre-operatively and post-operatively.

A surgical pause

Anaesthesia slows GI motility for 1 to 2 days following surgery. GI or abdominal surgery may hinder a return of full bowel function for 3 to 4 days. Decreased bowel motility may also result from the bowel's exposure to air and handling during the surgical procedure.

A painless pause

Opioids used to manage pain post-operatively can reduce bowel motility. Fear of pain upon defecation, especially if the patient has an abdominal incision, can also inhibit normal bowel function.

Altered bowel function

Alterations in bowel function include constipation, diarrhoea, distension, faecal impaction, faecal incontinence and flatulence.

Constipation

Constipation is most common in older patients. It can be caused by immobility, a sedentary lifestyle and certain medications. A patient who's constipated may complain of a dull abdominal ache and a full feeling. Hyperactive bowel sounds, which may signal irritable bowel syndrome, are sometimes present. A patient with complete intestinal obstruction won't pass flatus or stool, with an absence of bowel sounds below the obstruction.

Diarrhoea

Toxins, medications or a GI condition, such as Crohn's disease, can result in diarrhoea. Typical symptoms include cramping, abdominal tenderness, anorexia and hyperactive bowel sounds. Diarrhoea accompanied by a fever suggests a toxin as the causative agent.

Distension

Distension may result from gas, a tumour or a colon filled with stool. It can also suggest an incisional hernia, which may protrude when the patient lifts their head and shoulders.

Faecal impaction

Faecal impaction is a large, hard, dry mass of stool in the folds of the rectum or in the sigmoid colon. It's the result of prolonged retention and stool accumulation. Poor bowel habits, inactivity, dehydration, improper diet (especially inadequate fluid intake), the use of constipation-inducing drugs and incomplete bowel cleaning after a barium enema or barium swallow are all possible causes.

Faecal incontinence

Faecal incontinence is the involuntary elimination of faeces from the bowel and may result from watery or loose stool. In an elderly patient, faecal incontinence commonly follows loss or impairment of anal sphincter control.

Flatulence

Flatus is the accumulation of gas in the GI tract resulting from swallowing air, diffusion in the blood and bacterial action in the large intestine. Certain foods, such as cabbage and onions, large amounts of carbonated beverages, smoking and anxiety (which can cause excessive swallowing) can also produce flatus.

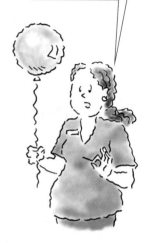

Do you sometimes feel like a balloon ready to pop?

Nursing interventions for bowel elimination

Nursing interventions for bowel elimination include stool specimen collection, testing the stool for occult blood, administering enemas, colostomy or ileostomy care and irrigating a colostomy.

Stool specimen collection

Stool is collected to determine if blood, ova and parasites, bile, fat, pathogens or ingested drugs are present. Stool characteristics, such as colour, consistency and odour, can reveal such conditions as GI bleeding and steatorrhoea.

Random or specific

Stool specimens are collected randomly or for specified periods such as for 72 hours. Proper collection requires careful instructions to the patient to ensure an uncontaminated specimen.

What you need

Specimen container with lid ✳ gloves and apron ✳ tongue blade ✳ paper towel ✳ bedpan or portable commode ✳ laboratory request form

Getting ready

• Inform the patient that a stool specimen is needed for laboratory analysis.
• Explain the procedure to the patient to ensure cooperation and prevent the disposal of timed stool specimens.

How you do it

Collecting a random specimen

• Ask the patient to notify you when they have the urge to defecate. Ask them to defecate into a clean, dry bedpan or portable commode. Instruct them not to contaminate the specimen with urine or toilet tissue because urine inhibits faecal bacterial growth and toilet tissue contains bismuth, which interferes with test results.
• Put on gloves and apron.

Stands out from the crowd

• Using a tongue blade or the spoon incorporated in the specimen container, transfer the most representative stool specimen from the bedpan to the specimen container, and cap the container. If the patient passes blood, mucus or pus with the stool, include this with the specimen.
• Wrap the tongue blade in a paper towel and discard it in the clinical waste. Remove and discard your gloves and apron, and wash your hands thoroughly *to prevent cross-contamination*.

Collecting a timed specimen

• Ensure that all nursing staff are aware on each shift and that it is documented that timed stool collection is in progress.
• After putting on gloves and apron, collect the first specimen, and include it in the total specimen.

Complete transfer

• Obtain the timed specimen as you would a random specimen. Remember to transfer all stool to the specimen container.
• If stool must be obtained with an enema, use only tap water or normal saline solution.
• Send each specimen to the laboratory immediately with a laboratory request form or, if permitted, refrigerate the specimens and send them all

when collection is complete. Remove and discard gloves and apron. Wash your hands.
• Make sure that the patient is comfortable after the procedure and has the opportunity to thoroughly clean their hands and perianal area. Offer assistance if help with perineal care is indicated.

Practice pointers
• Never place a stool specimen in a refrigerator that contains food or medication *to prevent contamination*. (See *Collecting a stool specimen*.)
• Notify the doctor if the stool specimen looks unusual. (See *Documenting stool collection*.)

Assessing stool for occult blood

Faecal occult blood tests are valuable for detecting occult blood (hidden GI bleeding), which may signal colorectal cancer, and can distinguish between true melaena and melaena-like stools. Certain medications, such as iron supplements and bismuth compounds, can darken stools to resemble *melaena*, which is black, tarry stool containing blood.

Look for blue

The Hematest (an orthotolidine reagent tablet) and the Hemoccult slide (filter paper impregnated with guaiac) are two common occult blood-screening tests. Both tests produce a blue reaction in a faecal smear if occult blood loss exceeds 5 ml in 24 hours. A newer test, Colocare, requires no faecal smear. These tests are also performed in the laboratory unless the clinical area has the screening kits available

Repeat three times

To confirm a positive result, the test must be repeated at least three times while the patient follows a meatless, high-residue diet. A positive result doesn't necessarily confirm colorectal cancer, but it does indicate the need for further diagnostic studies. GI bleeding can result from conditions other than cancer, such as ulcers and diverticula.

These tests are easily performed on collected specimens or smears from a digital rectal examination.

Enema administration

Enema administration involves instilling a solution into the rectum and colon. In a retention enema, the patient holds the solution for 30 minutes to 1 hour. In an evacuant enema, the patient expels the solution almost completely within 15 minutes. Both enemas stimulate peristalsis by mechanically distending the colon and stimulating rectal wall nerves.

Teacher's lounge

Collecting a stool specimen

If the patient is to collect a stool specimen at home, instruct them to collect it in a clean container with a tight-fitting lid, to wrap the container in a bag, and to keep it in the refrigerator (separate from food items) until it can be transported.

Take note!

Documenting stool collection

In your notes, be sure to record:

• date and time of specimen collection and transport to the laboratory
• colour, odour and consistency of the stool
• unusual characteristics
• whether the patient had difficulty passing the stool.

Enem-ies

Enemas are contraindicated after a recent colon or rectal surgery or a myocardial infarction and in a patient with an acute abdominal condition of unknown origin such as suspected appendicitis. They also should be administered cautiously to a patient with an arrhythmia.

> Enemas are contraindicated after some surgeries or MIs.

What you need

Patient's medicines administration record (MAR) ✳ prescribed solution ✳ bath thermometer ✳ enema ✳ gloves and apron ✳ absorbent pads ✳ bedpan with cover or bedside commode (if required) ✳ water-soluble lubricant ✳ toilet paper ✳ clinical waste bag ✳ soap and water if patient requires cleaning

Prep package

Pre-packaged disposable enemas are available in evacuant and retention types. (See *Understanding types of enemas.*)

Getting ready
- Check the patient's identity.
- Explain the procedure to the patient and gain verbal consent.
- Provide privacy.
- Wash your hands and bring all equipment to the patient's bedside.
- Prepare the enema as indicated.
- For administration to an adult, warm the solution to a comfortable temperature *to reduce patient discomfort.*

Understanding types of enemas

This chart outlines the preparation steps and purposes of common evacuant and retention enemas.

Solution	Preparation	Purpose
Evacuant enemas		
Phosphate	Single dose disposable enema	Constipation, bowel evacuation prior to surgery and abdominal procedures
Sodium citrate	Single dose disposable enema	Constipation
Retention enemas		
Arachis oil	Single dose disposable enema. *Refer to local policy regarding use, due to peanut allergy*	To soften impacted faeces

Ages and stages

Giving an enema to a child

Ensure that the child understands fully what will happen and that there is another person present to comfort the child, ideally a parent. Unless contraindicated, help the child onto their left side with their right knee bent up. After lubricating the end of the tube, separate the child's buttocks and push the tube gently into the anus, aiming it towards the umbilicus. Insert the tube 5.0 to 7.5 cm (for an infant, insert it 2.5 to 3.5 cm).

Try this solution

Avoid forcing the tube to prevent rectal wall trauma. If it doesn't advance easily, let a little solution flow in to relax the inner sphincter enough to allow passage.

A matter of degree

To avoid burning rectal tissues, don't administer an enema solution that's warmer than 37.8° C.

How you do it
- Check the patient's MAR and the enema.
- Assess the patient's condition.
- Provide privacy. If you're administering an enema to a child, familiarise them with the equipment and allow a parent or another relative to remain with them during the procedure. (See *Giving an enema to a child*.)
- Instruct the patient to breathe through their mouth *to relax the anal sphincter, which will ease insertion.*
- Wash your hands and put on gloves and apron.
- Assist the patient into left-lateral position with right knee bent up *to facilitate the solution's flow into the descending colon.* If contraindicated or if the patient reports discomfort, reposition them on their back or right side.

Prep procedures

- Place absorbent pads under the patient's buttocks *to prevent soiling the bed linen.*
- Have a bedpan or commode nearby and toilet tissue within the patient's reach. If the patient can use the bathroom, make sure that it's easily accessible.
- Remove the cap from the nozzle of the enema and then lubricate the end (if not pre-lubricated).

> If you're administering an enema to a child, familiarise it with the equipment and allow a parent or another relative to remain with it during the procedure.

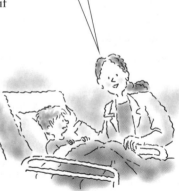

Contraction reaction

- Expel excessive air from the enema. Separate the patient's buttocks and touch the anal sphincter with the rectal tube or nozzle of enema *to stimulate contraction*. Then, as the sphincter relaxes, tell the patient to breathe deeply through their mouth as you gently advance the tube 10 to 12.5 cm.
- If the patient feels pain or if the tube meets continued resistance, notify the doctor. *This may signal an unknown stricture or abscess.*

Go with the flow

- Slowly introduce the fluid *to prevent stimulating peristalsis*. This is done by squeezing/rolling the bottle/pack from the bottom to the top *to prevent backflow*. Remove the enema nozzle from the patient and discard in clinical waste bag. For retention enemas keep the patient in bed and elevate the foot of the bed by 45 degrees *to aid retention of the enema for the period prescribed*.

Time frame

- For an evacuant enema, instruct the patient to retain the solution for 15 minutes, if possible.
- For a retention enema, instruct the patient to avoid defecation for the prescribed time.
- Position the patient on the bedpan with the call button within their reach. If they'll be using the bathroom or the commode, instruct them to call for help before attempting to get out of bed *because the procedure may make the patient, particularly an elderly patient, feel weak or faint*. Also instruct them to call if they feel weak or in pain at any time.
- When the solution has remained in the colon for the recommended time or for as long as the patient can tolerate it, assist the patient onto a bedpan or to the commode or bathroom.

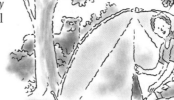

I like to have a little privacy when I'm camping in the middle of nowhere. So, imagine how much privacy your patient desires when he has an enema!

Wrapping it up

- Provide privacy. Instruct the patient not to flush the toilet.
- Assist the patient with cleaning, if necessary, and help them to bed. Place a clean absorbent pad under them *to absorb rectal drainage*.
- Observe the contents of the toilet or bedpan. Carefully note faecal colour, consistency, amount and foreign matter, such as blood, rectal tissue, worms, pus, mucus or other unusual matter.
- Send specimens to the laboratory, if required.
- Dispose of bedpan or and clean commode/bedpan holder as per local policy.
- Properly dispose of the enema equipment. Discard your gloves and apron, and wash your hands.
- Document in nursing records details of enema administration. (See *Documenting enema administration*, page 488.)

Practice pointers

- Schedule a retention enema before meals. A full stomach may stimulate peristalsis and make retention difficult.
- If the patient has haemorrhoids, instruct them to bear down gently during tube insertion *because bearing down causes the anus to open and facilitates insertion.*

Colostomy and ileostomy care

A patient with a colostomy or an ileostomy must wear an external pouch to collect emerging faecal matter. The pouch also helps control odour and protect the stoma and peristomal skin. Most disposable pouching systems can be used for 2 to 7 days, though some models exceed 7 days.

Half-full

An external pouch must be emptied when it's one third to one half full. Patients with an ileostomy may need to empty their pouch more frequently, four or five times daily. A pouch should be changed immediately if a leak develops.

After meals

The best time to change a pouching system is when the bowel is least active, usually 2 to 4 hours after meals. After a few months, most patients can determine which time is best for them.

A protective seal

The type of pouch selected depends on the stoma's location and structure, availability of supplies, wear time, consistency of effluent and personal preference. The best adhesive seal and skin protection for the individual patient should also be considered.

What you need

New appliance and scissors if not pre-cut ✻ stoma measuring guide ✻ disposable plastic bag ✻ water ✻ toilet or commode ✻ warm water ✻ gloves and apron ✻ soft wipes

Choices, choices, choices

Appliances may be drainable or closed-bottomed, disposable or reusable, adhesive-backed and one-piece or two-piece. (See *Comparing ostomy appliances.*)

Getting ready

- Explain the procedure to the patient.
- Wash your hands and bring all equipment to the patient's bedside.

How you do it

- Provide privacy and emotional support.

Take note!

Documenting enema administration

If you have administered an enema, be sure to record:

- date and time of administration
- type and amount of solution administered
- special equipment used
- retention time
- approximate amount of stool
- colour, consistency and amount of the stool
- abnormalities within the stool
- complications.

Comparing ostomy appliances

Available in many shapes and sizes, ostomy pouches are fashioned for comfort, safety and easy application. A disposable closed-end pouch may meet the needs of a patient who irrigates, wants added security or wants to discard the pouch after each bowel movement. Another patient may prefer a reusable, drainable pouch. Some commonly available pouches are described here.

One-piece disposable pouch

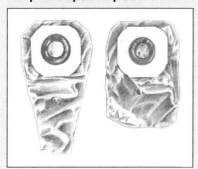

A one-piece closed-end pouch (left) is also disposable and made of odour-proof plastic. It may have a carbon filter for gas release. A patient with a regular bowel elimination pattern may choose this style.

Two-piece disposable pouch

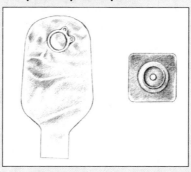

The patient who must empty their pouch often (because of diarrhoea or a new colostomy or ileostomy) may prefer a one-piece (bag with integrated baseplate attached), drainable, disposable pouch.

This odour-proof, plastic pouch comes with an attached adhesive seal. The bottom opening allows for easy draining. This pouch may be used permanently or temporarily, until stoma size stabilises.

A two-piece disposable drainable pouch with a separate baseplate (above) permits frequent changes and minimises skin breakdown. Also made of odour-proof plastic, this style usually snaps to the baseplate with a flange mechanism.

Fitting the appliance and skin barrier

• For a pouch with an attached skin barrier, measure the stoma with the stoma-measuring guide. Select the opening size that matches the stoma.

• For an adhesive-backed pouch with a separate skin barrier, measure the stoma with the measuring guide and select the opening that matches the stoma. Trace the selected size opening onto the paper back of the skin barrier's adhesive side. Cut out the opening. (If the pouch has pre-cut openings, which can be handy for a round stoma, select an opening that's 0.3 cm larger than the stoma. If the pouch comes without an opening, cut the hole approximately 3 to 4 mm wider than the measured tracing.) The cut-to-fit system works best for an irregularly shaped stoma.

• For a two-piece pouching system with flanges, see *Applying a skin barrier and pouch*, see page 490.

Applying a skin barrier and pouch

Fitting a skin barrier and ostomy pouch properly can be done in a few steps. Shown here is a commonly used two-piece pouching system with flanges.

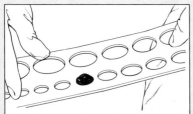 Measure the stoma using a measuring guide.

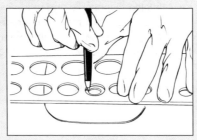 Trace the appropriate circle carefully on the back of the skin barrier.

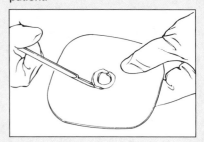 Cut the circular opening in the skin barrier. Bevel the edges to keep them from irritating the patient.

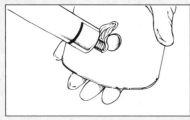 Remove the backing from the skin barrier and moisten it or apply barrier paste, as needed, along the edge of the circular opening.

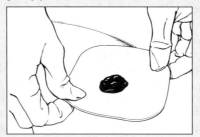 Centre the skin barrier over the stoma, adhesive side down, and gently press it to the skin.

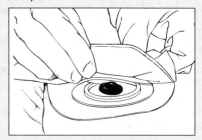 Gently press the pouch opening onto the ring until it snaps into place.

Can't feel a thing

- Avoid fitting the pouch too tightly because the stoma has no pain receptors. A constrictive opening could injure the stoma or skin tissue without the patient feeling warning discomfort. Also avoid cutting the opening too big *because this may expose the skin to faecal matter and moisture*.
- If the patient has a descending or sigmoid colostomy, has formed stools and has an ostomy that doesn't secrete much mucus, they may choose to wear only a pouch. In this case, make sure the pouch opening closely matches the stoma size.
- Between 6 weeks and 1 year after surgery, the stoma will shrink to its permanent size. At that point, pattern-making preparations will be unnecessary unless the patient gains weight, has additional surgery or injures the stoma.

Applying or changing the pouch
- Collect all equipment.
- Wash your hands and provide privacy.
- Explain the procedure to the patient because the patient will eventually perform the procedure themselves.
- Put on gloves and apron.

Out with the old

- Remove and discard the old pouch in a plastic bag. Wipe the stoma and peristomal skin gently with a soft wipe.
- Carefully wash the peristomal skin with mild soap and water and dry it by patting gently. Allow the skin to dry thoroughly. Inspect the peristomal skin and stoma. If necessary, shave surrounding hair (in a direction away from the stoma) *to promote a better seal and avoid skin irritation from hair pulling against the adhesive*.
- If applying a separate skin barrier, peel off the paper backing of the prepared skin barrier, center the barrier over the stoma, and press gently *to ensure adhesion*.
- You may want to outline the stoma on the back of the skin barrier (depending on the product) with a thin ring of stoma paste *to provide extra skin protection*. (Skip this step if the patient has a sigmoid or descending colostomy, formed stools and little mucus.)

I'm going to explain each step so that you can understand the procedure and, eventually, learn to do it yourself.

Peel and press

- Remove the paper backing from the adhesive side of the pouching system and center the pouch opening over the stoma. Press gently *to secure*.
- For a pouching system with flanges, align the lip of the pouch flange with the bottom edge of the skin barrier flange. Gently press around the circumference of the pouch flange, beginning at the bottom, until the pouch securely adheres to the barrier flange. (The pouch will click into its secured position.) Holding the barrier against the skin, gently pull on the pouch *to confirm the seal between flanges*.

Warm to the task

- Encourage the patient to stay quietly in position for about 5 minutes to improve adherence. The patient's body warmth also helps to improve adherence and soften a rigid skin barrier.
- Leave a bit of air in the pouch *to allow drainage to fall to the bottom*.
- Apply the closure clamp, if necessary.

Emptying the pouch
- Put on gloves and apron. Tilt the bottom of the pouch upwards and remove the closure clamp.

- Turn up a cuff on the lower end of the pouch and allow it to drain into the toilet or bedpan.
- Wipe the bottom of the pouch and reapply the closure clamp.
- If desired, the bottom portion of the pouch can be rinsed with cool tap water. Don't aim water up near the top of the pouch *because this may loosen the seal on the skin*.
- A two-piece flanged system can also be emptied by unsnapping the pouch. Let the drainage flow into the toilet.

Gas release

- Release flatus through the gas release valve if the pouch has one. Otherwise, release flatus by tilting the pouch bottom upwards, releasing the clamp and expelling the flatus. To release flatus from a flanged system, loosen the seal between the flanges.
- Never make a pinhole in a pouch to release gas *because doing so destroys the odour-proof seal*.

Practice pointers

- After performing and explaining the procedure to the patient, encourage self-care.
- Use adhesive solvents and removers only after patch-testing the patient's skin. Some products may irritate the skin or produce hypersensitivity reactions. Consider using a liquid skin sealant, if available, *to give skin tissue additional protection from drainage and adhesive irritants*.
- Remove the pouching system if the patient reports burning or itching beneath it or if there's purulent drainage around the stoma. Notify the stoma nurse of skin irritation, skin breakdown, a rash or an unusual appearance of the stoma or peristomal area.
- Use commercial pouch deodorants, if desired. Most pouches are odour-free, and odour should only be evident when emptying the pouch or if it leaks. Instruct the patient to avoid odour-causing foods such as fish, eggs, onions and garlic.
- Document the procedure according to local policy. (See *Documenting colostomy and ileostomy care*.)

Colostomy irrigation

Irrigation of a colostomy serves two purposes. It allows a patient with a descending or sigmoid colostomy to regulate bowel function, and it cleans the large bowel before and after tests, surgery or other procedures.

Colostomy irrigation may begin as soon as bowel function resumes after surgery. However, most clinicians recommend waiting until bowel movements are more predictable, which may take 4 to 6 weeks. Initially, the nurse (usually a stoma nurse or an experienced qualified nurse) or the patient irrigates the colostomy at the same time daily, recording the output and any spillage between irrigations.

Take note!

Documenting colostomy and ileostomy care

In your notes, be sure to record:

- date and time of the pouching system change
- characteristics of drainage, including colour, amount, type and consistency
- appearance of the stoma and peristomal skin
- patient teaching
- patient's response to self-care and evaluation of their learning progress.

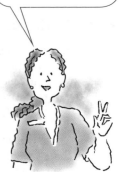

Colostomy irrigation serves two purposes.

Practice pointers

• Irrigating a colostomy to establish a regular bowel elimination pattern doesn't work for all patients. If the bowel continues to move between irrigations, try decreasing the volume of irrigant. Increasing the irrigant won't help because it serves only to stimulate peristalsis. Keep a record of results. Also consider irrigating every other day.

Regulation station

• Irrigation may help to regulate bowel function in a patient with a descending or sigmoid colostomy. A patient with an ascending or transverse colostomy won't benefit from irrigation, and a patient with descending or sigmoid colostomy who's missing part of their ascending or transverse colon may not be able to irrigate successfully.

Diet and exercise

• If diarrhoea develops, discontinue irrigations until stools regain form. Irrigation alone won't achieve regularity. The patient must also observe a nutritionally adequate diet and exercise regimen.

Quick quiz

1. What role does the epiglottis play in swallowing?
   A. Opens to allow air to enter
   B. Closes to prevent aspiration
   C. Opens or closes depending on the food type
   D. Rotates to aid in swallowing

Answer: B. The epiglottis, a thin flap of tissue over the larynx, closes during swallowing to prevent aspiration.

2. An adhesive-backed ostomy opening should be how much larger than the stoma?
   A. 1 to 2 mm
   B. 2 to 3 mm
   C. 3 to 4 mm
   D. 4 to 5 mm

Answer: C. In general, the opening should be 3 to 4 mm larger than the stoma itself. An opening that fits too tightly can injure the stoma. If the opening is too large, skin surrounding the stoma may come in contact with faeces, causing skin breakdown.

3. Which GI hormone stimulates gastric secretion and motility?
   A. Gastrin
   B. Gastric inhibitory peptides

C. Secretin
D. Cholecystokinin

Answer: A. Gastrin is produced in the pyloric antrum and duodenal end mucosa and stimulates gastric secretion and motility.

Scoring

☆☆☆   If you answered all three questions correctly, super! You've really digested this chapter.

☆☆   If you answered two questions correctly, great! Your functions (brain, that is) are all in line.

☆   If you answered fewer than two questions correctly, don't worry. Reread the chapter and you'll soon swallow all the facts you need!

Appendices and index

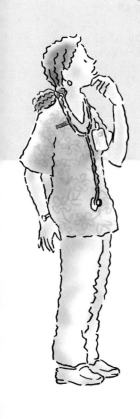

Glossary	496
Selected references	500
Index	503

Glossary

abduct: to move away from the midline of the body; the opposite of adduct

activities of (daily) living: (ADLs or ALs) activities performed every day, such as bathing, eating and toileting

adduct: to move towards the midline of the body; the opposite of abduct

advance directive: written legal document that identifies a patient's wishes in advance about the types of health care he desires should the patient be unable to decide for himself

aerobic: oxygen necessary for growth

affective: pertaining to emotions or feelings

agent: factor that by its presence or absence can lead to disease

agonist: drug that binds to a receptor to elicit a physiologic response

alopecia: loss of hair

alveolus: in the lung, a small sac-like dilation of the terminal bronchioles

anaerobic: oxygen not required for growth

anion: ion with a negative electrical charge

angina: pain that's felt in the chest region; typically associated with a heart attack

anorexia: loss of appetite

antagonist: drug that binds to a receptor but doesn't produce a response or blocks the response at the receptor

antibody: immunoglobulin produced by the body in response to exposure to a specific foreign substance (antigen)

antigen: foreign substance that causes antibody formation when introduced into the body

antiseptic: agent applied to living tissue to stop or slow the growth of microorganisms

anuria: urine output of less than 100 ml in 24 hours

aphasia: disturbance in the ability to communicate in speech, writing or reading

apnoea: cessation of breathing

arthrosis: a joint or articulation between bones; a degenerative disease of a bone; clean technique involving measures to reduce and control the number of microorganisms

assessment: first step in the nursing process; involves data collection

atrophy: wasting away

auscultation: listening to body sounds using a stethoscope

automaticity: ability of heart to generate its own electrical impulse

autonomy: degree of independence of action

bactericidal: ability to kill bacteria

bacteriostatic: ability to inhibit the growth of bacteria

basal metabolic rate: amount of energy used by the body at absolute rest when in an awake state

base: substance with the ability to combine with hydrogen ions; alkali

beneficence: doing good

bereavement: response to the loss or death of a significant person

blood pressure: force exerted by the blood on the walls of the vessels; expressed in millimetres of mercury (mmHg)

body image: feelings about one's body

body mechanics: use of body positioning or movement to prevent or correct problems related to activity or immobility

bone: dense, hard, connective tissue that composes the skeleton

bone marrow: soft tissue in the cancellous bone of the epiphyses; crucial for blood cell formation and maturation

borborygmi: loud sounds produced by the normal movement of air through the intestines (bowel sounds)

bradycardia: abnormally slow heart rate, usually fewer than 60 beats per minute

bradypnoea: abnormally slow respiratory rate, usually fewer than 10 breaths per minute

bronchiole: small branch of the bronchus

buccal: pertaining to the cheek

buffer: substance that helps to control pH through neutralisation

bursa: fluid-filled sac lined with synovial membrane

calorie: unit of heat

capillary: microscopic blood vessel that links arterioles with venules

carpal: pertaining to the wrist

cartilage: connective-supporting tissue occurring mainly in the joints, thorax, larynx, trachea, nose and ear

case management: multidisciplinary means of providing holistic care mainly for long-term conditions

cation: positively charged ion

central nervous system (CNS): one of the two main divisions of the nervous system; consists of the brain and spinal cord

cilia: small, hair-like projections on the outer surfaces of some cells

coeliac: pertaining to the abdomen

cognition: thinking and awareness

colloid: fluid containing starches or proteins

communication: exchange of information

complete protein: protein that contains the essential amino acids for body maintenance and growth

conceptual framework: formal explanation of how concepts are linked, with an emphasis on the relationship among them

confidentiality: maintenance of patient information as private

consciousness: state involving full awareness and ability to respond to stimuli

continuity of care: provision of services uninterrupted as the patient moves within the health-care system

contralateral: on the opposite side; the opposite of ipsilateral

coping mechanism: method used to manage stress

coronary: pertaining to the heart or its arteries

cortex: outer part of an internal organ; the opposite of medulla

costal: pertaining to the ribs

crystalloid: solution that's clear

critical thinking: process that's purposeful and disciplined and requires the use of reason and reflection to achieve insight and determine conclusions

cultural diversity: wide-ranging ideas and opinions of persons for behaviour that add to the fabric of society

culture: behaviour and beliefs of a specific group that's passed from one generation to the next

cutaneous: pertaining to the skin

cyanosis: bluish discoloration of the skin and mucous membranes

debridement: removal of dead tissue or foreign material from a wound

dehiscence: separation of a wound's edges

deltoid: shaped like a triangle (as in the deltoid muscle)

dermis: skin layer beneath the epidermis

diaphragm: membrane that separates one part from another; the muscular partition separating the thorax and abdomen

diarrhoea: frequent elimination of watery stool

diastole: resting portion of the cardiac cycle where the coronary arteries are filling with blood and the ventricles are relaxed

diffusion: movement of particles from an area of higher concentration to one of lower concentration

discharge planning: coordination and arrangement of the patient's transition from one health-care setting to another

disinfectant: solution used to kill microorganisms on inanimate objects

distal: far from the point of origin or attachment; the opposite of proximal

diuresis: formation and excretion of large amounts of urine

documentation: process of writing a record of patient information and care

dorsal: pertaining to the back or posterior; the opposite of ventral or anterior

duct: passage or canal

dyspnoea: difficulty or laboured breathing

empathy: process of putting one's self into the feelings of another

enema: instillation of fluid into the rectum and colon

endocardium: interior lining of the heart

endocrine: pertaining to secretion into the blood or lymph rather than into a duct; the opposite of exocrine

epidermis: outermost layer of the skin; lacking vessels

erythrocyte: red blood cell

ethics: professional standards of behaviour that indicate right and wrong

evaluation: last step of the nursing process; determines the effectiveness of nursing care

evidence-based care: approach that emphasises decision-making based on the best pertinent research-based evidence

evisceration: internal organ protrusion through an opening in a wound

exocrine: pertaining to secretion into a duct; the opposite of endocrine

extracellular fluid space: space outside of cells that contains fluid

extravasation: the escape of fluid into the surrounding tissue

febrile: state of temperature elevation

fistula: abnormal opening between organs or between an organ and body surface

flaccid: lacking muscle tone or resistance

flatus: gas or air in the GI tract

focused health assessment: data collection directly related to the patient's problems

foramen: small opening

fossa: hollow or cavity

fundus: base of a hollow organ; the part farthest from the organ's outlet

gait: characteristics associated with a patient's walking

gastric lavage: instillation and removal of solution into the stomach

gland: organ or structure of the body that secretes or excretes substances

glomerulus: compact cluster; the capillaries of the kidney

glycogenesis: formation of glycogen from glucose

goal: intended purpose; that which is to be achieved with the delivery of care

granulocyte: type of white blood cell, including eosinophils, neutrophils and basophils

haematuria: blood in the urine

haemoglobin: protein found in red blood cells that contains iron

haemoptysis: blood in the sputum

health: optimal state of well-being

health assessment: data collection focusing on the ability of the patient to perform activities

homeostasis: balance in the body

hormone: substance secreted by an endocrine gland that triggers or regulates the activity of an organ or cell group

hospice: provision of care to the terminally ill involving a family focus

host: person or thing that harbours a microorganism and allows it to grow

hypertension: elevated blood pressure

hypertonic: having a greater concentration than body fluid

hypotension: low blood pressure

hypotonic: having a lesser concentration than body fluid

hypoxaemia: state in which the blood contains a lower than normal amount of oxygen

hypoxia: state in which the tissues have a decreased amount of oxygen

implementation: fourth step of the nursing process in which the care plan is carried out

incomplete protein: protein that lacks sufficient amino acids to support growth

infarction: death of tissue due to ischaemia

infiltration: seepage or leakage of fluid into the tissues

informed consent: legal document that a patient or legal guardian signs giving permission for a procedure after the patient or guardian has demonstrated an understanding of the procedure

inferior: lower; the opposite of superior

inspection: assessment technique that involves systematic observation

interstitial fluid: fluid contained between the cells

intracellular fluid compartment: fluid contained within the cells

intravascular fluid: fluid contained within the blood vessels and lymphatics

ion: charged particle that forms when an electrolyte separates in solution

ipsilateral: on the same side; the opposite of contralateral

ischaemia: insufficient blood supply to a part

isotonic: having the same concentration as body fluid

joint: fibrous, cartilaginous or synovial connection between bones

justice: treatment of all patients fairly and equally

Korotkoff sounds: sounds heard when auscultating blood pressure denoting systolic and diastolic pressures

laceration: wound caused by tearing of the tissues

laws: standards for human conduct and enforced by the government

lacrimal: pertaining to tears

lateral: pertaining to the side; the opposite of medial

leukocyte: white blood cell

libel: injury to a person's reputation in written form

ligament: band of white fibrous tissue that connects bones

living will: advance directive that states the medical care that a person would want or would refuse should the person be unable to give consent or refusal

lumbar: pertaining to the area of the back between the thorax and the pelvis

lymph: watery fluid in lymphatic vessels

lymphocyte: white blood cell; the body's immunologically competent cells

maceration: tissue softening resulting from excessive moisture

malpractice: professional negligence

mammary: pertaining to the breast

manubrium: upper part of the sternum

meatus: opening or passageway

medial: pertaining to the middle; the opposite of lateral

membrane: thin layer or sheet

micturition: urination

mourning: behavioural process that occurs in a person after a significant loss, such as loss of health or the death of a loved one

muscle: fibrous structure whose contraction initiates movement

myocardium: thick, contractile layer of muscle cells that forms the heart wall

nephron: structural and functional unit of the kidney

nerve: cord-like structure consisting of fibres that convey impulses from the central nervous system to the body

networking: process of interacting with colleagues who share common interests

neutropenia: decreased number of neutrophils

neutrophil: white blood cell that removes and destroys bacteria, cellular debris and solid particles

nociceptors: nerve endings that respond to noxious stimuli

noncompliance: inability or unwillingness to adhere to a prescribed regimen

normal flora: organisms that inhabit the body but usually cause no harm

nursing process: systematic method for delivering nursing care

objective data: information that's observable and measurable and that can be verified and validated

oedema: accumulation of fluid in the interstitial space

olfactory: pertaining to the sense of smell

oliguria: urine output of less than 500 ml in 24 hours

ophthalmic: pertaining to the eye

osmosis: movement of water through a semi-permeable membrane from an area of higher water concentration (lower solute concentration) to a lower one (higher solute concentration)

outcome: end product of nursing care, that which is hoped to be achieved

palpation: use of touch to determine size, shape and consistency of underlying structures

parenteral nutrition: administration of nutrients I.V.

pathogen: organism capable of causing disease

pectoral: pertaining to the chest or breast

percussion: use of tapping on a body surface with fingers to determine density of underlying structure or area

peristalsis: wave-like movement to progress contents through the intestines

pericardium: fibroserous sac that surrounds the heart and the origin of the great vessels

phrenic: pertaining to the diaphragm

plantar: pertaining to the sole of the foot

plasma: colourless, watery fluid portion of lymph and blood

platelet: small, disk-shaped blood cell necessary for coagulation

pleura: thin serous membrane that encloses the lung

plexus: network of nerves, lymphatic vessels or veins

popliteal: pertaining to the back of the knee

posterior: back or dorsal; the opposite of anterior or ventral

primary source: patient

pronate: to turn the palm downwards; the opposite of supinate

proximal: situated nearest the centre of the body; the opposite of distal

pruritus: itching

pulse deficit: difference between the apical and radial pulse rates

purulent: pus-producing or pus-containing

range of motion: extent to which a person can move their joints or muscles

reflex: involuntary action

renal: pertaining to the kidney

respiration: exchange of carbon dioxide and oxygen in tissue and the lungs

role: expected function and behaviour of a person

sanguinous: referring to or containing blood

secondary source: anyone other than the patient who supplies information

self-concept: mental image that a person has of one's self

sensory deprivation: lack of exposure to appropriate sensory stimuli

sensory overload: state of increased arousal in which the patient is unable to manage incoming stimuli

serosanguineous: containing blood and serum

serous: serum-like, watery and thin

slander: verbal injury to a person's reputation

spasticity: sudden, involuntary increase in muscle tone or contractions

standard precautions: set of guidelines developed to protect against infection transmission

sternum: long, flat bone that forms the middle portion of the thorax

striated: marked with parallel lines such as striated (skeletal) muscle

subcutaneous: related to the tissue layer under the dermis

sublingual: under the tongue

superior: higher; the opposite of inferior

supinate: to turn the palm of the hand upwards; the opposite of pronate

surgical asepsis: sterile technique involving measures to keep an object free from all microorganisms

symphysis: growing together; a type of cartilaginous joint in which fibrocartilage firmly connects opposing surfaces

synapse: point of contact between adjacent neurons

systole: period of ventricular contraction

tachycardia: rapid heart rate; usually greater than 100 beats per minute

tachypnoea: rapid respiratory rate; usually greater than 20 breaths per minute

tendon: band of fibrous connective tissue that attaches a muscle to a bone

therapeutic communication: use of special techniques to interact, enabling a person to express feelings and work out problems

thrombus: blood clot

total parenteral nutrition: administration of highly concentrated nutrient solutions via a central intravenous site

transfusion: administration of whole blood or blood products directly into a person's circulation

urinal: metal or plastic device used by male patients for urinary elimination

values: personal beliefs that guide decision-making

valve: structure that permits fluid to flow in only one direction

venepuncture: insertion of a needle or catheter into a vein

ventilation: movement of air in and out of the lungs

ventral: pertaining to the front or anterior; the opposite of dorsal or posterior

ventricle: small cavity, such as one of several in the brain or one of the two lower chambers of the heart

viscera: internal organs

xiphoid: sword-shaped; the lower portion of the sternum

Z-track: technique of I.M. medication administration that prevents medication from seeping into the tissue

Selected references

Publications

Beauchamp, T., and Childress, J. (2001). *Principles of Biomedical Ethics*, 5th edn. New York: Oxford University Press.

Bennett, G., Dealey, C., and Posnett, J. (2004). The cost of pressure ulcers in the UK. *Age and Aging* 33: 230–235.

Complete Guide to Documentation. Philadelphia: Lippincott Williams & Wilkins, 2003.

Craven, R.F., and Hirnle, C.J. (2003). *Fundamentals of Nursing: Human Health and Function*, 4th edn. Philadelphia: Lippincott Williams & Wilkins.

Dealey. C. (2005). *The Care of Wounds: A Guide for Nurses*. 3rd edn. Oxford: Blackwell.

DeLaune, S.C., and Ladner, P.K. (2006). *Fundamentals of Nursing: Standards & Practice*, 3rd edn. Clifton Park, N.Y.: Thomson Delmar Learning.

Department of Health (1983). *Mental Health Act* (revised 2007). London: DH.

Department of Health (1990). *Access to Health Records Act*. London: DH.

Department of Health (1991). *The Patients' Charter*. London: DH.

Department of Health (1998). *Data Protection Act*. London: DH.

Department of Health (1999). *Our Healthier Nation*. London: DH.

Department of Health (DH) (2001). *National Service Framework for Older People*. London: DH.

Department of Health (2001). *The Essence of Care: Patient Focused Benchmarking for Health Care Practitioners*. London: DH.

Department of Health (2002). *Guidance on the Single Assessment Process for Older People*. London: DH.

Department of Health (2004). *Choosing Health: Making Health Choices Easier*. London: DH.

Department of Health (2004). *Standards for Better Health*. London: DH.

Department of Health (2005). *Mental Capacity Act*. London: DH.

Department of Health (2006a). *The Health Act 2006: Code of Practice for the Prevention and Control of Healthcare-associated Infections*. London: DH.

Department of Health (2006b). Health Technical Memorandum 0701: *Safe Management of Healthcare Waste*. London: DH.

Department of Health (2007). *Saving Lives: Reducing Infection, Delivering Clean and Safe Care* (revised edn). London: DH.

Department of Health (2009). *Prevention Package for Older People*. London: DH.

Finlay, T. (2004). *Intravenous Therapy*. Cambridge: Blackwell Scientific Publishers..

Gahart, B.L. and Nazareno, A.R. (2004). *Intravenous Medications: A Handbook for Nurses and Allied Health Professionals*, 21st edn. Philadelphia: Elsevier Science.

Hadaway, L.C. (October, 2003). Infusing without infecting. *Nursing 2003* 33(10): 58–63.

Harkreader, H. and Hogan, M.A. (2004). *Fundamentals of Nursing: Caring and Clinical Judgment*, 2nd edn. Philadelphia: W.B. Saunders Co.

Health and Safety Executive (HSE) (2004). *Manual Handling Operations Regulations 1992* (amended 2004). London: HMSO.

I.V. Therapy Made Incredibly Easy, 3rd edn. Philadelphia: Lippincott Williams & Wilkins, 2005.

Ignatavicius, D.D. and Workman, M.L. (2005). *Medical-Surgical Nursing Critical Thinking for Collaborative Care*, 5th edn. Philadelphia: W.B. Saunders Co.

Infusion Nurses Society, (2001). *Infusion Therapy in Clinical Practice*, 2nd edn. Philadelphia: W.B. Saunders Co.

Josephson, D.L. (2004). *Intravenous Infusion Therapy for Nurses: Principles and Practice*, 2nd edn. Clifton Park, N.Y.: Thomson Delmar Learning.

Just the Facts: I.V. Therapy. Philadelphia: Lippincott Williams & Wilkins.

Kasper, D.L., *et al.* (2005). *Harrison's Principles of Internal Medicine*, 16th edn. New York: McGraw-Hill Book Co.

Knibbe, H., *et al.* (2008). *The Handbook of Transfers*. Gloucester: Diligent.

Malkin, B. (2008) Are techniques used for intramuscular injection based on research evidence? *Nursing Times* 104 (50/51): 48–51.

Medicines and Healthcare Products Regulatory Agency (2005). *Patient Group Directions*. London: MHRA.

National Institute for Health and Clinical Excellence (2000). *Guidance on the Use of Inhaler Systems (devices) in Children Under the Age of 5 years with Chronic Asthma*. London: NICE.

National Institute for Health and Clinical Excellence (2003). *Clinical Guideline 7 Pressure Ulcer Prevention*. London: NICE.

National Institute for Health and Clinical Excellence (2003). *Infection Control: Prevention of Health-Care Associated Infections in Primary and Secondary Care*. London: NICE.

National Institute for Health and Clinical Excellence (2005). *The Prevention and Treatment of Pressure Ulcers*. London: NICE.

National Institute for health and Clinical Excellence (2006). *Nutrition Support in Adults: Oral Nutrition Support, Enteral Tube Feeding and Parenteral Nutrition*. London: NICE.

National Institute for Health and Clinical Excellence (2007). *Feverish illness in children: Assessment and initial management in children younger than 5 years*. London: NICE.

National Institute for Health and Clinical Excellence (2008). *Continuous Subcutaneous Insulin Infusion for the Treatment of Diabetes Mellitus*. London: NICE.

National Institute for Health and Clinical Excellence (2008). *Surgical Site Infection: Prevention and Treatment of Surgical Site Infection*. London: NICE.

National Patient Safety Agency (2007). *Promoting Safer Use of Injectable Medicines: NPSA Template Standard Operating Procedure for Use of Injectable Medicines*. London: NPSA.

National Patient Safety Agency (2008). *Right Patient, Right Blood: New Advice for Safer Blood Transfusions*. London: NPSA.

NHS Institute for Innovation and Improvement (2007). *Releasing Time to Care: The Productive Ward*. London: HMSO.

Nursing and Midwifery Council (2004). *Standards of Proficiency for Pre-registration Nursing Education*. London: NMC.

Nursing and Midwifery Council (2007). *Essential Skills Clusters (ESCs) for Pre-registration Nursing Programmes*. Annexe 2 to Circular 07/2007. London: NMC.

Nursing and Midwifery Council (2007). *Standards for Medicines Management*. London: NMC.

Nursing and Midwifery Council (2008). *Standards for Medicines Administration*. London: NMC.

Nursing and Midwifery Council (2008). *The Code: Standards of Conduct, Performance and Ethics for Nurses and Midwives*. London: NMC.

Nursing and Midwifery Council (2008). *The Prep Handbook*. London: NMC.

Nursing and Midwifery Council (2009). *NMC Record Keeping: Guidance for Nurses and Midwives*. London: NMC.

Nursing and Midwifery Council (2009). *Supply and/or Administration of Medicine by Student Nurses and Student Midwives in Relation to Patient Group Directions (PGD)*. Circular 05/2009. London: NMC.

Nursing Procedures, 4th edn. Philadelphia: Lippincott Williams & Wilkins, 2004.

Roper, N., Logan, W.W. and Tierney, A.J. (1998). *The Elements of Nursing*. Churchill Livingstone: Edinburgh.

Royal College of Nursing (2005). *Standards for Infusion Therapy*. London: RCN.

Royal College of Nursing (2007). *Standards for Assessing, Measuring and Monitoring Vital Signs in Infants, Children and Young People*. London: RCN.

Royal College of Nursing (2008). *Defining Nursing*. London: RCN.

Royal College of Nursing (2009). *The Recognition and Assessment of Acute Pain in Children*. London: RCN.

Royal Pharmaceutical Society of Great Britain (2005). *The Safe and Secure Handling of Medicines: A Team Approach*. London: RPSGB.

Scottish Executive (2001). *Guidance on the Single Shared Assessment for Community Care Needs*. Circular no. CCD 8/2001. Scottish Executive: Edinburgh.

Smith, J. (2005). *The Guide to the Handling of People*, 5th edn. BackCare: Middlesex.

Smith, P.E. (2005). *Taylor's Clinical Nursing Skills: A Nursing Process Approach*. Philadelphia: Lippincott Williams & Wilkins.

Smith, S. (2007). Assessing pain in people with dementia 2: The nurse's role. *Nursing Times* 103(30): 26.

Timby, B.K. (2005). *Fundamental Nursing Skills and Concepts*, 8th edn. Philadelphia: Lippincott Williams & Wilkins.

Timby, B.K. and Smith, N.E. (2005). *Essentials of Nursing*. Philadelphia: Lippincott Williams & Wilkins.

Vaccination Administration Taskforce (2001). UK Guidance on Best Practice in Vaccine Administration. London: Shirehall Communications.

Welsh Assembly Government (2006). *National Service Framework for Older People in Wales*. Cardiff: Welsh Assembly Government.

World Health Organisation (1992). *Basic Documents*. 39th edn. Geneva: WHO.

World Health Organisation (2002). *Activeaging: A Policy Framework*. Geneva: WHO.

Web Sites
BBC. *A Hard Night's Sleep*. Available at: *http://www.bbc.co.uk/science/humanbody/sleep/articles/sleepdisorders.shtml* (accessed 07 February 2010).

British National Formulary (2009). Available at: *www.bnf.org*. (accessed 25 October 2009).

Health and Safety at Work Act (1974). Available at: *http://www.opsi.gov.uk/RevisedStatutes/Acts/ukpga_19740037_en_1* (accessed 11 February 2010).

The Human Rights Act (1998). Available at: *http://www.opsi.gov.uk/ACTS/acts1998/ukpga_19980042_en_1* (accessed 11 February 2010).

International Council of Nurses (2005). *ICN code of ethics for nurses*. Available at: *www.icn.ch/icncode.pdf* (accessed 27th October 2009)

Lifting Operations and Lifting Equipment Regulations (1998). Available at: *http://www.opsi.gov.uk/si/si1998/19982307.htm* (accessed 11 February 2010).

The Management of Health and Safety at Work Regulations (1999). Available at: *http://www.opsi.gov.uk/SI/si1999/19993242.htm* (accessed 11 February 2010).

Manual Handling Operations Regulations (1992). Available at: *http://opsi.gov.uk/si/si1992/UKsi_19922793_en_1.htm* (accessed 11 February 2010).

National Patient Safety Agency (NPSA) (2009). *Oxygen Safety in Hospitals/Rapid Response Report*. Available at: *www.nrls.npsa.nhs.uk/alerts/?entryid45=62811* (accessed 29 October 2009).

Pratt, R.J. *et al*. (2007). *Epic2: National Evidence-Based Guidelines for Preventing Healthcare–associated Infections in NHS Hospitals in England*. Available at: *www.epic.tvu.ac.uk/Downloads/* (accessed 24 October 2009).

Provision and Use of Work Equipment Regulations (1998). Available at: *http://www.opsi.gov.uk/SIsi1998/19982306.htm* (accessed 11 February 2010).

Index

A

Abdomen, exercising, 337
Abdominal distension, 482
Abduction pillow, 322i
    applying, 321
Absorption, drug, 127
Absorption as skin function, 256
Accessory muscles, 93, 222
Access to Health Records
            Act 1990, 32
Acid–base balance, lungs and, 227
Active aging, 27
Active transport, solute movement
            and, 204
Activities of daily living, 78–79
Activity intolerance, 319
Acute illness, 24
Acute pain, 389–390
    physiologic and behavioural evidence
            of, 390t
    treating, 401–402
Adaptability, of verbal communication, 61
Adjuvant analgesics, 404
Administration, drug. *See* Drug
            administration
Admission assessment, 45
Adult health care, 26
Adults
    assisting, with feeding, 438–441
        practice pointers for, 441
        preparing for, 438–439
    sleep requirements for, 369–370
Advance decision, 77
Advance directives, 36, 77
Advocate, nurse as, 12
Age
    changes in gastro-intestinal system
            with, 428, 477
    effect of, on sleep, 369–370

as pressure ulcers risk factor, 295
as wound healing factor, 265
Aging, skin function and, 296t
Airborne transmission of infection, 105
Air-fluidised bed, 301
Airways, 219–221, 220i
Alcohol
    effect on sleep, 371
    in hand washing, 108, 109,
            111, 113
Aldosterone, 199
Alginate dressing, 280
    applying, 281
Alignment devices
    applying, 321
    purpose of, 321
    types of, 321, 322i
Alimentary canal. *See* Gastro-intestinal
            system; Gastro-intestinal tract
Allergy, medication error and, 142
Allied Health Professions Federation, 405
Alternating-pressure air mattress, 301
Alternative therapies
    for insomnia, 380
    for pain, 411–412
Ambulating patients, 327–333
    transfer techniques for, 328–331
    using proper body mechanics for,
            327–328
    using walking frame, 331, 332i, 333
Ampoule, withdrawing medication from,
            182–183
Anabolism, 417
Ankle, exercising, 336, 337
Anorexia, 436
Anticonvulsants, as analgesics, 404
Anti-diuretic hormone, 199, 453
Antrum, stomach, 427
Anxiety, urinary elimination and, 455
Apical pulse measurement, 88–89

Apical–radial pulse measurement,
            89–90
Apneustic, respiratory pattern
            for, 92t
Apnoea, respiratory pattern for, 92t
Apocrine glands, 253, 343
Argentaffin cells, 426i
Ascending colon, 421i, 430
Assessment, 44–47
    data collection in, 73
    health history and, 45, 73–80
    interview techniques for, 45–47
    obtaining data for, 47
    personal information, 47
    types of, 44–45
    of vital signs, 82–99
Assistive feeding devices, 440i
Asymptomatic infection, 102
Atrophy, 436
Auerbach's plexus, 422
Autonomic arousal, pain and, 388
Autonomic nervous system, 391
Axillary temperature, measuring, 83,
            85, 85t

B

Bacillus anthracis, 109
Back, exercising, 337
Bacteria as infecting organisms,
            102–103, 103i
    classification, 102–103
Ball-and-socket joints, 317–318, 318i
Barrier clothing, 112
Bed bath, 345–347
    performing, 345–347
    practice pointers, 347
    preparing for, 345
Bed making
    for occupied bed, 361–363
    for unoccupied bed, 359–361

Note: Page numbers followed by "i" refer to an illustration; "t" refer to a table.

Bedpan and urinal use, 458–460
   aftercare for, 459–460
   placing bedpan for, 459
   placing urinal for, 459
   practice pointers for, 460
Beds as pressure reduction devices,
   301–302
Bed to stretcher/trolley transfer,
   328–329
   pat slide and slide sheet, 328–329
   performing, 329
   preparing for, 328–329
Bed to wheelchair transfer, 329–331
   preparing for, 330
   procedure for, 330
Behavioural approaches, for pain
   management, 413
Bile, 432, 473
Biliary duct system, 421i, 424t,
   432, 474
Biofeedback
   insomnia and, 378
   as pain-relieving technique, 413
Biographic data, collecting, 76–77
Black wound, caring for, 270–271, 271t
Bladder, 451
Blanchable erythema as sign of tissue
   damage, 306
Blood administration, I.V. therapy and,
   208–209
Blood pressure, 93
   diastolic, 93
   effect of age on, 94
   measuring, 94, 95i, 96–97, 96i
      correcting problems of, 98t
      sites contraindicated for, 94
   as pressure ulcer risk factor, 297
   systolic, 93
Body, stomach, 427
Body fluids, loss of, urinary elimination
   and, 453
Body language, 63
Body mass index, 418–419
Body mechanics
   for lifting and carrying, 328
   for pushing and pulling, 327–328
   for stooping, 328

Body position
   bowel elimination and, 478
   urinary elimination and, 452
Body temperature, 83
   factors that affect, 83
   measuring, 83–86
      in infant, 86
      methods for, 85t
Bone, drug storage in, 128
Bones, 316, 317i
Bowel elimination, 471–493
   digestion and, 474–478
   factors affecting, 478–481
      body position, 478
      exercise and activity, 478
      faecal diversion, 478–479, 479i
      fluid intake, 479
      ignoring urge to defecate, 480
      lifestyle, 480
      medications, 480
      nutrition, 480–481
      surgery, 481
   nursing interventions for, 482–493
      colostomy. See Colostomy
      enema administration.
         See Enemas
      ileostomy. See Ileostomy
      stool specimen collection. See
         Stool specimen collection
   patterns of, 478
Bowel function, altered, 481–482
   constipation, 481
   diarrhoea, 481
   faecal impaction, 482
   faecal incontinence, 482
   flatulence, 482
Braden scale, 298
Bradycardia, pulse pattern for, 89t
Bradypnoea, respiratory pattern for, 92t
Brain injuries, effect of, on mobility, 319
Breathing, mechanics of, 221–222,
   222i. See also Respiration
Breathing-related sleep disorders,
   373–374
   treatments for, 377
Breath sounds, assessing, 91–92
Brief pain inventory, 395

British Association for Parenteral and
   Enteral Nutrition, 419
Bronchi, 220–221, 220i
Buccal drug administration, 120

C

Caecum, 421i, 430
Calcium
   functions of, 201t
   imbalances of, 201t
Caldicott Guardian, 32
Cancer pain, 391–392
   treating, 402
Capacity to consent, 41
Capillary-filling pressures, pressure
   ulcers and, 291
Capillary filtration and reabsorption, fluid
   movement and, 204–205
Capsules
   administering, 145–147
   teaching about giving, 147
Cardia, stomach, 427
Cardiac arrest, dealing with, 35–38
Cardiac glands, 426i
Cardiopulmonary resuscitation, 35
Caregiver, nurse as, 11–12
Care pathways, 52–53, 52t
Care plans
   care pathways and, 52–53, 52t
   formulating, 47–48
   implementing, 48–49
   individualised, 52
   standardised, 51–53
   traditional, 50–51
Cartilage, 316
Case manager, 14
Casey's model, 16t
Catabolism, 417
Cataplexy, 374
Catheterisation, 463
Catheter specimen of urine, 468
Central nervous system, 390
Cephalic phase, of digestion and
   absorption, 424–425, 424t
Chair scale, 97
Change agent, nurse as, 13
Chest drainage. See Thoracic drainage

Note: Page numbers followed by "i" refer to an illustration; "t" refer to a table.

Chest physiotherapy, 232
Cheyne–Stokes respirations, pattern
  of, 92t
Children. *See also* Paediatric patient
  administration of enema to,
    486, 486i
  overweight, 436
  pain assessment of, 396
  sleep requirements for, 369
Chlamydiae as infecting organisms, 104
Chloride
  functions of, 201t
  imbalances of, 201t
Cholecystokinin, 432, 433t
Cholinergic medications, 454
Chronic illness, 24
Chronic pain, 390–391
  causes of, 390
  treating, 402
Chronopharmacotherapy, 377
Chronotherapy, 376
Circadian sleep disorders, 371–373
  delayed sleep phase, 373
  jet lag, 373
  shift-work, 373
  treatments for, 376–377
    chronopharmacotherapy, 377
    chronotherapy, 376
    luminotherapy, 376–377
    melatonin, 377
Clarity, of verbal communication, 60
Clear-liquid diet, 439
Clinical nurse specialist, 14
Closed chest drainage system,
    246–247. *See also* Thoracic
    drainage
Closed-ended questions, 46, 62
Closed-wound drain management,
    288–289
  documenting, 289
  performing, 288–289
  practice pointers, 289
  preparing for, 288
Closed-wound drain system, 288–289
Clostridium difficile, 109
Clostridium perfringens, 429, 476
Clothing, protective, 113

Code of conduct, NMC, 6–10
Code of ethics for nurses, 31
Cognitive approaches, for pain
    management, 413
Cognitive therapy, insomnia and, 379
Cold therapy, for pain management,
    408–410
  mechanics of, 408–409
  methods of, 408, 409i
  special considerations for,
    409–410
  uses for, 408
Collagen fibers, 252
Colocare, faecal occult blood
    testing, 484
Colonised infection, 102
Colostomy, 479, 479i
  documenting care for, 492
  irrigation of, 492–493
    practice pointers for, 493
    purpose of, 492
  pouching systems for, 488, 489i
    applying or changing, 490i,
      491–492
    emptying, 491–492
    fitting, 489–490
    practice pointers, 492
    preparing to care for, 488
Communication, 59–71
  blocks to, 67–70, 68i
  cultural barriers, 64
  documentation and, 71
  with elderly patients, 69–70, 80
  non-verbal, 63–64
  with paediatric patients, 68–69
  therapeutic relationships and, 64–67
  with unconscious patient, 70
  verbal, 59–63
Complementary therapies
  for insomnia, 380
  for pain, 411–412
Confidentiality, 31–32
Constipation, 481
Contact transmission of infection, 105
Continuous positive airway pressure,
    obstructive sleep apnoea
    syndrome, 377

Contraction, wound healing process
    and, 262
Contracture, wound healing process
    and, 262
Contrast therapy, 408. *See also*
    Cold therapy, for pain
    management
Controlled drug, 140
Coping strategies for pain, 386–387
Coughing exercises, 228
Credibility, of verbal communication, 61
Culture, dietary habits and, 437
Cyanosis, 92–93
Cystocele, 452

D

Data Protection Act 1998, 32
De-afferentation pain, 391
Debridement, 311
Deep-breathing exercises, 228–229
Defecate, ignoring urge to, bowel
    elimination and, 480
Dehiscence as wound healing
    complication, 267, 267i
Delayed sleep phase sleep
    disorder, 373
  chronotherapy for, 376
  luminotherapy for, 376–377
Dementia, people with, pain assessment
    for, 396
Denture care, 357–358. *See also*
    Mouth care
Dermis, 252–253, 342, 342i
Descending colon, 421i, 430
Developmental theories, 17–18
Diabetic foot care, 355
Diaphragm, 221
Diarrhoea, 481
Diastolic blood pressure, *vs.* systolic
    blood pressure, 93
Dietary guidelines, 420
Dietary restrictions, culture and beliefs
    and, 437
Diet as tolerated, 439
Diffusion, 225–227
  gas exchange and, 225–226,
    226i

Note: Page numbers followed by "i" refer to an illustration; "t" refer to a table.

Digestion and absorption
  accessory organs of, 431–434,
    473–474
    biliary duct system, 432
    liver, 431
    pancreas, 432–434
  cephalic phase of, 424–425, 424t
  gastric phase of, 425–427, 426i
  gastro-intestinal tract and, 420,
    474, 475i, 476–477
  intestinal phase of, 428–430
  purpose of, 420
  in small intestine, 429, 472, 474,
    475i, 476
Digital scale, in weight
    measurement, 98
Discharge planner, nurse as, 13
Disease
  development of, 23
  drug response and, 130
  effect of, on mobility, 318–319
Disposal of waste, 114
  EWC and, 114
Distension, abdominal, 482
Diuretics, urinary elimination and, 454
Documentation
  communicating by, 71
  importance of, 41–42
  of I.V. therapy, 214–215
  passive ROM exercises, 336
  pulse oximetry, 239
  tracheostomy care, 242
Dormant infection, 102
Droplet transmission, 105
Drug absorption, 127
Drug administration. See also Drugs
  age as factor in, 131
  common errors in, 140–143
  controlled drug, 140
  guidelines for, 139
  I.V. therapy and, 208
  pharmacokinetics and, 125–130
  procedures for, 134–140
  record, essential criteria of, 132i
  routes of, 118–125, 124–125t
  underlying diseases and, 130
Drug chart, 131

Drug distribution, 127–129
  body storage of drug and, 128
  factors that affect, 128–129
Drug metabolism and excretion,
    129–130
Drug nomenclature, 117, 118
Drug prophylaxis, infection prevention
    and, 108
Drugs. See also Drug administration
  expiration date for, 139
  legal aspects of, 116–117, 117t
  legislations related to, 117t
  professional aspects of, 117
  storage and preparation
    guidelines, 138
Duodenum, 421i, 428
Dyspnoea, signs of, 92
Dysuria, 456

E

Ear drops, 119
  instilling, 164–166, 165i
    in paediatric patient, 166
    positioning in, 165i
    practice pointers for, 166
    teaching about, 166
Eccrine glands, 253, 342i, 343
Economic resources, altered nutrition
    and, 437
Educational preparation for nursing,
    10–11
Elastin, 252
Elbow, exercising, 334, 337
Elderly patient
  assessing respirations in, 91
  communicating with, 80
  communication with, 69–70
  drug action in, 131
  intramuscular medication
    administration and, 192
  normal blood pressure in, 94
  wound healing in, 265
Electrolytes, 200. See also Fluid and
    electrolyte balance
  functions of, 201–202t
  signs and symptoms of imbalances
    of, 201–202t

Electronic vital signs monitor, 95i
Emergency assessment, 45
Emotional by-products of pain, 399–400
End-of-life decisions, 33–34
Endogenous infection, 102
Endotracheal tube
  drug administration and, 120
Enemas
  administration of, 484–488
    to child, 486, 486i
    documenting, 488
    preparing for, 485, 486
  contraindications for, 485
  evacuant, 484, 485t, 487
  practice pointers for, 488
  retention, 484, 485t, 487, 488
Enemas, medicated
  administering, 171
  contraindications for, 171
  retention, 171
Energy as metabolism by-product, 417
Enteral administration, 121
Enterobacter aerogenes, 429, 476
Enterogastric reflex, 474
Environment, effect of, on sleep
    quality, 370
Epic2: National Evidence-based
    Guidelines for Preventing
    Healthcare-associated
    Infections in NHS England, 107
EPIC2 guidelines, 107, 111
Epidermis, 250–251, 341, 342i
Epidural infusion, 124t
Epiglottis, 219, 220i, 472
Epithelial tissue, 307
Errors in drug administration, 140–143
Escherichia coli, 429, 476
Essence of Care, The, 417–418
Essential Skills Clusters, 10
  domains of, 11
Ethics, 30–38
  code of, for nurses, 31
  committee to addresses issues of, 34
  conflicts related to, 33–35
  decisions related to, 32–33
  principles of, 30
Eupnoea, respiratory pattern in, 92t

Note: Page numbers followed by "i" refer to an illustration; "t" refer to a table.

European Waste Catalogue Codes, 114
Evaluation, 49–50
Evidence-based care, 19
Evisceration as wound healing complication, 267, 267i
Excretion, of drugs, 129–130
Excretion as skin function, 256
Exercise, bowel elimination and, 478
Exercises
    active range-of-motion, 336
    coughing, 228
    deep-breathing, 228–229
    isometric, 336–337
    passive range-of-motion, 333–334, 336
Exogenous infection, 102
Expiration date, drug, 139
Extracellular fluid, 198
Eye care, 349–350
    performing, 349–350
Eye drops
    instilling, 158–160
        practice pointers for, 160
    minimising systemic reactions to, 160
    sensing instillation of, 161
    teaching about, 161

F

Face mask in preventing infection, 111
Faecal diversion, bowel elimination and, 478–479, 479i
Faecal impaction, 482
Faecal incontinence, 482
Faecal occult blood testing, 484
    Hematest reagent tablet test for, 484
    Hemoccult slide test for, 484
Family, effects of illness on, 24
Family history, obtaining, 76
Fat, drug storage in, 128
Federation of Holistic Therapists, 405
Feeding, assisting adult with, 438–441
    practice pointers for, 441
    preparing for, 438–439
Feeding tube. See also Gastric feeding
    contraindications for, 442
    indications for, 441–442
    types of, 442

Female
    perineal care for, 348
    urethra, 451
Fingers and thumb, exercising, 336
Fistula formation as wound healing complication, 268
Five rights of drug administration, 135–138
Flatulence, 482
Floating ribs, 221
Flood warning, 208
Flow incentive spirometer, 230, 230i
Fluid and electrolyte balance, 202–205
Fluid intake
    bowel elimination and, 479
    urinary elimination and, 452–453
Fluid intake and output, recording, 442
Fluids, 197. See also Fluid and electrolyte balance
    extracellular, 198
    functions of, 198–199
    gains and losses of, 199i
    identifying imbalances of, 200
    intracellular, 198
    maintaining balance of, 198
    movement of, 203–205
    regulating volume and concentration, 199
Foam dressing, 280
    applying, 281
Foam mattress, 301, 302
Foley catheter. See Indwelling urinary catheter
Foot care, 354–356
    for diabetic patients, 355
    performing, 355
    practice pointers, 356
    preparing for, 354
Foot cradle, 301
Forearm, exercising, 334
Friction as cause of pressure ulcers, 294–295
Full-liquid diet, 439
Full-thickness wounds, 269i, 270, 310i
Fundus, stomach, 427
Fungi as infecting organisms, 104

G

Gall bladder, 424i, 432, 473
    functions of, 424i, 432
Gas exchange, 225–226, 226i
Gastric feeding. See also Feeding tube
    delivering, 443–444
    discontinuing, 444
    documenting, 446
    practice pointers, 445–446
    preparing for, 443
Gastric glands, 426i
Gastric inhibitory peptides, 433t
Gastric medication administration, 150–152
    performing, 151–152
    practice pointers for, 152
    preparing, 150–151
Gastric phase, of digestion and absorption, 425–427, 426i
Gastric secretion, sites and mechanisms of, 426i
Gastrin, 427, 433t
Gastro-intestinal hormones, 433t
Gastro-intestinal system. See also Gastro-intestinal tract; specific accessory organs
    age-related changes, 428, 477
    structures of, 421i
Gastro-intestinal tract, 471–473
    digestion and absorption and, 420, 474, 475i, 476–477
    innervation of, 423
    structures of, 421–423
    substances secreted by, 423
    vascular structures of, 474
Gastrostomy tube, administering medication through, 150–152
Gate-control theory about pain, 384, 385i
Gauze dressings, 280
Gel pads, 301
Gloves, contaminated, removal techniques for, 113
Goserelin, 122
Granulation tissue, 307
Guide to the Handling of People, the, 323

Note: Page numbers followed by "i" refer to an illustration; "t" refer to a table.

H

Haematuria, 456
Haemorrhage as wound healing
    complication, 267
Haemostasis as wound healing phase,
    259i, 260
Hair, 343
Hair care, 350–352
    frequency of, 350
    performing, 350–351
    practice pointers for, 351–352
Handling and disposal of sharps
    in preventing infection, 112
Hand roll, 322i
    applying, 321
Hand washing
    alcohol in, 108–109, 111, 113
    effective technique for,
        109–111, 110i
    infection prevention and, 108–109
Head box as oxygen delivery system in
    children, 235i
Health
    definition of, 21–22
    factors that affect, 22
Health Act 2006: Code of Practice for
    the Prevention and Control
    of Healthcare-associated
    Infections, The, 107
Health and Safety at Work
    Act (1974), 324
Health-care-associated infections,
    105–107
    control precautions of, 107
    incidence of, 105–106
    preventing, 106
    risk of, 106
    transmission of, 105
Health-care waste, disposal of, 114
    EWC and, 114
Health history, 73–80
    conducting interview for, 75–76
    general health review and, 76–79
    interview techniques for, 45–46,
        74–75
    obtaining data for, 47

    personal information, 47
    purpose of collecting, 73
Health-illness continuum, 21–24
Health promotion, 25–27, 417–418
Health Protection Scotland,
    109, 111
Heat therapy, for pain management,
    407–408
    mechanics of, 407
    special considerations for, 408
    uses for, 407
Height, measuring, 97, 98–99
Helminths as infecting organisms,
    104–105
Hematest reagent tablet test, 484. *See*
    also Faecal occult blood
    testing
Hemoccult slide test, 484. *See also*
    Faecal occult blood testing
Hepatocytes, 431
Hip, exercising, 336, 337
HOP 5. *See Guide to the Handling of*
    People, the
Hospital hygiene, 114
HSWA 74. *See Health and Safety at*
    Work Act (1974)
Human need theories, 17
Human Rights Act (1998), 324–325
Hungry to be heard: The scandal of
    malnourished older people in
    hospital, 419
Hydrochloric acid, 427
Hydrocolloid dressing, 280
    applying, 280–281
Hydrogel dressing, 280
    applying, 281
Hydrotherapy, 406–407
    forms of, 406
    indications for, 406
    mechanics of, 406–407
    potential hazards of, 407
Hygiene, 339. *See also* Self-care
    body and, 341–344
      oral cavity, 344
      skin, 341–344
    factors that influence practices
      of, 339

    performing common practices
      of, 344
    bed bath, 345–348
    eye care, 349–350
    foot care, 354–356
    hair care, 350–352
    mouth care, 356–359
    occupied bed making, 361–363
    perineal care, 348–349
    shaving patient, 352–354
    unoccupied bed making,
      359–361
Hyperalgesia, 389
Hypercalcaemia, 201t
Hyperchloraemia, 201t
Hyperkalaemia, 202t
Hypermagnesaemia, 201t
Hypernatraemia, 202t
Hyperphosphataemia, 202t
Hypertonic solutions, 206i,
    207–208, 207t
Hyperventilation, 227
Hypnosis, as pain-relieving
    technique, 413
Hypocalcaemia, 201t
Hypochloraemia, 201t
Hypodermis, 253–254
Hypokalaemia, 202t
Hypomagnesaemia, 201t
Hyponatraemia, 202t
Hypophosphataemia, 202t
Hypotension, urinary elimination
    and, 453
Hypotonic solutions, 206i, 207t, 208
Hypoventilation, 227
Hypoxaemia, causes of, 233

I

Ileostomy, 479, 479i
    documenting care for, 492
    pouching systems for, 488, 489i
    applying or changing, 490i,
      491–492
    emptying, 491–492
    fitting, 489–490
    practice pointers, 492
    preparing to care for, 488

Note: Page numbers followed by "i" refer to an illustration; "t" refer to a table.

Ileum, 421i, 428
Illness
    definition of, 23–24
    effects of, 24
        on family, 24
    types of, 24
Immobility
    as pressure ulcer risk factor, 295
    treating, 319, 320i, 321, 322i
Implementation, 48–49
Incentive spirometry, 229–232
    benefits, 230–231
    devices used for, 229–230, 230i
    performing, 231–232
    practice pointers for, 232
    preparing for, 231
Incontinence, as pressure ulcer risk
        factor, 295
Indwelling urinary catheter, 463
    care of
        documenting, 467
        performing, 466
        practice pointers for, 468
    insertion of, 463–466
        documenting, 466
        in female patients, 464, 466
        positioning elderly female
            for, 464
        practice pointers, 466
        preparing for, 463
        preventing problems with, 465
    removal of
        documenting, 467
        performing, 467
        preparing for, 467
    urine collection from
        performing, 468
        practice pointers, 469
        preparing for, 468
Infection, 101–114
    control precautions, 107
    factors that increase risk of,
        101–102
    health care-associated, 105–106
        preventing, 106
    microorganisms that cause,
        102–105, 103i

as pressure ulcer risk factor, 297
    preventing. See Prevention of
        infection
    transmission of, 105
    types of, 102
    urinary elimination and, 453
    as wound healing complication, 267
    as wound healing factor, 264–265
Inflammation as wound healing phase,
        259i, 260–261
Inflammatory response, 259i, 260–261
Informed consent, 40–41
Infusion rates, 211–213
    calculating, 212i
    checking, 212–213
    regulating, 211–212
Infusions, specialised, 124–125,
        124–125t
Initial assessment, 45
Injection
    intradermal, 183, 183i
    intramuscular, 187–193, 190i, 191i
    preparing, 177–183, 178i–179i
        practice pointers, 181, 183
    subcutaneous, 184–187, 185i, 186i
    Z-track, 193–194, 194i
Insomnia
    alternative and complementary
        therapies for, 380
    behavioural interventions for,
        378, 379
    cognitive therapy for, 379
    patient history of, 376
    pharmacologic options for, 380, 381t
    relaxation techniques for, 378
    sleep hygiene for, 378, 379
Insulin delivery options, 185. See also
        Subcutaneous medication
        administration
Insulin syringe, 178i
Intentional torts, 39
Intercostal muscles, 221
Interdisciplinary team, for pain
        management, 401
International Council of Nurses code
        of ethics, 31
Interstitial fluid, 198

Intestinal phase, of digestion and
        absorption, 428–430
Intra-articular infusion, 125t
Intracellular fluid, 198
Intradermal drug administration,
        122–123, 183, 183i
    implant and, 122–123
    indications for, 183
    injection sites for, 183i
Intramuscular medication administration,
        123, 187–194
    aspiration for blood and, 189
    complications of, 193
    disadvantages of, 123
    in elderly patients, 192
    injection sites for, 190i
        in infants and children, 191i
    practice pointers for, 192, 193
    precautions for, 188
    Z-track method of, 193–194, 194i
Intramuscular needle, 179i
Intraosseous infusion, 125t
Intraperitoneal infusion, 125t
Intrapleural infusion, 125t
Intravascular fluid, 198
Invasive procedures, infection and, 102
Irregular pulse pattern, 89t
Ischaemia, 306
Isolation equipment, how to use,
        112–113
Isometric exercises, 336–337
Isotonic solutions, 206–207, 206i, 207t
I.V. drug administration, 123–124.
        See also I.V. therapy
    disadvantages of, 123–124
I.V. therapy, 196–215
    benefits of, 196–197
    delivery of, 210–211, 211i
    documenting, 214–215
    fluids, electrolytes and, 197–210,
        199i, 201–202t, 206i, 207t
    infusion rates and, 211–213, 212i
    professional and legal standards
        for, 213
    risks of, 197
    teaching about, 215
    uses of, 208–210

Note: Page numbers followed by "i" refer to an illustration; "t" refer to a table.

J

Jejunum, 421i, 428
Jet lag sleep disorder, 373
    chronopharmacotherapy for, 377
Joint motion, types of, 335i
Joints, 316–318, 318i

K

Kidneys, 448–450
    anatomy of, 448–450, 449i
    functions of, 450
    nephron and, 450
Knee, exercising, 336, 337
Korotkoff sounds, 96, 97
Kussmaul respirations,
        pattern of, 92t

L

Lactobacillus bifidus, 429, 476
Large intestine
    elimination and, 476–477
    functions of, 424t, 429, 473
    segments of, 429–430, 473
Larynx, 220, 220i
Latent infection, 102
Lateral position, 320i
Laws, nursing and, 38–39
Leader, nurse as, 12
Legal aspects of, drugs,
        116–117, 117t
Lifestyle
    bowel elimination and, 480
    effect of, on sleep, 370
    habits, and altered nutrition, 437
Lifting Operations and Lifting Equipment
        Regulations (1998), 324
Liquid medication, administration,
        147–149
    in infants, 149
    practice pointers for, 148
Liver, 421i, 431, 473
    functions of, 424t, 431, 473
Living will, 36, 77
Lobule, 431
Local Education Authority, 420
Low-air-loss bed, 301

Luminotherapy, 376–377
Lungs, 219–221, 220i
    acid-base balance and, 227
Lymphatic system, 254

M

Maceration, pressure ulcers and, 295
Magnesium
    functions of, 201t
    imbalances of, 201t
Male
    perineal care for, 348
    urethra, 451
Malnutrition, 419
Malnutrition Advisory Group, 419
Malnutrition Universal Screening
        Tool, 419
Malpractice, 39
Management of Health and Safety at
        Work Regulations (1999), 324
Manual Handling Operations Regulations
        (1992), 323
Maslow's hierarchy of needs, 17, 17i
Massage therapy, for pain
        management, 411
Mattresses as pressure reduction
        devices, 301–302
Mattress overlays as pressure reduction
        devices, 301–302
Maturation as wound healing phase,
        259i, 263
McGill pain questionnaire, 395–396
Medical futility, determining, 34–35
Medical history
    obtaining, 77–78
    pain assessment and, 397
Medical interpreter, 75
Medication calculations, safeguards for,
        135, 136
Medication errors, 140–143
    administration route and, 142–143
    allergy alert and, 142
    MAR errors, 142
    procedural safeguards against,
        138–140
    reducing through patient
        teaching, 141

    similar names and, 140–141
Medication history, pain assessment
        and, 398
Medications. See also Drugs
    bowel elimination and, 480
    effect of, on sleep patterns, 371
    urinary elimination and, 454
    as wound healing factors, 266
Medicines administration record,
        131, 134
    errors, 142
Meditation, as pain-relieving
        technique, 413
Meissner's plexus, 422
Melatonin, as sleep disturbance
        treatment, 377
Mental Capacity Act 2005, 37, 77, 325
Mental Health Act 1983, 41
Metabolic acidosis, 227
Metabolic alkalosis, 227
Metabolism
    of drugs, 129–130
    nutrition and, 416–417
    as skin function, 256
Metered-dose inhaler
    how to use, 175–176
    practice pointers for, 176
Meticillin-resistant Staphylococcus
        aureus, 106
Mixed opioid agonist–antagonists, 404
Mobility. See also Immobility
    definition of, 315
    factors that affect, 318–319
Moisture, excessive, as cause of
        pressure ulcers, 295
Mononeuropathy, 391
Mouth, 344
    dry, causes of, in older adults, 425
    role of, in digestion, 424t,
        425, 471
Mouth care, 356–359
    dentures and, 357–358
    performing, 357, 358–359
    preparing for, 356
Moving and handling
    devices, 301
    principles of, 325–326

Note: Page numbers followed by "i" refer to an illustration; "t" refer to a table.

Mucosa, of gastro-intestinal tract, 422–423
Multidisciplinary team, 53–54
Muscles, 318
Muscle sprain, applying cold to, 409i
Muscle tone, decreased, urinary elimination and, 452
Muscle wasting, 436
Musculoskeletal system
    anatomy and physiology, 316–318, 317i
    factors that affect function of, 318–319
Myenteric plexus, 422, 423
My 5 Moments for Hand Hygiene, 109

N

Nails, 343–344
    trimming of, 355
Names, in medication error, 140–141
Narcolepsy, 374–375
Nasal administration, 119, 167
Nasal cannula as oxygen delivery system, 233, 234i
Nasogastric tube, administering medication through, 150–152
National Institute for Health and Clinical Excellence
    guidelines, 52
National Patient Safety Agency, 109, 111, 208, 233
National Service Frameworks, 26
Neck, exercising, 334, 337
Necrotic tissue, 307–308
Needles, types of, 178i–179i
Negligence, 39
Neonates, sleep requirements for, 369
Nephron, 450
Neuman's model, 16t
Neurogenic bladder, 454
Neurologic injury
    and urinary incontinence, 454
Neurologic injury, urinary elimination and, 454
Neuropathic pain, 391

NHS Institute for Innovation and Improvement, The, 418
Nil by mouth, 439
Nocturia, 456
Non-blanchable erythema as sign of tissue destruction, 306–307
Non-narcotic analgesics, 403
Non-nursing theories
    developmental theories, 17–18
    human need theories, 17
    systems theories, 15
Non-opioid analgesics, 403
Non-pharmacological pain management, 405–413
    alternative and complementary therapies, 411–412
    cognitive and behavioural approaches, 413
    physical therapies
        cold, 408–410
        heat, 407–408
        hydrotherapy, 406–407
        massage, 411
        TENS, 410–411
Non-rapid-eye movement sleep, 366
    functions of, 368
Non-steroidal anti-inflammatory drug, 403
Non-synovial joints, 316
Non-verbal communication, 63–64
    strategies for, 64, 75–76
Normal pulse pattern, 89t
Norton scale, 298
Nose drops, instilling, 167
    practice pointers for, 167
Nosocomial infections. *See* Health-care-associated infections
Numerical rating scale, 393, 394i
Nurse educator, 14
Nurse practitioner, 14
Nurse researcher, 14
Nurses. *See also* Nursing
    functions of, 11–13
    roles of, 13–14
Nursing
    code of conduct, 6–10
    educational preparation for, 10–11

historical evolution of, 3–4
laws and, 38–39
legal issues that affect, 40–42
practice guidelines for, 6–11
as a profession, 4–11
professional organisations and unions, 11
research and, 18–19
Royal College of Nursing's definition of, 5
theories of, 14–15, 16t
Nursing and Midwifery Council, 418
    code of conduct, 6–10
    recommendations, 39
    role of, 6
    Standards of Proficiency for Pre-registration Nursing Education, 10
Nursing model, 74
Nursing practice, regulation of, 39–40
Nursing process, 43–54
Nursing research, 18–19
    evidence-based care, 19
    steps in process of, 18
Nutrients, 416
    standards for, 420
    types of, 416
Nutrition, 415–446
    altered, 434–437
        preventing, 437–446
    balanced diet and, 418–420
    bowel elimination and, 480–481
    defined, 415
    digestion and absorption. *See* Digestion and absorption
    health promotion and, 417–418
    metabolism and, 416–417
    nutrients and, 416
    as pressure ulcer risk factor, 297
    urinary elimination and, 454
    as wound healing factors, 263–264
Nutritional status, 418–420
    assessing, 418–419
    evaluating assessment findings in, 435t
    good nutrition, 419
    poor nutrition, 419–420

Note: Page numbers followed by "i" refer to an illustration; "t" refer to a table.

O

Objective data, 73
Obstructive sleep apnoea
    syndrome, 373
    treatments for, 377
Occupied bed making, 361–363
    performing, 362–363
    practice pointers for, 363
    preparing for, 361–362
Oesophagus, 421i
    role of, in digestion, 424t,
        425, 472
Older adults health care, 26–27
Open-ended questions, 46, 62
Ophthalmic administration, 119,
    158–163
    documenting, 163
    teaching about, 161, 163
Ophthalmic ointment
    administering, 160–163
        practice pointers, 163
    teaching about, 163
Opioid agonists, 403
Opioid antagonists, 403–404
Optimal nutrition, 419
    promoting, 437–438
Oral cavity, 344. *See also* Mouth
Oral medication administration,
    120–121, 145–149
    disadvantages of, 121
    documenting, 147
    paediatric patient and, 149
    practice pointers for, 147, 148
Oral temperature, measuring,
    83–84, 85t
    contraindications for, 87
Orem's self-care model, 16t
Organ donation, 37–38
Orientation phase, of therapeutic
    relationships, 65–66
Ostomies, types of, 479i
Ostomy appliances, 489i
Our Healthier Nation 1999, selected
    objectives, 25
Outcome statements, writing, 49
Oxybutynin, 454

Oxygenation as wound healing
    factors, 264
Oxygen supply, limited, effect of, on
    mobility, 319
Oxygen therapy, 232–237
    delivery systems, 233,
        234–235i, 235
        paediatric patient and, 235i
    in home setting, 236–237
    monitoring patient receiving, 236
    practice pointers for, 235–236
    preparing for, 235
    temperature measurement and, 87

P

Padding, 301
Paediatric patient
    assessing respirations in, 91
    communication with, 68–69
    drug action in, 131
    ear drop administration and, 166
    inhalation medication administration
        and, 176
    intramuscular medication
        administration and, 191i
    normal blood pressure in, 94
    oral medication administration
        and, 149
    topical medication administration
        and, 153
Pain
    alternative therapies for, 411–412
    assessment of, 388–392
        documenting findings of, 395
        people with dementia, 396
        tools for, 394–396
    autonomic arousal and, 388
    beliefs about, 384, 386–388
    children's, assessment of, 396
    complementary therapies for,
        411–412
    coping strategies for, 386–387
    as fifth vital sign, 392
    non-pharmacological management
        of. *See* Non-pharmacological
        pain management
    patient history and, 397–399

    pharmacological management of.
        See Pharmacological pain
        management
    psychological characteristics of,
        399–400
    rating scales for, 392–394
        numerical rating scale, 393, 394i
        pain intensity rating scale,
            393, 393i
        verbal descriptor scale, 393, 394
        visual analogue scale, 393, 393i
    self-efficacy and, 387
    theories about, 383–384, 385i
    threshold of, 383, 389
    tolerance of, 383, 389
    treatment for
        goals of, 400–401
        specific types of, 401–402
    wound healing and, 276–277
Pain intensity rating scale, 393, 393i
Pain rating scales, 392–394
    numerical rating scale, 393, 394i
    pain intensity rating scale, 393, 393i
    verbal descriptor scale, 393, 394
    visual analogue scale, 393, 393i
Pancreas, 421i, 432, 433–434, 473
    endocrine function of, 424t, 433
    exocrine function of, 424t, 432, 433
Pancreatic duct, 434
Paradoxical intention, insomnia
    and, 378
Paraplegia, 319
Parenteral nutrition, 209–210
Parietal peritoneum, 422
Partial-thickness wounds,
    269–270, 269i
Patient group directions, 133–134
Patient history, pain assessment and,
    397–399
Patient interview
    conducting, 74–75
    overcoming obstacles to, 75
    pain assessment and, 397
    techniques for, 45–46, 74–75
Patient rights, 40–41
Patients' Charter, The, 40
Patient-specific direction, 130–131

Note: Page numbers followed by "i" refer to an illustration; "t" refer to a table.

Penile sheath, 461–463
  application of
    performing, 462, 462i
    practice pointers, 463
    preparing for, 462i
  catheterisation, 463
  removal of, 462
Peplau's person-centred approach, 16
Pepsin, 427
Perineal care, 348–349
  for female patients, 348
  for male patients, 348
  performing, 348–349
  practice pointers for, 349
  preparing for, 348
Peripherally inserted central
    catheter, 210
Peripheral parenteral nutrition,
    209–210
Peristalsis, 423, 427
Personal information, obtaining,
    76–77
Personal values, 29
Phagocytosis, 260
Phantom pain syndrome, 391
Pharmacodynamics, factors that
    influence, 126i
Pharmacokinetics, 125, 127–130
  drug administration and,
    125–130
  factors that influence, 126i
Pharmacological pain management,
    403–404
  adjuvant analgesics, 404
  mixed opioid agonist–antagonists, 404
  non-opioid analgesics, 403
  opioid agonists, 403
  opioid antagonists, 403–404
Pharmacologic classes, 118
Pharmacology, 117
Pharmacotherapeutics, factors that
    influence, 126i
Pharynx, 421i, 425
  role of, in digestion, 472
Phosphorus
  functions of, 202t
  imbalances of, 202t

Physically impaired patient, positioning,
    319, 320i
Physical therapies, 406–411
  cold, 408–410
  heat, 407–408
  hydrotherapy, 406–407
  massage, 411
  TENS, 410–411
Polyneuropathy, 391
Polyuria, 457
Positioning
  for ear drops, 165i
  in gastric medication
    administration, 152
  patient in bed, 299–300, 299i
  seated patient, 300–301
Post-registration education and practice
    standards (PREP), 40
Postural drainage, 232
Potassium
  functions of, 202t
  imbalances of, 202t
Practice guidelines for, 6–11
Pre-interaction phase, of therapeutic
    relationships, 65
Pre-prepared syringe, 178i
Pressure
  as cause of pressure ulcers,
    291–293, 292i
  devices to reduce, 301–302
  managing, to prevent pressure ulcer
    formation, 298–303, 299i
Pressure gradient, 292, 293i
Pressure ulcers, 289–313
  assessing for, 305–309
  causes of, 290–295
  clinical manifestation of, 290
  closed, 309
  costs associated with, 290
  grading for, 309, 310i
  incidence and prevalence of,
    289–290
  locations for, 291
  preventing, 298–304, 299i
  risk factors, 295, 297–298
    assessing, 297–298
  treatment of, 311–313

Prevention of infection, 107–114
  hand hygiene and, 108–111, 110i
  hospital hygiene and, 114
  isolation procedures and, 112–113
  prophylactic antibiotics in, 108
  protective equipment, personal
    and, 111
  safe handling and disposal of sharps
    in, 112
  waste disposal and, 114
Primary intention wound healing,
    257–258
P.R.N. medication orders, 133
Professional aspects of, drugs, 117
Professional attitude, maintaining,
    79–80
Professional organisation, 11
Professional responsibilities, 324
Proliferation as wound healing phase,
    259i, 261–263
Prone position, 320i
Protection as skin function, 255
Protective clothing, 113
Protective equipment, personal, 111
Protective isolation, 112
Protozoa as infecting organisms, 104
Provision and Use of Work Equipment
    Regulations (1998), 324
Psychogenic pain, 399
Psychosocial history, obtaining, 78
Pulmonary perfusion, 225
Pulse, 86
  apical measurement of, 88–89
  apical–radial measurement of,
    89–90
  documenting, 90
  patterns of, 89t
  radial measurement of, 88
  sites for assessing, 87, 87i, 88
Pulse oximetry, 237–239
  documenting, 239
  mechanics of, 237, 238i
  performing, 237–238
    in infants, 238
  practice pointers for, 238–239
  preparing for, 237
Pyloric glands, 426i

Note: Page numbers followed by "i" refer to an illustration; "t" refer to a table.

Q

Quadriplegia, 319
Questions, open-ended *vs.* closed, 46,
  61–62

R

Radial pulse measurement, 88
Range-of-motion exercises
  active, 336
  passive
    contraindictions for, 333
    documenting, 336
    indications for, 333
    performing, 334, 336
    preparing to perform, 334
Rapid-eye movement sleep, 366,
  367–368
  functions of, 368
Rapid Response Report, 233
Reactive hyperaemia as signs of
  ischaemia, 306
Rectal drug administration, 121–122
  disadvantages, 121–122
Rectal medication administration,
  168–171, 170i
Rectal suppositories
  administering, 168–170
    in adult, 170i
    in paediatric patients, 169
    practice pointers for, 170
  contraindications for, 170
Rectal temperature, measuring, 83, 85t
  contraindications for, 87
Rectum, 421i, 430
Red wound, caring for, 270–271, 271t
Registration, 39–40
Rehabilitation, beliefs about pain and,
  387–388
Relaxation response, as pain-relieving
  technique, 413
Relaxation techniques, as sleep
  disturbance treatment, 378
*Releasing Time to Care: The Productive
  Ward*, 418
Religious practices, dietary restrictions
  and, 437

Renal cortex, defined, 450
Researcher, nurse as, 13
Respiration, 90
  accessory muscles use during, 222
  accessory muscle use during, 93
  documenting, 93
  effect of age on, 91
  as function of respiratory system,
    222–227
  measuring, 90–93
  mechanics of, 221–222, 222i
Respiratory medication administration,
  119–120, 174–176, 175i
  paediatric patient and, 176
Respiratory muscles, 221–222
Respiratory patterns, types of, 92t
Respiratory rate, 90
Respiratory system
  anatomy and physiology, 219–222,
    220i, 222i
  functions of, 223–227, 226i
  therapy for altered function, 227–247
Restrictive diets, 439
Retention enema, 171
Ribs, 221
Rickettsiae as infecting organisms, 104
Right dose, confirming, 135
Right drug, confirming, 135
Right patient, confirming, 136
Right route, confirming, 137
Right time, confirming, 136–137
Risk assessment, 79–80
Rogers' humanist approach or person-
  centred approach, 16t
Roper, Logan and Tierney's model, 16t
Routes, drug administration, 118–125,
  124–125t
  medication error and, 142–143
Royal College of Nursing, 11
  definition of nursing of, 5
Roy's adaptation model, 16t
Rugae, 472

S

*Saving Lives: Reducing Infection,
  Delivering Clean and Safe
  Care*, 107

Scalene muscles, 222
Sebaceous glands, 253, 342i, 343
Secondary intention wound healing, 258
Secretin, 433t
Self, therapeutic use of, 67
Self-care, 339. *See also* Hygiene
  ability to perform, 340
  factors affecting, 340
  normal patterns of, 340
Self-efficacy, belief in, 387
Semi-prone position, 320i
Semi-recumbent position, 320i
Sensory perception as skin function, 255
Shaving patient, 352–354
  performing, 352–354
  practice pointers for, 354
  preparing for, 352
  using electric or battery razor for,
    353–354
  using straight or safety razor for,
    352–353
Shearing force as cause of pressure
  ulcers, 293–294, 294i
Shielded needle, 179i
Shift-work sleep disorder, 373
  chronopharmacotherapy, 377
Shoulder, exercising, 334, 337
Sigmoid colon, 421i, 430
Silent infection, 102
Simple mask as oxygen delivery system,
  233, 234i
Simplicity, of verbal communication, 60
Sinusoids, 431
Skin, 249–257, 341–344
  age related changes in, 252, 296t
  blood supply to, 254
  drug storage in, 128
  functions, 250, 254–257
  functions of, 341
  layers of, 250–254, 341–343, 342i
  lymphatic system of, 254
  managing integrity of, 303–304
  structural supports for, 252
Sleep, 365
  factors affecting, 369–371
    age, 369–370
    environment, 370

Note: Page numbers followed by "i" refer to an illustration; "t" refer to a table.

lifestyle, 370
medications, 371
stages of, 366–368, 367i
functions of, 368
neurologic regulation of, 368
Sleep disorders, 365, 371–376
breathing-related, 373–374
circadian rhythm. *See* Circadian
sleep disorders
narcolepsy, 374–375
pharmacologic therapy, 375
primary hypersomnia, 375
primary insomnia, 375–376
secondary causes of, 365–366
treatments for, 376–380, 381t
Sleep hygiene, 378
Sleep restriction, insomnia and, 378
Small intestine
digestion and absorption in, 429,
472, 474, 475i, 476
divisions of, 428, 472
functions of, 424t
Smoking as wound healing factors,
266–267
Social communication as skin function,
256–257
Social history, pain assessment and,
398–399
Sodium
functions of, 202t
imbalances of, 202t
Soft diet, 439
Source isolation, 112
Special diets, 439
Specificity theory about pain, 384
Sphygmomanometer, how to
use, 96t
Spinal cord injuries, effect of, on
mobility, 319
Spirochaetes, 103
Spirometry incentive. *See* Incentive
spirometry
Staff nurse, 13
Standardised care plan, 51–53
Standard precautions, 107
Standards for Better Health, 418
Standards of nursing care, 6–10

Standards of Proficiency for
Pre-registration Nursing
Education, NMC, 10
Standard syringe, 178i
Standing scale, 97, 98
Stat medication orders, 131
Sternocleidomastoid muscles, 222
Stertor, 91
Stimulus control, insomnia and, 378
Stomach, 421i
emptying of, 428, 474
functions of, 424t, 472
role of, in digestion, 426–427
sites and mechanisms of gastric
secretion in, 426i
Stool
assessment of, for occult
blood, 484
characteristics of, 477, 478
Stool specimen collection, 482–484
documenting, 484
patient teaching for, 484
practice pointers, 484
random, 483
times, 483–484
Storage and preparation guidelines,
drug, 138
Stratum corneum, 341
Stratum germinativum, 341
Stress, urinary elimination and, 455
Stridor, 91
Subclinical infection, 102
Subcutaneous medication
administration, 122,
184–187
disadvantages of, 122
indications for, 184
injection sites for, 185i
in paediatric patient, 187
practice pointers for, 187
preparing for, 184, 186
teaching about, 187
technique for, 186i
Subcutaneous needle, 178i
Subcutaneous tissue, 253–254
Subjective data, 73
Sublingual drug administration, 120

Submucosa, of gastro-intestinal
tract, 422
Submucosal plexus, 422, 423
Supine position, 320i
Support aids and cushions, 301–302
for sitting, 302–303
Suppositories, rectal. *See* Rectal
suppositories
Surgery
bowel elimination and, 481
urinary elimination and, 455–456
Surgical history, pain assessment
and, 397
Surgical wound management, 283–288
applying fresh dressing in, 287
caring for wound in, 285–286
dressing wound with drain in, 287
practice pointers, 287–288
preparing for, 283–284
removing old dressing in, 285
Sustained maximal inspiration, 231
Sustained-release drugs, 138
Sweat glands, 342i, 343
Sweat glands, 253
Sympathetic pain, 391
Synovial joints, 316–318, 318i
Syringe, types of, 178i
Systems theories, 15
Systolic blood pressure, *vs.* diastolic
blood pressure, 93

T

Tablets
administering, 145–147
scored, how to break, 146
teaching about giving, 147
Tachycardia, pulse pattern for, 89t
Tachypnoea, respiratory pattern in, 92t
Teacher, nurse as, 12
Teeth, 344
Telephone medication message
accuracy, 134
Temperature, body. *See* Body
temperature
Termination phase, of therapeutic
relationships, 66
Tertiary intention wound healing, 258

Note: Page numbers followed by "i" refer to an illustration; "t" refer to a table.

Theories
  non-nursing, 15, 17–18
  nursing, 14–15, 16t
Therapeutic relationships, phases of,
    64–67
Therapeutic use of self, 67
Thermometers, types of, 84i
Thermoregulation as skin function, 255
Thoracic drainage, 245–247
  clamping alert, 247
  closed systems, managing, 246
  practice pointers, 247
  preparing for, 245–246
Thorax, 221
TILE acronym, 323
Timing and relevance, of verbal
    communication, 60–61
Toddlers, sleep requirements for, 369
Topical medication administration, 119,
    152–157
  advantages of, 119
  paediatric patients and, 153
Torts, 38–39
  intentional, 39
  unintentional, 39
Total parenteral nutrition. See Parenteral
    nutrition
Tracheal suction, 241–245
  aftercare for, 245
  complications of, 245
  documenting, 245
  performing, 242–245
  practice pointers, 245
  preparing for, 242
  purpose of, 241
Tracheostomy care
  changing fixation device/ tapes, 240
  changing tracheostomy dressing and
    tapes, 239–240
  changing tracheostomy inner tube,
    240–241
  cleaning stoma and outer cannula
    in, 240
  concluding, 241
  documenting, 242
  goals of, 239
  preparing for, 239–240

Tracheostomy tube, types of, 239
Traditional care plan, 50–51
Transcutaneous electrical nerve
    stimulation therapy, 410–411
  indications for, 410
  mechanics of, 410
  special considerations for, 411
Transdermal medication administration,
    153–157, 154i
  documenting, 157
  practice pointers, 156
  preparing for, 155
  teaching about, 157
Transdermal ointment, applying,
    155–156
Transdermal patch, 154i
  applying, 156
  defibrillator paddle and, 157
Transfer techniques
  from bed to stretcher/trolley,
    328–329
  from bed to wheelchair transfer,
    329–331
Translingual drug administration, 120
Transmission, of infection, 105
Transparent film dressing, 280
  applying, 281
Transverse colon, 421i, 430
Trapezius muscles, 222
Trauma, effect of, on mobility, 318–319
Trochanter roll, 322i
  applying, 321
Tube feeding. See Gastric feeding
Tunica muscularis, 422
Tunnelling, wound assessment and,
    274–275
Tympanic temperature, measuring, 83,
    84i, 85–86

U

Unconscious patient, communication
    with, 70
Undermining, wound assessment and,
    274–275
Undernutrition, 419
Unintentional torts, 39
Unison, 11

United Kingdom Central Council, 6
Universal precautions, 107
Unoccupied bed making, 359–361
  performing, 359–361
  practice pointers for, 361
  preparing for, 359
Ureters, 450–451
Urethra, 451
Urinal use. See Bedpan and urinal use
Urinary elimination, 448–469
  factors affecting, 452–456
    body position, 452
    decreased muscle tone, 452
    fluid intake, 452–453
    hypotension, 453
    infection, 453
    loss of body fluids, 453
    medications, 454
    neurologic injury, 454
    nutrition, 454
    obstruction of urine flow,
      454–455
    psychological, 455
    surgery, 455–456
Urinary frequency, 457
Urinary hesitancy, 457
Urinary incontinence, 457
  neurologic injury and, 454
Urinary system, 448–451, 449i
  abnormalities in, 456–457
  bladder, 451
  kidneys. See Kidneys
  ureters, 450–451
  urethra, 451
Urinary tract infection, 453
Urinary urgency, 457
Urine, 450
  obstructed flow of, 455–456
Urine specimen collection
  documenting, 461
  from indwelling catheter, 468–469
  random, 460–461
    performing, 460–461
    practice pointers for, 461
    preparing for, 460
  from specific gravity
    measurement, 461

Note: Page numbers followed by "i" refer to an illustration; "t" refer to a table.